What Really Works in Natural Health

www.**booksattransworld**.co.uk

WHAT REALLY WORKS IN NATURAL HEALTH

The Only Guide You'll Ever Need

SUSAN CLARK

BANTAM PRESS

LONDON • NEW YORK • TORONTO • SYDNEY • AUCKLAND

TRANSWORLD PUBLISHERS
61–63 Uxbridge Road, London W5 5SA
a division of The Random House Group Ltd

RANDOM HOUSE AUSTRALIA (PTY) LTD
20 Alfred Street, Milsons Point, Sydney,
New South Wales 2061, Australia

RANDOM HOUSE NEW ZEALAND LTD
18 Poland Road, Glenfield, Auckland 10, New Zealand

RANDOM HOUSE SOUTH AFRICA (PTY) LTD
Isle of Houghton, Corner of Boundary Road & Carse O'Gowrie,
Houghton 2198, South Africa

RANDOM HOUSE PUBLISHERS INDIA PRIVATE LIMITED
301 World Trade Tower, Hotel Intercontinental Grand Complex,
Barakhamba Lane, New Delhi 110 001, India

Published 2004 by Bantam Press
a division of Transworld Publishers

A catalogue record for this book is available
from the British Library.
ISBN 9780593049211

Typeset 11/16 pt Sabon by
Falcon Oast Graphic Art Ltd.

Printed in Great Britain by
Mackays of Chatham plc, Chatham, Kent

3 5 7 9 10 8 6 4

Papers used by Transworld Publishers are natural, recyclable products made from
wood grown in sustainable forests. The manufacturing processes conform to the
environmental regulations of the country of origin.

Note

**The advice in this book is intended to help you make an informed choice about your health.
It is not to be treated as a substitute for medical advice either from your family doctor or a
qualified health practitioner such as an accredited nutritionist, naturopath or medical herbalist.
This is important because natural medicines, such as herbs, can be every bit as powerful as
prescription drugs (which is, of course, why they work) and are likely to interact with existing
medication. In my experience, medical practitioners who are sympathetic to complementary
medicine are better able to advise on the likelihood and the consequences of such interactions.
To find practitioners in your locality, see Useful Contacts on page 447.**

For Gill Goose – who really can fly without wings!

Contents

Preface

This book is for anyone who has more than a passing interest in natural health but who finds it hard to keep track of what works, what to take and why. I wrote it not only because there is so much good (if fragmented) information on natural medicine out there, but also because in the six years I have been reporting exclusively as a journalist in the *Sunday Times* about developments in the field, the topic has moved on considerably, with mainstream science catching up with folklore and anecdotal evidence to prove that these remedies work and explain how.

The fact is that few doctors have the time to keep up with a topic so vast – there are some 30,000 ready-made supplements on the market, and with more than 1000 new launches each year, finding the right one for you can be hard work. It can be tempting to mix remedies ad hoc every time you read another article about another super-supplement, but the key to using natural remedies safely and effectively to maintain good health is to use a good quality range that has done the mixing for you.

I believe this new book will help you make your own best health choices, and my motivation for writing it is to pass on the extensive knowledge I have gained around a topic that, while it so often deserves the kicking it gets for bad science and hyperbole, equally deserves a mainstream platform for the good stuff.

I am completely passionate about the topic. For five years I never read a novel because there was always a herbal textbook or university research paper in my hands. I travel widely – from sailing up the Amazon to look for rainforest herbs to tramping through the New Zealand bush searching for Maori plants – and have become an expert in natural health along the way.

The signs were always there. I grew up in Devon making dandelion remedies to get rid of my sister's freckles, experimenting in cooking with flowers and brewing elderberries and stinging nettles into various healing potions, and while I followed an academic route through the sciences at university, that feeling of being close to nature and thinking about how plants, for example, can serve us has never left me.

I am not a doctor or a practitioner and don't pretend to be anything other than a journalist with a genuine interest in this subject and a brief to find out more. Six years ago, when I first started writing the *Sunday Times*'s 'What's The Alternative?' column, I walked into a consumer minefield of claims, counterclaims, hyperbole, pseudoscience and dross, and knew I had found the job for me. I have a science degree and have been a health journalist for twenty years and, if nothing else, this background gives me the skills to work out what works and why.

If I can find double-blind, placebo-controlled trials proving the efficacy of a herbal remedy, then great, I will report them, but I also believe it is arrogant in the extreme to ignore what we call empirical evidence, which is simply that we know something works because thousands of patients tell us so.

I am not a zealot and it is not a case of being what is derisively called 'an alternativist'. I practise yoga, work out with a fitness trainer, give the dog homeopathic remedies and dose my daughter with elderberry if she is sickening. But if I collapsed tomorrow, I would want my husband to call the ambulance, and, equally, after three days in hospital, I would want the herbalist, nutritionist or homeopath on hand to help me recover.

I believe you can only make a truly informed choice about your health and well-being when you know all your options – allopathic and natural – and this book, which is my fourth in a series, will help you do just that.

If you want to read it cover to cover, it will take you on a journey through nature's most astonishing miracle – the human body – and help you work out how to use natural remedies to stay well. If you are sick and looking for specific information, simply use the index and follow the cross-referencing to give yourself the best chance you will ever have of recovering fully.

The topic is so huge – and growing all the time – that I could have written a tome ten times the size but I do not have that luxury so I have distilled everything I have researched and discovered down to what you need to know and what works.

As a writer I take the view that if something catches my attention it will likely catch yours too, and so I have included information on research trials, which now tell us how traditional remedies work, plus reports on more cutting-edge theories which may work, we just don't know how or why yet. Whatever their outcome, they deserve their place in this book because, if nothing else, they make us think about how the body works and, more importantly, how much we still do not know. In other words, we need to keep an open mind.

If you have my earlier books, what you will find here is all the information that has emerged since those were first published; if you like, this really is the cutting edge. Where appropriate, I have also included supplier and resource and dosage details, and even specific brands so that those of you in a hurry can get hold of the remedies you need.

To anyone still asking how I can believe in this stuff, I reply that in a recent survey of UK scientists, researchers at the University of Exeter's Department of Complementary Medicine found that four out of ten of the country's leading scientific brains use natural remedies and complementary health treatments themselves. This is twice the number of lay people thought to be interested (although I would dispute this figure and put it much higher), so maybe those scientists already know something the rest of us are only just catching on to.

Finally, the other question I get asked from time to time is whether I get paid by companies to recommend certain products, and the answer is, of course, no. I have been a journalist longer than a natural health specialist and that independent way of thinking and looking at the world is now very much a part of me. I wouldn't know who I was without it. That's just who I am.

Susan Clark

PART ONE

CHAPTER ONE

Healthy Skin, Hair, Nails and Eyes

The eyes might be the windows to the soul, but it is your skin that acts like a mirror to tell the world what is really going on inside your body. An over-burdened liver, a sluggish digestive system or hormones that have gone into spin will all eventually take their toll on your skin, which means, unless you address these underlying problems, the topical lotions and creams you may be using can never really work.

Skin Deep

The skin, which is the largest organ in the body and comprises 12–15 per cent of your total body weight, has three functions: to protect the inner body from invasion by foreign matter, to control temperature and moisture content, and to help the internal systems eliminate waste. What this means is that this organ, which can vary in thickness from just 0.6mm on the eyelids to 3mm on the palms of the hands and soles of the feet, is also the dumping ground for an overworked lymphatic system (that part of the immune system that clears toxins from the body's internal tissues, see pages 6 and 260).

Just as we judge the health of our family pets from the state of their coats, we can judge our own health from the appearance of the skin, hair, nails and eyes, and when there is a problem, you may need to turn health detective to work out what is going on inside and, more importantly, why.

So the message, if you suffer from skin problems, is simple: you have to treat the problem from the inside out, starting with the digestive system.

To make sense of this approach, think of it this way: everything you ingest can have a positive or negative effect on your skin once it has been broken down (by the digestive system), processed (by the liver) and, if not needed, disposed of (by the lymphatic and excretory system). So all these different parts need your help.

Going Down – Digestion

Chapter 2 will tell you everything you need to know about your digestive system and, if you have any kind of skin problem, you need to turn to that chapter now and then come back to learn how the liver is important and why you need to support it.

If you have troublesome skin, you need to learn how you can cleanse the digestive tract, kick-start it back to normal functioning and then support it on a daily basis to maintain its ability to absorb the nutrients essential for good skin.

Going Deeper – the Liver

Think of this organ as the body's chemical-processing plant. Everything you eat, drink and swallow must eventually pass through the liver, which is why, along with the brain and heart, it is one of the hardest-working organs in the body. In fact, the only substance you can ingest without taxing the liver in any way is water and, even then, if you are drinking tap water, the liver will have to deal with contaminants.

The good news about this organ is that it is also one of the most forgiving in the body. In other words, whatever your lifestyle to this point, you can (unless it has already become diseased) start supporting it now and you can expect it to recover and keep working for you. This is because liver cells have the extraordinary ability, with the right support and over time, to regenerate themselves. This will not, of course, happen overnight. It can take up to two years for the regenerative process to take place.

The single most important natural remedy that will assist this process is a herb called **milk thistle**. This plant provides four active agents, which are collectively known as silymarin, and in trials researchers have shown these become even more effective when bound with a compound that combines fat (lipid) and phosphate called phosphatidycholine. So, if you plan to take a supplement, find one that recognizes this and combines both. Take as directed on the label.

There are many other herbs that can support the liver, including dandelion, but the advantage with milk thistle is that there is no known toxicity. In animal trials, even high doses administered over a long period of time did not trigger unwelcome side effects. Prescription medications and heavy alcohol consumption can also inflame the liver and preliminary evidence suggests milk thistle can help protect against this damage too.

Methionine is a sulphur-containing amino acid which helps prevent the accumulation of fat in the liver. People do take it in supplement form (500mg a day with food) but it can increase levels of homocysteine – a by-product of the metabolism of protein that has been recognized as being a better indicator of the risk of heart disease than cholesterol levels – so this is not good. It is better to source your methionine from such foods as fish and meat, and dairy products such as milk, cheese and yoghurt.

A better nutraceutical* support for the liver is **Lecithin,** a phospholipid sourced commercially from soy, which lots of people take to control cholesterol levels but which also works to support the liver thanks to the presence of phosphatidycholine (see milk thistle, above). If you want to take this supplement, look for a product that contains 90 per cent phosphatidycholine and take 350–500mg, three times a day. Your health store may try to persuade you that this is a cholesterol-lowering agent but the research to support this has been heavily criticized and there are better agents, such as **red yeast** (see Chapter 3: Heart, Blood and Lungs).

Going Out – the Lymphatic System

Unlike blood, which has a heart to pump it around the body, the lymphatic system, which circulates waste material, toxins, bacteria, the body's own disease-fighting white blood cells and excess water, relies on movement to keep flowing. When it becomes sluggish, the skin becomes the dumping ground.

In fact, the lymph system is a crucial component of the immune system, the body's natural defence mechanisms, which play a key role in keeping skin healthy and resisting infections. For every-

---

* 'Nutraceutical' is used to describe a compound with a chemical action that is drawn from a natural source such as a nutrient.

thing you need to know about supporting the immune system, go to Chapter 5.

To keep the lymph flowing, take regular exercise and buy a trampoline or mini-rebounder. If these are outside your budget, get a skipping rope (which will also help build bone density, see Chapter 4). I applaud the Ayurvedic position on exercise which abhors the macho 'no pain no gain' principles. The body's pain response is there for a reason – to stop you from hurting yourself – so you should exercise comfortably and with respect to your age, fitness levels and body type. Walking the dog each day for 20 minutes will help keep your lymphatic system working.

Natural healers recommend alternating hot and cold showers in the morning to keep the lymphatic system healthy but, for most of us, this is just too grim to contemplate. Invest instead in a long-handled skin-brushing brush (available from health stores for this purpose) and after towelling yourself dry after a shower or bath, brush the skin in circular motions from the legs up, taking care to avoid the area over the heart. Brush vigorously enough that the skin reddens but not so hard it hurts.

The One to Watch – Red Clover

Since the skin is a mirror to your whole health, the truth is there is not one single system that does not affect its functioning, and anyone past the age of puberty already knows how hormones play a critical role. For a more detailed explanation of how the body's own chemical messengers get thrown out of balance and what you can do to bring that balance back, see Chapter 6. Here, I want to talk about a humble roadside weed whose flower contains over 100 different chemicals, a plant I believe has enormous and, to date, mostly untapped potential in keeping hormone-related skin problems under control.

Red clover has been enjoying the spotlight as one of the more important phytoestrogens now incorporated in supplements designed to help alleviate the worst symptoms of the menopause. Phytoestrogens, as the name implies, are plant chemicals which have an oestrogenic action* in the body but only – and this is the bit that proves nature to be cleverer than any scientist – if the body needs it. In other words, if oestrogen levels are low, red clover will increase them, but if they are high, red clover will reduce them. This is not the same action as synthetic hormone-replacement chemicals, not least because phytoestrogens are much weaker than the real thing – and remember, in natural health, it is not always a case of the stronger the dosage the better.

What is rarely discussed is that red clover is also a rich source of all the nutrients needed to support healthy skin, including vitamin A, the B vitamins, calcium, magnesium, iron and selenium. It also has a potent blood-cleansing action in the body (see page 29), and if I were in the business of formulating an acne remedy for adult men and women, this would be the herb I would start with.

If you suffer from either eczema or psoriasis, you can use a topical salve from Green People, which combines hemp oil with red clover (see page 37). The salve was formulated for infants but is just as effective for adult skins. To treat skin problems, use the Acne Tincture from the Organic Pharmacy (020 7351 2232; www.TheOrganicPharmacy.com), which combines red clover with liver-detoxifying dandelion, hormone-rebalancing agnus castus and immune-boosting echinacea. If you prefer a supplement, take the new Doctor's A–Z Red Clover Combination (from Victoria Health – 0800 389 8195; www.victoriahealth.com) which combines all the above with liquorice and sarsaparilla, a herb that is used to remedy both skin and digestive disorders.

---

* The oestrogenic action of red clover makes it an unsuitable herb for teenage boys coping with troubled skin. Saw palmetto is a better male hormone-balancing alternative.

Feeding Your Skin

If you have dry, tired skin, you are not getting enough **essential fatty acids** in your diet, which is easily remedied by adding a teaspoon of liquid flaxseed oil to your breakfast cereal. If you hate the taste, then use one of the new sprinkle sachets (again from Green People) which combine omega-3 and omega-6 fatty acids in the correct healthy ratio and which you can scatter over cereals or salads or blend into smoothies made with yoghurt or soya milk and soft fruits such as bananas.

Zinc is another crucial skin nutrient. You can tell if you are already deficient by looking at your fingernails, where white flecks across the nailbed are a telltale sign. Remedy this by taking a supplement, which provides 30mg of zinc a day.

Vitamin A can help with skin disorders but is potentially more harmful than other vitamins since it is fat-soluble and can build up to toxic levels in the body. The safer way to take it in supplement form is as **betacarotene**; sometimes called provitamin A since the body converts it to provide the vitamin A it needs for you.

B-complex combines all the B vitamins, which work best when taken together and are known as 'nature's stress-busters'. They also improve the absorption of other nutrients so make sure you are taking a supplement or getting enough in the diet. B-rich foods include poultry, wholegrain breads, nuts, legumes (see page 81) and meats.

Probiotics provide millions of replacement live micro-organisms to rebuild levels of the healthy bacteria that live in the gut and aid digestion. I cannot stress enough how important it is to take a probiotic if you have troublesome skin, but the real problem is: how do you know which of the hundreds on the market to buy? With all the claims and counterclaims, and with many of these supplements failing miserably to provide anything like the promised billions of replacement live bacteria they claim on the label, this really is a minefield.

My advice is: keep it simple.

What we do know is that in independent tests the **Lactobacillus acidophilus** strain came out tops. And while the colon bacteria should be predominantly (85 per cent) this strain, this is rarely the case in adults. Also, the only two strains of bacteria currently established on the US GRAS (Generally Regarded As Safe) list are the Lactobacillus acidophilus and bifidobacteria species, which are both normal inhabitants of the human digestive tract, so stick with these strains and do not be tempted by any new (often more expensive) cultures that have no history of safe usage in humans.

The UK-based company that has been supplying Lactobacillus acidophilus, in powder form, for both infants and adults for many years is Biocare (0121 433 3727). Since it is available in powder form, you can easily blend it into smoothies (see below).

If you have an underlying digestive or skin complaint, you should also investigate taking a combined pre- and probiotic supplement (see page 65).

Tried and Applied

To make a delicious banana smoothie, blend one banana with a glass of live yoghurt, two teaspoons of honey, half a teaspoon of cinnamon and the same again of probiotic Lactobacillus acidophilus powder.

A–Z of Skin-nourishing Foods

I would love it if supermarkets sold foods with labels that told us their true nutritional and health benefits. Imagine pushing your trolley around and knowing that the sweet potato you plan to bake for tea is a rich source of the antioxidant vitamins A, C and E, which can help protect the skin and other body tissues from pollutants, or that mushrooms are high in both zinc and the B vitamins that are also important for healthy skin. It might take twice as long to get to the checkout, but with that kind of information at your fingertips, in no time at all you would know that for healthier skin you need to pile your trolley high with the following foods.

A is for avocados, apricots, almonds and apples. Apples are a good food source of quercetin, an anti-inflammatory and anti-viral agent that can protect the skin and prevent viral conditions, including shingles.

B is for broccoli, beetroot, bananas, butternut squash. Bananas are the very best natural probiotic, selectively feeding up the good bacteria in the gut to support the digestive system.

C is for carrots, celery, cantaloupe melon, cherries, chicken. Poultry is a good source of the B vitamins, nature's stress-busters. These keep digestion healthy and support the immune system.

D is for dandelion, a brilliant liver detoxifier. Harvest the young leaves and toss into green salads.

E is for vitamin E, a skin-protecting antioxidant present in sunflower seeds, brazil nuts, leafy green vegetables and sweet potatoes. Endive lettuce is also rich in antioxidant nutrients. Check out the lettuce facemask from Lush (01202 668 545; www.lush.co.uk), which you use twice a week and keep in the fridge.

F is for figs, fish and the crucial skin-boosting essential fatty acids present in flaxseed or cold-water oily fish such as salmon or mackerel.

G is for garlic, green vegetables, vitamin-C-rich guava. Garlic can help change the overly acid body-chemistry of psoriasis sufferers (see page 48) back to a mostly alkaline pH to help boost immunity and prevent symptoms.

H is for horseradish, a decongestant which helps break down the fibres in meat you've eaten so the body can absorb nutrients more readily.

I is for blood-building iron, important for good skin tone. The best food sources are red meats, asparagus, nuts, beans, dried peaches, egg yolks, molasses and oatmeal.

J is for juicing, the fastest way to get a rich source of nutrients and live enzymes into the digestive system to help keep skin clear, eyes bright, hair glossy and nails strong (see superjuice for skin, page 14).

K is for kiwi fruit, which has a higher vitamin C content than oranges, and vitamin K, a nutrient found in cauliflower, egg yolks, green leafy vegetables and soybeans, which can help prevent spider and broken veins.

L is for detoxifying lemons, lentils, leafy greens and also lycopene, the antioxidant in tomatoes, which increases when you cook them.

M is for millet, melons, milk (which is a good source of vitamin A) and methionine. Methionine is a nutrient that helps prevent the accumulation of fat in the liver and is found in all fish and meats, plus dairy products such as milk, cheese and yoghurt.

N is for skin-protecting niacin (vitamin B3) found in crabmeat, chicken, sesame seeds, pork, avocados, dates, prunes, figs, whole-wheat foods and roasted peanuts.

O is for vitamin-C-rich oranges, calcium-rich okra, which is good for the skin, and antioxidant-rich olive oil, which can help suppress the herpes virus.

P is for pumpkin, pumpkin seeds, prunes, papaya, peaches, vitamin-B-rich poultry, vitamin-C-rich potatoes and iron-rich parsley.

Q is for quercetin, an anti-inflammatory agent to help sensitive skins, found in apples, onions, shallots and yellow peppers.

R is for red grapes, brown rice, red peppers and raisins, which counter the effects of acid-producing foods in the digestive tract.

S is for sweet potatoes, spinach, sea vegetables, squash, soybeans, salmon, immune-boosting shiitake mushrooms and strawberries. Strawberries, as well as being antioxidant, act as antiviral agents which can prevent the herpes cold-sore virus.

T is for tofu, a good source of calcium for vegetarians, and tuna which provides vitamin D, plus tomatoes, which when cooked supply an even better source of the antioxidant, lycopene.

U is for vitamin U, a nutrient present in cabbage juice which can help soothe an upset stomach and kick-start a sluggish digestive tract.

V is for vanadium, a trace element nutrient similar to zinc and found in most body tissues. It is present in fish, dill, vegetable oils, seafoods and meats but is rapidly used up by the body and not easily absorbed.

W is for wheat (one to avoid if you have digestive and skin problems) and walnuts, which provide vitamin A in the diet. Watercress provides betacarotenes for the body to make the vitamin A it needs.

X is for Xylitol, a naturally occurring plant sugar found in raspberries, strawberries, plums and mushrooms. It increases the activity of the antimicrobial enzymes in saliva and so, as well as protecting from tooth plaque, can help prevent pathogens (bad or harmful disease-causing bacteria) from entering the digestive tract.

Y is for yellow fruits and vegetables, which are another good source of skin-loving vitamin A and live or active yoghurt which provides calcium and, if you buy the right brand, probiotic acidophilus.

Z is for zinc, which is present in shellfish, pumpkin seeds, eggs, mushrooms, meats and (non-leavening) brewer's yeast.

Tried and Applied

Superjuice: Juice organic apples, carrots and beetroots and add a splash of lemon juice and 20 drops each of milk thistle, goldenseal, dandelion and yellow dock organic herbal tinctures to make a juice that will decongest the liver and digestive system to support the skin. This is also an excellent hangover cure.

Ancient Wisdom, 21st-century Healing

Traditional Chinese Medicine (TCM)

TCM practitioners see the skin as the body's 'third kidney', which means they treat it as an organ of elimination. TCM is complex and not for the faint-hearted. A whole treatment regimen will include tongue diagnosis, pulse and even face reading, acupuncture or acupressure, plus the prescribing of highly sophisticated combinations of herbs in the form (most commonly) of teas which you brew yourself or as broths, washes, ointments, poultices, porridges and even pillows.

For maximum therapeutic benefits, you should find an accredited practitioner in your area. To do this, contact the Register of Chinese Herbalists on page 448.

One of the things I love about TCM are the names of the

remedies – who can forget a formulation called Little Green Dragon Decoction for chronic asthma, Five Seed Decoction to boost sperm vitality, or the Laughter Decoction for stomach ulcers, which was first written up in a Ming Dynasty Chinese herbal called Harmonious Medical Prescriptions?

Traditionally, many of the herbs used to remedy skin complaints were dissolved in lard rendered from suckling pigs, since this encouraged the rapid absorption of the herbs through the skin, but there are other less taxing ways to brew your herbs, disguise the foul taste and still get all the benefits.

Herbal porridges are the 21st-century solution, not least since they are nutritious in their own right and soothing to the digestive tract. The porridge is served for breakfast and could not be easier to make: simply boil your prescribed herbs together with wholegrains in either water or chicken broth until the grains are soft and the medicinal properties of the herbs have been extracted.

Try eating this for breakfast for a few months and notice how it is not only your skin that improves but your overall health and vitality too.

Tried and Applied

Chinese herbal porridge for healthy skin using ginger, jujube and brown rice: Soak two cups of rice overnight and then bring to the boil the following morning with eight cups of water. Add 5g of fresh or dried ginger and 6 Chinese jujubes* (crushed).
*Jujubes, also known as Chinese dates, are used in Chinese medicine to counter bloating and slow down the skin's ageing process. You can buy them in Asian supermarkets or by mail order from Creative Nature on 020 8941 7485.

Ayurvedic (Indian) Remedies

I love Ayurveda, which is often described as the science of living wisely, and which is the ancient Indian philosophy of health and well-being that introduced the world to yoga. I travel often to India to investigate the incredible hands-on treatments available as well as the healing properties of the herbs that families use there.

Although complex, the basic premise with Ayurveda is that people can be classified (and treated) according to three energy types: pitta (fire), vata (air) and kapha (earth). The fact is, we all have all three types of energy, or doshas, but one or two will dominate and thus affect our health and well-being. Pitta types, for instance, are fiery and likely to suffer more inflammation and heat-related disorders in the body than kapha types, who have a heavier constitution, suffer more lethargy and operate at a slower pace.

An experienced Ayurvedic practitioner will take the pulses in your wrist to determine your dominant energy types and prescribe accordingly. The key to the treatment programme, which can involve nutritional changes, herbal remedies and the prescription of yoga practices, is to rebalance the three energies to attain perfect health.

The food you eat will also affect your health, depending on your dosha. Vata people, for example, do well on rice but should avoid couscous. They are fine with fish but may have problems if they eat lamb, and they should eat cooked spinach but avoid cabbage.

Pitta types are better off drinking beer than wine, should choose white turkey meat and avoid tuna steaks, and can eat lots of carrots but not fresh corn.

Kapha people need to give cucumber a miss but will do well on broccoli and aubergine. They can eat basmati rice but not oat bran or pasta and need to avoid very cold drinks.

To rebalance your three energies, you need to eat – or avoid – certain foods. Too many raw vegetables and uncooked foods will aggravate vata types. Signs of trouble include arthritis, constipation, rheumatic pains, abnormal blood pressure and mental problems.

Heavy drinking, coupled with eating too many hot and spicy foods, exacerbate pitta energy – so will not drinking enough water (you need to aim for eight glasses a day). Signs of disturbance include skin disorders, getting angry quickly and a yellow tinge to the eyes.

Ice cream and other cold foods and drinks do kapha people no favours. Wet weather and cat-napping in the afternoons also make this energy-type worse. Flabby muscles, tiredness, impotence, feeling weak and feeling run down are all warning signs.

If you can get to an authentic Ayurvedic spa, book in for a Podikizhy treatment, where two therapists will massage your entire body using detoxifying and skin-rejuvenating herbs wrapped into a muslin bundle, which is then dipped in warm water before it is applied. The treatment, which also exfoliates the whole body, takes about an hour. Once you are covered entirely in oil (and no longer in control of your slippery body), you will discover what it must feel like to be a wet fish and you will emerge from the treatment room feeling, quite literally, the cleanest you have ever been.

In the meantime, you can raid your own kitchen cupboard for a traditional Ayurvedic skin remedy that could not be simpler (or cheaper) to make. And all you need is a humble potato!

Tried and Applied

Simply grate a large potato and squish the pulp and juices into a sticky poultice that you apply and leave on the skin overnight. The theory is that this simple remedy creates a nourishing skin

> food that regenerates skin tissue at the cellular level to leave it looking clear of blemishes and completely revitalized.

Rich in skin-rejuvenating silicon and vitamin C, **strawberries** also contain ellagic acid, a cancer-protecting chemical that has the extraordinary ability to repair DNA. The only strawberry face cream I have ever found is an Ayurvedic one that I recently brought back from one of my regular fact-finding trips to India. My Lakme strawberry silk crème smells good enough to eat. I hide my supplies from visitors but if you want to track it down, it is made by Hindustan Lever Ltd, a company based in Mumbai (Bombay).

To learn more about this complex but rewarding system of healing, and to determine your own dosha or type, check out the UK practitioner Sebastian Pole's excellent Ayurvedic Zone on my website, www.whatreallyworks.co.uk or visit www.thenaturalhealthclub.com.

Native American Remedies

The medicinal properties of many of the more popular herbs on sale in the west, including immune-boosting echinacea, were known to the Native American shaman healers long before 21st-century scientists were able to tell us what was in them and why they worked.

Goldenseal (Hydrastis canadensis) was the herb the tribes used as a general skin tonic (they would boil the root in water and use the liquid as a skin wash) and even to help heal arrow wounds.

Now considered a 'wonder remedy' with a range of uses, including strengthening the immune system, maintaining healthy digestion and warding off microbes and viruses, it is widely on sale in tincture form and really can help support healthy skin from the inside out. Be warned, though: this herb is bright yellow and needs handling with care since it will stain anything it comes into contact with.

You can now buy goldenseal tea bags in good health stores but to make your own brew (which you can also allow to cool and use as a herbal facewash), see making an eyewash with eyebright (page 38).

Native New Zealand Remedies

If ever there was a country designed to promote natural health it has to be New Zealand. I try to visit as often as I can, not least because there are over 2000 herbs which the Maori know how to use, most of which we have never even heard of.

One remedy that has made waves outside New Zealand is **manuka honey**, which is a superior wound-healing agent and probiotic. If you live there, you can afford to buy family-size jars in the supermarket to keep in the bathroom and use to cleanse your face at night. Unfortunately for those who have to buy this honey in health stores elsewhere, there is a premium on it, making this an expensive face-cleansing option.

What is now available is the excellent and organic **Living Nature** range which includes manuka honey and which is formulated by New Zealand biochemist Suzanne Hall, who lives on North Island. For daily cleansing, moisturizing and eyecare, this range is hard to beat. To benefit from the anti-bacterial and probiotic properties of manuka honey internally, use the new **Kiwiherb** range which is formulated by UK-trained medical herbalist Phil Ramussen, who now lives in New Zealand too, and which combines various Maori herbs with manuka honey.

Still Using Commercial Deodorants?

Nobody has yet established a proven link between an increased risk of breast cancer and the use of chemical-laden underarm deodorants, but what I can report is that one of the UK researchers currently investigating this proposition has stopped using commercial antiperspirants, and that discovery, several years ago, was enough for me to switch to more natural alternatives for good.

The single most natural way to kill off the bacteria that cause underarm body odour while still allowing the skin to perspire is to use a natural crystal. **Deokrystal** from Green People (01444 401444; www.greenpeople.co.uk) is made from **alunite,** a mineral whose deodorizing properties were first used by ancient Egyptian and Chinese populations. It costs under £10 for a 100g chunk, and to use it you simply wet the crystal in hot water and rub it under the arms. (The crystal will break if you drop it, but otherwise it should last a year and you can't get better value than that.) If the thought of a crystal is too wacky for you, the same company makes a roll-on deodorant from rosemary, grapefruit-seed extract and witch hazel, which also includes alunite in the preparation.

Get your teenagers to switch to one of the funky Krysztals deodorant bars from Lush (01202 668 545; www.lush.co.uk). I like the Oxeo cube that combines elderflower, marigold, honey and rose. For the more mature, who may favour something more traditional-looking but still more natural, check out the aluminium-free jasmine and rose Fresh Deodorant from beauty specialists Martha Hill (01780 470 140; www.marthahill.com).

Animal Testing . . . would you do this to your pet?

If you have not taken a cruelty-free stand, then take it now. Some 30,000 animals are killed in the name of cosmetic testing every year in Europe alone and the proposed EC marketing ban on cosmetics that have been animal-tested has now been postponed indefinitely.

To test for skin irritability, researchers shave the fur off the backs of rabbits before the chemical is applied. This is often so strong it burns right through the skin. In the 'Draize' test, the substance under investigation is smeared under the eyelids or squirted into the eyes. Again, rabbits are the preferred victims since their large eyes make it easier to see the ulceration of the eyeballs and they cannot produce enough tears to wash away the irritants.

We already know that up to 8000 cosmetic ingredients are safe to use on humans. If you are not already asking why we need more, and thus more animal suffering, ask that question now.

There are humane alternatives and you can *vote with your purse* by only buying cosmetic and skincare products from cruelty-free companies, such as The Organic Pharmacy (020 7351 2232; www.TheOrganicPharmacy.com) or Farmacia Urban Healing (020 7831 0830); two excellent companies that now specialize in only 100 per cent natural ranges.

To help stop animal testing for good, contact the British Union for the Abolition of Vivisection (BUAV) on 020 7700 4232.

Cruelty-free Skincare Shopping

If you are ever in London's fashionable Kings Road area, make sure you visit the Organic Pharmacy, tucked away at number 396. The brainchild of qualified pharmacist and homeopath Margo

Marrone, the shop, which offers on-site complementary treatments and therapies in the downstairs clinic, specializes in natural
skincare ranges and substitutes the conventional 'pharmacy' offering
with all-natural alternatives. In other words, you can buy everything that is on sale in your local chemist shop, from acne creams
to nappies, but here all the items on sale are natural and, where
possible, organic too. Check it out (www.TheOrganicPharmacy.com)
and do not leave the store without a jar of the carrot butter
cleanser and the rose and jasmine night conditioner. The organic
rose in this range is harvested by hand from a village at the
foothill of a range of mountains in Iran. Jasmine is symbolic
because its flowers open at night, which is, of course, when this
cream does its work.

Top Three Skincare Products

Skin disorders are distressing because you cannot hide them from
the world. I know of psoriasis and acne rosacea sufferers who
have hidden themselves away at home for years before chancing
on one of my columns or books and finding remedies which not
only worked to help manage their symptoms but which gave them
back a 'normal' life.

If you simply don't have time for liver cleanses, digestive detoxifying programmes or an in-depth consultation with a practitioner
to get to the underlying causes of your complaint, the following
over-the-counter remedies offer a temporary quick fix. Actually,
there is no such thing as a quick fix in natural health, since it can
take a herbal remedy a month to kick in and you should persevere
for at least three months to get the full benefits and confirm you
are taking the right remedy for you. What I should say is that if
you don't have time to delve deeper into the problem, here are my
top three remedies and skincare regimens that all offer holistic
support for the skin.

Sher Skin Support

Helen Sher, who calls herself a skin psychologist, has spent over fifty years in the beauty business, a career that eventually brought her to the door of natural health. She specializes in ranges for acne and acne rosacea skins and recently joined forces with the UK supplement-maker Higher Nature to produce this excellent skin support remedy. It combines detoxifying herbs such as burdock and dandelion with essential skin nutrients including zinc, calcium and vitamin A, plus a probiotic to work from the inside out and boost skin health. For details, visit www.sher.co.uk.

Solgar Skin, Nails & Hair

Solgar is the upmarket brand leader in the vitamins, minerals and herbal supplements market, and every time I recommend this product, the company's phonelines get jammed. It provides 1g of methylsulphonylmethane (MSM), an organic form of sulphur originally developed to relieve arthritis but which users reported also dramatically improved the health of hair, skin and nails. The formulation also includes zinc (15mg), lysine (50mg) and silicon (50mg).

Carrot Butter Cleansing and Organic Rose Serum

Margo Marrone, the pharmacist and homeopath founder of the Organic Pharmacy in London, is passionate about finding cruelty-free and 100 per cent natural alternatives to the synthetic-laden mainstream cosmetics most of us have grown up with. Her organic skincare regime, which features a carrot butter cleanser, an organic rose serum, an antioxidant day cream and antioxidant capsules to support skin health from the inside too, is brilliant. For details, visit www.TheOrganicPharmacy.com.

Get Out in the Sun

Holidays really are crucial for your health, and researchers have finally proved what people have known all along: that a good break can do wonders for your health and well-being. A survey by the State University of New York took this premise a stage further by revealing that regular holidays lowered the risk of premature death by almost 20 per cent among men aged 35–57, and in women aged 45–64 the risk was halved.

That said, while Vacation Deficit Disorder (as it is now called) may be bad for your health, so too are the risks of overexposure to the sun, especially if you live in a climate where intense sunshine is not an everyday fact of life.

Sunbathing has had a bad press for a long time now yet we all know we feel and look better with a glowing tan and I have long argued that the benefits of safe and protected sunbathing far outweigh the risks. The key words here are **safe** and **protected.**

Betacarotenes – the natural chemicals which protect plants from sun damage – can do the same for humans too, especially when combined with **vitamin E**. In adult trials, reported in the journal *Proceedings of the Society for Experimental Biology and Medicine*, twenty-two men and women were given increasing doses of betacarotenes over twenty-four weeks while researchers measured the sensitivity of their skin to sunlight. They found that as the dosages increased the skin became more protected from sunburn.

A second study, published in the *American Journal of Clinical Nutrition*, found that taking vitamin E (500 IUs) along with betacarotenes (25mg) for 12 weeks increased this protection even more.

Companies that specialize in natural bodycare products are now harnessing the sun-protecting properties of plants to formulate sun creams and screens for adults and children. One of my favourites is Green People's range that features **edelweiss**, a plant which grows so high it has its own built-in SPF (sun protection factor).

If you or the kids do burn, aloe vera gel can minimize the damage. I never travel without it and on those occasions when my daughter has spent the day in the swimming pool and burned her face (because she's wiping the cream away with the water from her eyes faster than I can reapply it), I have been staggered by the combination of aloe vera gel and a seven-year-old skin's ability to rejuvenate itself.

Safe sunbathing means building up your exposure by 20 minutes a day, staying out of the more intense midday sun and using natural creams and blocks to screen out the more harmful rays. **Living Nature** (see pages 19 and 32) also make skin protection creams including a popular coffee and wild pansy lotion which is worth investigating.

Supporting Ageing Skin

I hate the term anti-ageing. What's the point of fighting what can only be a losing battle? Age has its own psychological advantages – more self-confidence; an acceptance, finally, of the way you look; pride in your achievements to date – and if you look after your skin, you can soften some of the harsher changes that might be making you wish you could turn the clock back.

There are thousands of books devoted to the idea of cheating biology when, in reality, you need to be working with those changes, not against them. When you boil it all down, there are just three remedies that will help protect your skin as it matures, and not one of them, to my knowledge, has yet been hijacked by the big cosmetic companies.

Pycnogenol: This is one of the plant chemicals known as

flavonoids, which, since they are water-soluble, offer better antioxidant protection than vitamin antioxidants against the free radicals that would otherwise ravage and damage both your skin and your internal organs. The body is also better able to absorb and utilize flavonoids, making them more 'bioavailable', the term we use to describe this property. Clinical tests show that Pycnogenol, which is the trademark name for pine-bark extract, is 50 times more potent than vitamin E and 20 times more protective than vitamin C.

Flavonoids work to strengthen and repair connective tissue inside and outside the body (i.e. the skin) and to slow down the ageing process, which is why they are now being used in natural cosmetics.

For example, one new face cream on the market combines Pycnogenol with astaxanthin, an even more impressive antioxidant sourced from yeast and microalgae and said to be 500 times stronger than vitamin E. (You can also get Pycnogenol in capsule form but it is expensive and I would only use it this way for serious conditions such as recovery from stroke, see page 171, or, since it also has an anti-inflammatory action in the body, to help alleviate the symptoms of endometriosis, see page 428.)

Tried and Applied

Astaxanthin & Pycnogenol Age-Defying Protection Cream is the one the cosmetic giants won't want you to know about. Why? Because it is cheaper and more effective than many of the less natural agents they include in their formulations and charge you a small fortune for. It is now on sale in the UK at Victoria Health stores (mail order 0800 389 8195; www.victoriahealth.com). Don't be put off by the carrot-colour; use this cream at night and to protect the skin or help it recover from sun damage.

Rosa mosqueta: This South American herb was investigated for its incredible skin regeneration properties, such as to help reduce scarring after surgery and accidents, but the people using it noticed it helped fade and soften wrinkle lines too. You can try the oil, which is inexpensive and works on facial lines, acne or eczema scars, but it can leave you feeling as though you smell like a chip. A better everyday solution has arrived in the form of a new beauty range from New Zealand called **Trilogy**, which harnesses the rejuvenating properties of this wonderful plant. For more details of this range, visit my website www.whatreallyworks.co.uk.

Silica: This is the trace element that works in the body to support the connective tissues, including the skin, and to improve elasticity. The **Harmony Health Formulation (HHF) organic silica skincare gel** I have written about in my columns has proved popular with older readers looking for a topical face cream, but you can get similar benefits using a herbal horsetail tincture, which is another excellent source of silica. If you want to try the gel, it is available from Revital (0800 252875; www.revital.com) where it costs £24.99. Horsetail is widely on sale in good health stores.

Homeopathy for Skin, Hair, Nails and Eyes

Classical homeopaths, who may have trained for up to seven years, believe homeopathy works best when you have what is called a **constitutional diagnosis** with a qualified practitioner who will prescribe the right remedy for you. To find a doctor who is also a qualified homeopath, and to find out how to get homeopathy on the NHS, call the British Homeopathic Association on 020 7935 2163. For other qualified homeopaths, call the Society of Homeopaths on 01604 621400.

What I am really saying is that, for the very best results, you should consult a qualified homeopath to make your constitutional diagnosis and prescribe for you accordingly.

Flower Power Remedies

I once had a letter from a reader whose doctor had advised her to stop taking the Australian Bush Flower remedy Woman Essence, since he feared it may have been causing liver toxicity. While I am the first to emphasize the importance of safety, the letter made me laugh, since were he to send this remedy to a laboratory for analysis they would have sent it back saying there's nothing in it, just brandy.

The brandy is used as a preservative, by the way, and the reason no other active agents would be found is that, unlike herbal remedies which provide dosages of the chemical constituents of plants, either via a standardized extract in a capsule or the whole plant harvested to make a herbal tincture, flower remedies simply capture the 'essence' or 'potency' of the plant and are made quite differently.

The theory, and this will be a leap for some of you, is that the finished remedy carries the healing vibration or energy of the plant so that it is working at a much more subtle level.

The essence will be a thousand-fold dilution of a plant that has been left in distilled water and sunlight to 'potentiate' the liquid with this vibration and, as with homeopathy, the idea is that the more dilute the final remedy, the more potent it is. There are no clinical trials to support this theory one way or the other but there is a great deal of anecdotal evidence from practitioners and clients who will generally be using a flower essence as an adjunct to other remedies and therapies to address the emotional or energetic issues that may underlie a physical complaint.

This is not as bonkers as it sounds. Ayurvedic practitioners, for example, who draw inspiration from the spiritual teachings of the yogis, believe that a physical problem is the last sign of an illness which manifests itself first in the outer etheric or auric sheaths of the body, and if you have studied yoga in any depth you will already know there are five of these so-called sheaths, which you can think of as an energy field around a person.

If you are interested in flower essences – and there are now very many different types on the market – you are spoilt for choice. I like the very contemporary Bush essences because they work fast, but that doesn't mean the more established ranges, such as the excellent Bach flower essences, don't work.

Remember, the purpose of flower essences is to address the underlying emotional and energetic causes of chronic conditions. This means, for best results, they should be used as an *adjunct* to other treatments.

Springclean Your Cells

Blood cleansers are used to help treat all conditions but are especially useful for skin disorders and for chronic conditions that have developed over years. Just as you springclean each room in your house, so you can springclean your blood and your cells to strengthen and boost your core health.

Combining herbs is an art, as well as a science, and unless you are confident about brewing your own remedies, I suggest you find a herbalist who can make your remedies for you. The National Institute of Medical Herbalists (01392 426022) can make a referral.

Tried and Applied

Alfalfa, dandelion root and kelp: This herbal cleanser will build the immune system and strengthen hair, skin and nails. Juicing is not an exact science and I never measure quantities. What you must remember is that you always need more vegetables than you think to get enough juice to make it worth the effort. Use your own taste buds to decide what works for you. You are not aiming for a therapeutic dose of these ingredients but the release of the live enzymes and other active agents that work inside the body to bolster health. You must drink your juice as soon as you make it to gain the maximum health benefits.

What Really Works for Skin, Hair, Nail and Eye Complaints

I could recommend some thirty different remedies for almost any chronic condition you care to suggest but what good is that? You need to know what really works and which of these thirty to try so here are my 1, 2, 3 . . . Easy Steps for everyday skin, hair, nail and eye complaints.

Acne

If you've never had acne, count your blessings because you've had a lucky escape. The single most common of all skin disorders, it affects up to 85 per cent of those aged between twelve and twenty-four, and while it is more frequent in males, it is more persistent in females.

Acne has nothing to do with poor hygiene or eating greasy foods and everything to do with a complex and poorly understood mechanism involving hormones, a bacterial infection and a genetic predisposition. Junk diets will not help because they stress the digestive system, but the only foods that have been linked with triggering an outbreak are salt (so cut back on this in your diet) and kelp, an iodine-rich seaweed supplement which is sold in health stores and which you need to avoid.

Acne sufferers have been found to have lower levels of zinc than non-sufferers and more gut toxins (probably as a result of taking antibiotics), which means any natural treatment programme must include a **zinc supplement** and a **probiotic**. For women, the contraceptive pill is often prescribed to control acne but this will only work if it is an oestrogen-rich formulation, which can have other, unwanted side effects, such as weight gain.

The herb that can help prevent the hormone disturbances which have been identified as one of the critical underlying causes of acne is **saw palmetto**, an anti-androgen currently better known for helping prevent prostate problems in older men. In test-tube trials, it has been shown to help prevent the conversion of the male hormone testosterone to a less helpful form called dihydrotestosterone (DHT), a process that has now been implicated in triggering acne flare-ups.

Lots of patients are already successfully using a retinol cream to prevent acne recurrences but, again, there are often side effects, ranging from dryness and irritation to more alarming reports of mood changes and severe depression. A natural remedy that has performed better than conventional antibiotic treatments in clinical trials but which most acne sufferers will never have even heard of is **guggul** (also known as guggulu or Indian Bdellium tree), a plant that is related to myrrh and widely used in Ayurvedic medicine for chronic skin complaints.

This agent is more commonly promoted as a cholesterol-lowering remedy but in American trials that compared it with the antibiotic Tetracycline in the treatment of acne, it was found to perform better, with sufferers reporting less inflammation, and with fewer relapses, especially among those with oily skins.

1, 2, 3 . . . Easy Steps to Stop or Control Acne Skin Conditions
Take the anti-androgenic herb, saw palmetto (250mg a day).

Add zinc (30mg a day), plus a good quality probiotic.

Introduce the Ayurvedic herb, guggul (25mg a day). If not on sale in your local health store, mail order Guggul Bolic from Victoria Health on 0800 389 8195; www.victoriahealth.com.

Lots of commercial cosmetics and face creams will exacerbate acne-troubled skin. Switch to more natural creams and check out the acne kit developed by Living Nature (www.livingnature.com), which specializes in organic, natural skincare products incorporating antibacterial manuka honey (see page 19). I also rate the Acne Tincture from the Organic Pharmacy (020 7351 2232; www.TheOrganicPharmacy.com) since it includes red clover (see page 8), dandelion, nettles and echinacea.

Acne Rosacea

Although treated as the poor relation to acne vulgaris, acne rosacea is not the same as acne and so will not respond to the exact same treatment regimen. It is much more common in women and often does not flare up until middle age. Characterized by facial flushing – caused by the sudden dilation of the tiny capillary blood vessels supplying facial tissue – this condition is always exacerbated by alcohol, spicy foods and temperature fluctuations in the environment.

Again, there is a brand new remedy that few sufferers will have even heard of. **Azelaic acid,** which occurs naturally in wheat, rye and barley, has both antibacterial and anti-inflammatory properties and in clinical trials, where forty rosacea patients were told to apply azelaic-acid cream to one side of their face and Metrogel antibiotic cream to the other, researchers found that after fifteen weeks of treatment the facial lesions (pustules) treated by azelaic-acid cream reduced by 78.5 per cent and those treated by the conventional drug reduced by 69 per cent. They concluded that the natural cream was 'significantly more effective'.

Although approved* by the FDA in America in 1995, it is currently a prescription-only medicine in the UK, where it is sold as **Skinoren.**

If you want to stick with a DIY natural regimen, the one that has proven most successful to date (anecdotally, since there are no clinical trials) is a combination of a form of vitamin C called **ester C** with antibacterial **grapeseed extract.** This combination has excellent anti-inflammatory properties and will work to strengthen the blood vessel walls and decrease swelling of the affected areas. The dosage of both is dependent on your body weight. If you weigh under 150lb (that's 70kg, or 10½ stone), work up to 1g of ester C and 200mg of grapeseed extract, three times a day. Over this weight, aim for 2g of ester C and 200mg of grapeseed extract, three times a day. (Be warned: these high doses of vitamin C can cause temporary stomach upset.)

1, 2, 3 . . . Easy Steps to Stop or Control Acne Rosacea

Helen Sher/Higher Nature skin support (see page 23). Also try the acne rosacea tincture from the Organic Pharmacy (see page 23) since it combines liver-cleansing milk thistle, calcium-rich red clover, capillary-supporting bilberry and hormone-rebalancing dong quai.

---

*Approval of a natural remedy is a tricky subject. Sometimes an agent is not for sale over-the-counter because of safety issues, but, more commonly, it is not available because the makers have been making medical claims for its efficacy when they have no licence to do so. The fact that natural agents cannot be patented is a major annoyance to the pharmaceutical industry, which must spend millions on research and development before bringing an approved drug to market (while small companies can produce pills from natural agents and sell them relatively cheaply, but not make the same claims for efficacy). The safety argument is a valid one but so is the argument that natural remedies should not be withdrawn simply because they pose a threat to the profits of the pharmaceutical giants.

Take vitamin C with grapeseed extract (as above).
Ask your doctor to prescribe azelaic-acid cream.

Boils and Spots

What is a spot and how does it form? And what is the real difference between a spot, a boil and a blackhead? Think of the appearance of a spot or boil as another simple three-step process. First, for whatever reason, the sebaceous glands that surround the many hair follicles in the skin begin to produce an excess of sebum, the oily substance the body produces naturally to lubricate the skin and hair and to retain moisture.

Secondly, dead skin cells start to become trapped in that sebum which is now building up in the follicle canal (or comedo). Nearby cells (which produce keratin, the protein that forms hair, the outer skin and nails), are also triggered to overproduce and begin to play their part in forming the blockage. Until the blockage is complete, what you see is a blackhead. Once the process is finished, you will have the type of spot people call a whitehead.

Thirdly, at this point, if the micro-organism Propionibacterium acnes is present, it revs up to break down this sebum blockage, a process which itself causes redness, soreness and inflammation.

1, 2, 3 . . . Easy Steps to Treat or Stop Spots

Paint your face – literally! Lots of cleansers now incorporate tea tree oil – a natural disinfectant that is five times more potent than household detergents yet still safe to put on your skin. For my money, manuka honey from New Zealand is even more powerful, so check out the Kiwiherb range which includes a manuka paint.

Zinc supports the skin and the immune system so, if you are over fifteen, take 30mg a day. (Under this age, check my website www.whatreallyworks.co.uk for safe age-related dosages.)

There's a new kid on the block that you won't find on sale in

Boots. Wild Chinese violet (Viola yesoensis) is used in Chinese medicine to treat boils and all other skin infections. If you can get the powder (try East West Herbs on 01608 658862), make a poultice or cold facemask by slowly mixing the herb with cold water to the consistency of thick porridge. If you can't be bothered to do that, mail order the new skin-clearing Derma E range from Victoria Health (0800 389 8195; www.victoriahealth.com).

Tried and Applied

For emergency spot treatments, mix a paste with sweet wheatgrass powder (one of the foul-tasting immune-boosting green superfoods) and warm water. Apply and leave overnight.

Check with your doctor that recurrent boils are not a sign of diabetes or, if you are female, that you do not have polycystic ovary syndrome (PCOS), which can cause acne-like lumps and bumps on the face, especially around the chin and brows. For more on this condition, see page 399.

Cold Sores

At the first sign of a tingle, dab tea tree oil at the site, which should help prevent an outbreak. Repeat this several times a day. Stress and sunlight can both trigger cold sores, so to prevent them in the future, support the immune system with elderberry to suppress the herpes simplex 1 virus which is causing them. If you don't like the smell of tea tree oil, use Bio-propolis gel from Bioforce; (www.bioforce.co.uk).

This virus is activated by an amino acid called arginine, which is present in chocolate, nuts and most cereal grains, so cut these out. Another amino acid, called lysine, will inhibit the absorption of arginine to suppress the virus. This is present in dairy products, potatoes and brewer's yeast, so eat more of these.

1, 2, 3 . . . Easy Steps to Stop or Relieve Cold Sores

Take zinc (30mg a day).

Take a lysine supplement (1g three times a day). This is sold in health stores as L-lysine.

Boost the immune system with astragalus – a Chinese herb which stimulates the antiviral immune-system protein called interferon, produced by white blood cells, and which, unlike echinacea, does not lose its potency if you take it long term (500mg a day). For children prone to cold sores, use elderberry (sold as Sambucol) to boost the immune system instead. Sambucol for Kids disguises the taste of the herb in a blackcurrant-flavoured tincture.

Eczema

Very few people are born with eczema and for many sufferers outbreaks will come and go throughout their lives. I have a girlfriend who did not suffer at all until her mother died unexpectedly, at which point the eczema outbreak on her hands was so extreme she had to wear gloves for two months.

Treating eczema with hydrocortisone creams from your doctor will clear the symptoms but is no better than turning a blind eye to the problem. To work out why you have an outbreak, you will need to think back several weeks, even months, to what was happening in your life that triggered the current bout.

Clinical studies confirm that repeated exposure to food allergens will trigger eczema; the worst of these allergens are cow's milk, eggs, wheat and fish. So if you have an outbreak, stop eating these foods for at least six weeks. Environmental allergens can also trigger a bout or worsen an existing outbreak; these include dust mites, animal dander and pollens, so again, try to limit your exposure to these allergens if you are a sufferer.

Eczema is increasingly common in very young children and lots of mums spend a small fortune on creams that don't really work.

The salve you should be using is an organic cream from Green People (mail order 01444 401444; www.greenpeople.co.uk) which combines hemp with anti-inflammatory calendula, lavender, red clover, sunflower oil and beeswax.

I know it sounds odd to be using cannabis (hemp) in an eczema cream but the resin in hemp oil does not contain cannabinone, which is found only in the flowering tops of the plants, and which is the substance responsible for the drug-related side effects people associate with this plant. The oil, used in this cream, is made from the seeds, which do not contain cannabinone. Hemp is also rich in the omega oils that are crucial to healthy skin and, in fact, provides the perfect topical ratio (2:1) of omega-3 and omega-6 fatty acids.

If you are an eczema sufferer and want to avoid passing your risk on to your kids – allergy-inducing antigens get transferred in breast milk – you need to take preventative steps in pregnancy. Firstly, cut out the food allergens that trigger an outbreak while breastfeeding, and, if you are currently pregnant, take a probiotic supplement from the third trimester (24 weeks) and continue for six months, including during breastfeeding.

1, 2, 3 . . . *Easy Steps to Stop or Relieve Eczema*
Increase your intake of essential fatty acids (see page 9), which support normal skin functioning.

Take a good quality probiotic.

Take 40–50mg of zinc daily (adult sufferers have been diagnosed with low levels of this nutrient), plus a good multisupplement to provide skin-protecting vitamins A and E.

Tried and Applied
To treat eczema itching, use starflower cream, which contains borage (rich in essential fatty acids) plus soothing chamomile and chickweed.

Eye Problems

In Chinese medicine, the eyes are linked with the liver and so any stress on the liver (see page 5) will take its toll on the health of your eyes. Prescription drugs, including steroids and tricyclic anti-depressants, can accelerate macular degeneration, which is the leading cause of loss of vision in the over-55s, but the eyes can also suffer an onslaught from everyday pollutants including allergens, household cleaners, tobacco smoke and sprays.

In natural health, sometimes the name of a plant is all you need to get started, and for most eye complaints look no further afield than **eyebright,** a remedy now on sale in health stores specializing in homeopathic and herbal remedies, to clean and protect the eyes. It has been used since medieval times when herbalists believed the bloodshot appearance of its petals was a sign – something they called the 'doctrine of signatures' – that it should be used for the eyes.

You can make a herbal eyewash with this vitamin-C-rich herb to gently bathe eyes that are irritated because of infection or an allergic reaction such as hayfever. This works because vitamin C is a natural antihistamine, so the wash will lessen the severity of the eye's reaction to an allergen. Eyebright also contains vitamin E, an antioxidant which can promote the healing of wounds and infections, including styes.

Tried and Applied

Eyebright is also rich in sulphur and so can help maintain healthy hair, fingernails and skin. To make an eye or facewash, first brew a herbal tea by boiling one tablespoon of the herb in a cup of water. Allow this to cool and use the liquid as an eye or facewash (or drink as a tea).

Forget chomping on carrots (although carrots, celery and parsley all supply nutrients to the eyes). Two more important nutrients for maintaining good eyesight are plant chemicals **lutein** and **zeaxanthin**. A diet containing high levels of both has now been linked to a much lower risk of a range of eyesight problems, including macular degeneration and cataracts, in later life.

Both chemicals are found in dark green foods such as **spinach** and **broccoli,** and also in **eggs,** but for a therapeutic dosage, which really will provide protection, you need to take a supplement. These two phyto (plant) chemicals will also help tired eyes recover from the strain of spending all day, every day at a computer screen.

1, 2, 3 . . . Easy Steps to Protect Your Eyes

Springfield's Macuvite (mail order from the NutriCentre: 0800 587 2290; www.NutriCentre.com) combines lutein with zeaxanthin.

To tackle fine lines around the eyes, use the Enchanted Eye Cream from Lush (01202 668 545; www.lush.co.uk).

To clear eye infections, including styes, make an eyewash with the herb eyebright or order a ready-made tincture from the Organic Pharmacy (020 7351 2232; www.TheOrganicPharmacy.com).

Research alert: American scientists are now developing a light-sensitive microchip retinal implant containing 1000 mini electrodes that will stimulate the neural pathways to convey visual images to the brain. This technology will help restore better vision to those suffering from macular degeneration and retinitis pigmentosa and although the images will come more slowly than normal, according to those leading the project, 'those that are blind . . . will see!' But not before the end of the decade

– the projected timescale for the clinical application of this technology is seven years from now.

Fungal Infections . . . including Thrush, Athlete's Foot and Ringworm

Fungal infections are always a sign of an impaired immune system since the body's natural defences are designed, when working optimally, to resist the organisms responsible for the infection. The immune system is complex but clever. It can 'remember' past infections and can make the antibodies to fight off organisms it has encountered before, but this is only part of the picture. (For a more detailed account, see Chapter 5.)

With fungal infections, antibodies are irrelevant. What's more important is the production of T lymphocytes (T-cells), a type of white blood cell that co-ordinates immune response and is responsible for cell-mediated immunity, i.e. all those defence mechanisms not related to the production of antibodies.

To address this holistically, you have to take another step back and understand that the gland responsible for the production of fungal-fighting T-cells is the thymus and so recurring fungal infections are a likely sign of a thymus gland that is working under par. You can buy thymus extract supplements in health stores, but since the active agents have been sourced from sheep, I would recommend using the immune-boosting Asian mushrooms – maitake, reishi, cordyceps and shiitake – that will do the same thymus-supporting job.

The two best antifungal herbs are **pau d'arco**, which comes from the bark of a South American tree, and **horopito**, a native New Zealand herb which has now been incorporated in the Kolorex* range for fungal infections, including candida (thrush). In preliminary trials in New Zealand, the new intimate care

*Kolorex is a trademark name.

(horopito) cream produced an 88 per cent improvement in the symptoms of vaginal thrush, making it an excellent alternative to the over-the-counter conventional treatment, Canesten cream.

Be careful if you are using pau d'arco bark to brew your own tea. Not all supplies are equal and more unscrupulous makers will substitute useless mahogany wood shavings for the native herb. If you want the raw herb, get it from Creative Nature on 020 8941 7485. You can also get good quality capsules and even pau d'arco tea bags from reputable supplier Rio Trading (01273 570987; www.riohealth.co.uk).

Colloidal silver can help disable the enzymes many forms of bacteria, fungi and viruses need to replicate to maintain an infection. This is now available in cream or spray form but you can safely take it internally too. (A colloid, incidentally, is a substance that consists of ultra-fine particles suspended in a different medium, which in this case is water. These particles are so small – from just 0.0001 of a micron in diameter – that colloidal silver is safe to swallow.)

Fungal infections love damp climates so you can further bolster your defences by changing the conditions fungi thrive on. Use **silica**, which has a drying action on damp skin. Take this either in liquid form or as one of the biochemic tissue salts now widely on sale which bypass the digestive system for better absorption.

1, 2, 3 . . . Easy Steps to Stop or Relieve Fungal Infections
Horopito (take Kolorex capsules internally and use the cream topically; mail order from the NutriCentre – 0800 587 2290; www.NutriCentre.com – if not on sale locally).

Mighty mushrooms . . . One of the best immune-boosting mushroom combination supplements on sale is New Chapter's Host Defence; mail order from Victoria Health (0800 389 8195; www.victoriahealth.com) if not on sale in your local health store.

Take a good quality probiotic, plus silica.

Hair (including hair loss)

For stronger, glossier hair take an iodine-rich **kelp** supplement plus **tyrosine** (see Fungal Infections/Sea vegetables, pages 40 and 71).

The sad truth is that most types of hair loss have no 'miracle' cure – conventional or natural – but that is not going to stop people from wanting a solution, scientists from trying to find one or the more unscrupulous from exploiting sufferers' distress.

In clinical trials, hair-loss patients taking **vitamin A** (18,000 IUS) in the form of retinal, along with 70mg of an amino acid called **L-cysteine** and 700mg of **gelatin** (an unsavoury by-product of the slaughterhouse) for six months, were deemed to suffer less overall hair loss than the control group.

It is a shame that there is a price premium on those products that do come along and that people who are worried about hair loss have to fork out £40 or more a month to try to tackle the problem. If you are determined to find a ready-made formulation, the new **Folligrow** programme from Denmark is again backed by clinical trials but expensive to maintain. In studies using this programme, 65 per cent of participants reported a moderate improvement in hair regrowth and 18 per cent reported a very clear improvement. This is a two-pronged approach, where you use a topical spray containing **saw palmetto**, which helps prevent the conversion of the male hormone testosterone into one of the androgens that causes hair loss (it would be cheaper to take this herb in supplement form by itself to do the same job), and then take capsules containing **fenugreek** to promote better circulation to the scalp, and a combination of **B vitamins** to nourish the hair follicles. Again, you can buy a good B complex and stimulate the follicles the Ayurvedic way by washing the hair in cold water and giving the scalp a vigorous massage every day.

Another ready-made remedy getting a lot of attention is Nourkrin. Formulated and tested by the Institute for Dermatological Research in Helsinki, it is an all-natural supplement which provides nutrients to stimulate the regrowth of hair follicles. It is, in effect, a protein compound extracted from the cartilage of deepsea fish which is then combined with trace minerals, vitamins and organic silica.

In Sweden, ninety-seven members of the Swedish Alopecia Association, who had all unsuccessfully tried other treatments, volunteered to use Nourkrin for twelve months so researchers could monitor its effects. Some fourteen participants withdrew after three months claiming no benefits at all, but of those that remained in the trial, 14 per cent reported 100 per cent regrowth of their hair and the majority reported regrowth of around 75 per cent.

There are, as you can imagine, different types of hair loss. Alopecia areata is the term used to describe sudden hair loss from a specific part of the body and Nourkrin has been shown to help remedy this in the majority of patients taking it. Alopecia universalis is a rarer condition where all the body hair is lost. The Swedish researchers found that Nourkrin had no impact on patients suffering from this more extreme form of alopecia.

1, 2, 3 . . . Easy Steps to Make Your Hair Your Crowning Glory

Biotin, which can also strengthen nails, can help counter greasy hair, dandruff and seborrhoeic dermatitis caused by excessive oiliness by improving the metabolism of scalp oils. Take 25mg a day.

Kelp and L-tyrosine supplements will give you stronger, glossier hair and slow down the rate of hair loss.

If you want to try either of the ready-made programmes (see above) you can mail order Nourkrin from Lifes2Good (www.lifes2good.com) and Folligrow from Victoria Health on 0800 389 8195; www.victoriahealth.com.

Research alert: Early double-blind, placebo-controlled clinical trials suggest saw palmetto really can make a difference. Sixty per cent of balding men given 400mg a day of liposterolic extract of saw palmetto (equivalent to 4g a day of the berry) were rated as having significant improvement to hair growth.

> ### Tried and Applied
>
> Herbavita is a new organic and ammonia-free hair colour range from Italy, which you can still use even if your hair has been chemically coloured. (If this is the case, your hair will be more porous so choose one shade lighter than the colour you want to end up with.) Designed to cover grey and increase shine, there are 30 different colours to choose from. To find your perfect colour, visit www.herbavita.co.nz.

Herpes

Too embarrassing to discuss with your best friend but not something you should ignore. As with cold sores, the herpes virus hides itself deep in the DNA of the nerve cells where it can, unless triggered, remain inactive for weeks, even months.

The good news is that flare-ups should become less severe with time, but the triggers can be everyday factors – stress, other infections, even a trip to the dentist – which are hard to avoid.

Lysine will help keep the virus dormant (for an explanation, see Cold Sores, page 35) and in clinical trials **melissa (lemon balm)** was shown to help herpes blisters heal more rapidly and prevent further flare-ups. Among fifty-eight trial participants, twenty-four of those using melissa reported a complete recovery within five days. This compared with just fifteen of the fifty-eight volunteers who were given a placebo treatment.

To prevent repeated outbreaks, you need to support the immune system too. Again, as with cold sores, use the Chinese herb **astragalus** (500mg daily), which you can safely take every day.

Take L-lysine (1g, three times a day).

One of the best antiviral skin creams you can use topically combines St John's wort with melissa (lemon balm) and chamomile because although St John's wort is better known as a natural anti-depressant, it has fantastic antiviral properties too, as does melissa. FSC's St John's wort cream costs just £3.99 for 50g, and, if not on sale at your local health store, is available by mail order from Revital (0800 252875; www.revital.com).

Olive leaf extract has antiviral properties which act specifically against the herpes virus. You can take it as a tea (steep two teaspoons of the dried leaf in 150ml of boiling water for 30 minutes, strain and drink three or four cups a day) or use a lotion (from Revital, as above) on your lesions.

Shingles

This is a viral condition caused by the varicella zoster virus (VZV), which can trigger chickenpox in children and painful shingles in adults.

The theory is that after a childhood infection the virus lies dormant in the nerve ganglia until reactivated in later life. The pain of an infection is followed by lesions, which may only appear for between three and five days, and while the duration of an outbreak is between seven and ten days, it can take up to a month for the skin to completely recover. In adults over the age of fifty, pain can persist for up to six weeks after the outward symptoms have cleared. This is known as postherpetic neuralgia.

Since the majority of people have chickenpox in childhood but not everyone suffers from shingles in later life, it makes sense to conclude a healthy immune system can keep the dormant virus suppressed, and researchers now link shingles with weakened immunity.

In trials the remedy that has performed well to reduce the pain of postherpetic neuralgia in shingles patients is **reishi (granoderma lucidum)**, an Asian mushroom that is rich in anti-inflammatory polysaccharides which has now been shown to have impressive antiviral properties in test-tube studies.

1, 2, 3 . . . Easy Steps to Stop or Clear Shingles

Take reishi mushroom capsules to boost your immune system and prevent recurrence. (Market leader in the supply of Asian mushroom supplements is a company called JHS in America. In the UK, mail order reishi available from the NutriCentre on 0800 587 2290; www.NutriCentre.com.)

Use Kiwiherb's Manuka Paint to soothe lesions during an outbreak.

Take anti-inflammatory quercetin, which has antiviral properties too.

Splitting and Broken Nails

You would be amazed to learn how many of the natural supplements on sale in health stores and supermarkets we have animals to thank for. One example is probiotics, which were first used in animal feeds to improve growth and yield. Another is biotin, a B vitamin only vets used to strengthen horses' hooves until someone had the bright idea of asking whether it would work on humans too.

The answer to which was a resounding yes! Swiss researchers gave 2.5mg of biotin every day to women complaining of brittle nails and reported that, after six months, nail thickness had increased by 25 per cent. In another study, 63 per cent of Americans taking the exact same dosage showed significant improvement in splitting and in the condition of the nail bed.

The other key nutrient if you want to strengthen nails is methylsulphonylmethane (MSM) or organic sulphur. This is present in rainwater so it is naturally a part of our food chain, but it is easily destroyed by cooking and food processing, making supplementation a safer bet. It works by strengthening the sulphide bonds in keratin, the protein that forms nails.

Strong nails also require a good dietary source of protein, which may be a problem if you are vegetarian and missing out on the sulphur-containing amino acids, cysteine and methionine. MSM will remedy this, and so will making sure your diet is rich in natural sources, including onion, garlic, sunflower seeds, fish and eggs.

1, 2, 3 . . . *Easy Steps to Strengthen Splitting Nails*

Biotin (2.5mg a day for six months will increase nail thickness by 25 per cent).

Methylsulphonylmethane (MSM), which is now sold in capsule, cream and powder form. Mail order in the UK from specialist company Higher Nature (01435 882880).

US supplement maker Nature's Plus has produced a cruelty-free nail strengthener called Ultra Nails, which you can now buy in the UK too. Designed to strengthen nails and cuticles, it combines cucumber and aloe vera with calendula, lavender and tea tree in a protein- and vitamin-enriched formula.

Psoriasis

What is happening here is that skin cells have gone into a frenzy of overdrive. In non-sufferers, it takes 47 to 48 days for the outside layer of skin (the epidermis) to replace itself. In psoriasis, this process takes just a few days and results in a build-up of dead skin cells and the formation of thick scales.

The most commonly affected areas are the elbows, knees, scalp and buttocks, and in 50 per cent of patients the fingernails are affected too. There is almost always a history of this condition in the family and it is now known to be linked to an abnormal immune response (for more on the immune system and how it works, see Chapter 5).

What is less well known is that psoriasis sufferers often have an overly acidic body chemistry, caused by overconsumption of acid-forming foods. Returning the body chemistry back to an overall alkaline pH is important because if it is too acidic this has a detrimental effect on the immune system and your ability to absorb nutrients.

So the first positive step you can take back to normal skin is to read Dr John Pagano's book, *Healing Psoriasis: The Natural Alternative*, and to eat more of the foods that will help the body return to a healthier slightly alkaline pH. These include carrots, celery, garlic, spinach, sprouts, watercress, cooked apples, grapes, pineapple and prunes. His theory is that you aim for the following ratio: for every four foods you eat, three should be plants that grow above the ground, and only one should grow in the ground. (Meat, for example, would increase acidity.)

Alcohol consumption is known to exacerbate psoriasis so moderate your intake and take this as a sign that the liver must be playing a role too. Alcohol increases the absorption of toxins from the digestive tract and many psoriasis patients show impaired liver function. Go to pages 61–3, 83 and 86 to see how you can cleanse the bowel, keep it healthy and support your liver.

The other thing that is going on (and nobody will have told you this) is a process called angiogenesis. This is the tightly controlled process of new blood-vessel formation from existing blood vessels, which normally only occurs under rare conditions such as wound healing and embryonic development. (It also takes place in cancer where new blood vessels feed the tumorous growths, but this does not mean that if you have psoriasis you have a higher risk of cancer. I am simply explaining what this process is.)

Psoriasis has now been linked with a dilation of capillaries (the earliest stage of angiogenesis), and much of the work in finding a holistic treatment is now focused on natural agents that block this process. One of these is the humble and much hated hedgerow weed, bindweed, which is being investigated by the Allergy Research Group in America where it has been shown to have promising angiogenesis properties – so watch out for development in that area.

In the meantime, animal studies have shown that cartilage extracts can do the same job. The extracts used are usually shark cartilage (which is expensive) but the results have been promising enough to give it serious consideration as a topical treatment for this distressing condition.

To begin to manage psoriasis, you must understand that no single treatment is going to work for what is clearly a multifactoral condition. You will need to change your diet, tackle the digestive and liver issues and use a topical cream/liquid or gel which has anti-angiogenesis properties.

1, 2, 3 . . . Easy Steps to Help Control or Prevent Psoriasis

Cleanse the colon with a herbal cleanser such as Nature's Secret Super Cleanse (from Victoria Health: 0800 389 8195; www.victoriahealth.com) and then rebuild digestive health with a good quality probiotic.

Support liver functioning by using milk thistle (see page 5), and cut down on, or cut out, alcohol, which makes psoriasis worse.

Allergy Research Group's liquid shark cartilage is sold as CarTcell. For details, visit www.allergeryresearchgroup.com.

Roll Out Your Yoga Mat

I like yoga because it is clever. You might think it is all about looking good in tight clothes and being able to fold the body in two, but actually each posture or *asana* is designed to work on three levels, physical, mental and spiritual, which means you can tailor a daily practice to your current health needs.

If, for example, digestive problems are causing related skin complaints, incorporate the shoulderstand (*Sarvangasana*), which will stimulate both the liver and the digestive tract.

Here are my **1, 2, 3 best yoga asanas** for keeping the digestive organs and the liver toned, which, in turn, will keep your skin looking good.

Sarvangasana (Shoulderstand)

Don't attempt this posture unless you have some experience of yoga, and even then, remember to take the time to avoid straining your neck by folding your mat to make padding for your shoulders.

Lie on your back with your arms alongside the body, palms on the yoga mat. Bring the knees into the chest and, in one fluid movement, propel both legs up straight. The most important thing with this posture is to support the back with your hands. To do this, you will need to keep the elbows tight into your sides. There should be no tension on your neck. Hold the posture for as long as you feel comfortable then come slowly down by bending the knees, still supporting the back, and allowing the spine to roll up.

Counter this posture and soothe the spine by spending five minutes in the **pose of the child** (so called because of its child-like simplicity) afterwards. To do this posture, kneel on your mat, place your forehead on the floor, let your arms rest alongside and allow the chest to release down onto the knees.

Dhanurasana (The Bow)

Lie flat on the stomach with the legs and feet together, arms and hands alongside the body. Bend the knees to bring both heels close to the bottom. Put your chin on your yoga mat and then reach back and take hold of both ankles. Now tense the leg muscles, push the feet up and away from the body, arch the back and lift the head and chest. Rocking back and forth in this position, which massages the digestive organs and liver, will increase the benefits.

Maintain this pose for as long as you feel comfortable, and afterwards counter with the pose of the child, as for the shoulderstand (above).

Pascimottanasana (Back-stretching Pose)

Although this pose will give the back a stretch, the action of folding the body forwards over itself massages the entire abdominal region, including the liver. It may look simple but it is one of the most difficult poses to master because it requires a relaxed mind and, according to the yogis, an attitude of complete surrender of the will.

Sit on your mat with your legs stretched out in front, feet together and hands on the knees. Slowly bend forwards from the hips, allowing the hands to slide down the legs and, if you can, gently take hold of your big toes with your fingers and thumbs. If this is impossible, take hold of a lower part of the leg and make sure your attitude to this posture stays relaxed. The more you strain, the less likely your body will fold over itself to allow the head to rest on the knees, which is what you are aiming for.

Yoga for Stiff Bodies

There is no substitute for a yoga class or one-to-one tuition if you are new to the practice, but if you are over forty and know your body is stiff, don't launch enthusiastically into a strenuous Iyengar or Astanga yoga class. Instead, investigate the little-known form of Vini yoga, which recognizes that the western body has its limitations, and that in the hands of the wrong teacher you can end up doing more harm than good.

Vini yoga is usually taught on a one-to-one basis, incorporates a therapeutic approach to remedy underlying health problems and acknowledges that what is going on in your life will also be affecting your body and overall health.

For more information on this brilliant system, visit www.viniyoga.co.uk or call 0117 944 2994. For other types of yoga, contact the British Wheel of Yoga on 01529 306851.

CHAPTER TWO

Healthy Digestion

With almost every chronic health complaint, from persistent tiredness to a low libido, there is only one place to start to get rid of the symptoms and get well again.

The gut.

In fact, throughout this book, I will be sending you back to this crucial chapter again and again, because unless your digestive system is working optimally, you cannot expect the full therapeutic benefits from any of the natural remedies you are using for any condition you are trying to treat.

We have already seen in Chapter 1 how you cannot hope to improve your skin if you ignore what's going on inside and the same holds true for every other health complaint you may be suffering from or anxious to avoid.

You may think you interface with the world through the outside of your body – your face, your form, your skin – but the real interaction takes place inside, with the digestive tract. Parts of the surface of the perforated intestinal lining are as thin as your eyelid and since there are so many open spaces in the body (the mouth, the nose, the ears . . . and that's just the top of the body), this is the only real physical barrier you have to the onslaught of pollutants, both environmental and dietary, and pathogens trying to get in.

To understand how to support this system holistically, you need a basic knowledge of what it does. The digestive system has four crucial jobs.

- To receive and break down foods into nutrients; the process we call digestion.
- To absorb nutrients into the bloodstream for transport to organs and tissues.
- To eliminate indigestible parts of food from the body.
- To host the so-called 'friendly' bacteria that help make nutrients that support these processes and the immune system.

Going In

From the time a food or any other substance enters your mouth to the time it leaves the body, it will pass through a complex series of mechanical (e.g. chewing) and chemical (e.g. the breakdown of fats by bile) processes, involving several different organs, and known collectively as the digestive system.

Rapid transit foods, such as fruits and wholegrains, can pass through this entire system within as little as ten hours. Foods that require more work to break down and digest, red meats for instance, can hang around for days.

Saliva contains special enzymes which start this process of digestion in the mouth, and the very act of chewing your food not only cuts food into more easily digestible particles which are then coated in the digestive enzymes present in saliva, but also sends a signal to the other digestive organs to swing into action.

Between meals, the flow of saliva helps wash away bacteria that would otherwise cause tooth decay. For details on how to use natural remedies to protect your teeth and maintain strong, healthy gums, see Chapter 4.

Going Down

Everything you ingest will find its way into the bean-shaped stomach where it can spend as little as one and as long as six hours. So, if you have breakfast at seven in the morning, you will naturally be ready to eat again at 1 p.m. If, however, you've had a later brunch, at around 11 a.m., you won't really need to eat again until 5 p.m. Just knowing this simple fact can help you stop yourself from overeating and putting an unnecessary burden on the digestive system.

In the stomach your food is churned around with the digestive juices and it will not leave this chamber until it is in a semi-liquid state known as chyme. This is also the first place you can support the digestive system by taking **digestive enzymes** (see page 85) or a supplement form of **hydrochloric acid** (which the body produces naturally to break down protein food solids) called **betaine hydrochloride,** which is derived from beets.*

It is estimated that 30 per cent of adults produce insufficient hydrochloric acid, which can affect the body's ability to absorb nutrients. Natural healers make a link between this problem – known in medical circles as hypochlorhydria, where there is a deficiency in the production of hydrochloric acid in the stomach, or achlorhydria, where none is produced at all – and numerous

---

* While the supplement betaine hydrochloride is extracted from beets, eating the raw vegetable will not provide therapeutic levels.

chronic conditions, including asthma, atherosclerosis, candida yeast infections, gastritis and rheumatoid arthritis, and while there is to date no clinical evidence to support this link, it makes sense when you consider the digestion as a holistic part of the whole.

If you plan to take a betaine hydrochloride supplement, watch the dosage. Too much can cause heartburn; if you have this side effect, drink several large glasses of water, which will dilute the acid concentration in the stomach. The safe therapeutic dosage is between 325mg and 650mg a day, with food. The other reason it is worth considering the value of this supplement is that proper gastric acidity is crucial for preventing pathogens (bad bacteria) from entering the rest of the digestive tract.

The Small Intestine

Semi-liquid food (chyme) moves out of the stomach down into the small intestine. Here the process of absorbing the nutrients you need to keep you well begins. The first nutrients to be absorbed are the minerals, including iron, magnesium, calcium and zinc. These are all absorbed at the start of this 6.5-metre/21-foot long tube in a section known as the duodenum, which receives pancreatic enzymes from the pancreas and bile from the liver. This is also where peristalsis – the wave-like action that moves food and waste through the gut, aiding digestion and absorption by churning it up with enzymes and intestinal secretions – starts.

The first few inches of the lining of the duodenum are smooth but the remainder has folds and pockets that serve to increase the surface area over which nutrients can be absorbed. The intestinal wall secretes mucus to lubricate the intestinal contents, and water to help dissolve digested food particles and reduce acidity as the contents move to the end of this section of the gut. Here, in the latter part, carbohydrates (sugars), proteins and fats are digested with the aid of more enzymes and of bile salts, which originate from the liver but will have been stored in the gallbladder.

By the time the intestinal contents pass out of the small intestine and into the large one (the colon) they will be a fluid mass of nutrients, water, mucus, bile salts and digestive enzymes.

Related Organs – Liver, Pancreas and Gallbladder

These three organs all work to support the digestive process. Think of the **liver** as the body's high-speed chemical processing plant: *everything* you ingest must pass through this large and extraordinary organ, and so its main challenge is to avoid toxic overload.

Nutrients absorbed into the bloodstream through the wall of the intestine are then passed via the portal vein into the liver for processing in two ways. Bacteria and foreign particles that have been absorbed are screened out, and many of the nutrients that have been absorbed from the gut are further metabolized and broken down.

The liver also makes about half the body's cholesterol (the rest comes from food), and 80 per cent of this 'homegrown' cholesterol is used to make bile, which the liver secretes into the gallbladder for storage.

The condition of the liver is critical to your overall health and well-being. In fact, naturopaths who treat health problems without resorting to allopathic drugs, drawing instead from a range of disciplines including homeopathy, herbal and detoxification programmes, believe almost all diseases are caused by colon and liver congestion. The theory is that when the liver becomes congested, toxins, which would otherwise have been screened and removed, circulate round the body in the blood, causing damage to its tissues and systems.

Signs of a congested liver include frequent headaches, digestive disturbances, insomnia, feeling sluggish when you wake up in the morning and a yellowy tinge to the skin. Emotional clues include feeling angry, impatient and irritable, when these would not be your normal reactions to everyday events.

You can easily give the liver a rest by cutting out meat, fats, refined foods, white sugar, flour products and alcohol. Stop eating these foods for a week and see how your energy levels and digestion improve.

For a discussion on liver-supporting herbs, go back to Chapter 1 (page 5).

Tried and Applied

Start the day with the fresh juice of half a lemon or lime dissolved in warm water. This can help both heal and clean a congested liver. Eat your main meal of the day before 3 p.m. to give the liver a chance to rest and repair itself, and allocate one day for a simple juice-only fast. Make your own Liver Superjuice using carrots, celery, parsley and apples.

The **pancreas** produces both digestive enzymes and hormones including insulin, which lowers blood sugar levels, glucagons, which raise blood sugar levels, and somatostatin, which prevents the other two hormones from being released.

There are remedies that can help support the pancreas (see Diabetes, page 92) and, while I am against using animals in this very cruel way, it is worth reporting that in trials on depancreatized dogs, the use of a decoction of **bilberry leaves** given orally was shown to help reduce hyperglycaemia, the telltale symptom of diabetes. This happened even when glucose, which would normally produce a blood sugar-level surge, was simultaneously injected into the dogs.

The active ingredient responsible for this insulin-like effect is an anthocyanoside called myrtillin. It is weaker than insulin but far less toxic and, in animal trials, a single therapeutic dose of just 1g a day was shown to bring about an improvement lasting for several weeks. **That said, if you have been diagnosed with a pancreatic disorder, do not try to self-treat. Instead, ask your health advisors about the role of natural remedies in supporting this organ.**

A trickle of bile flows continuously out of the liver and into the **gallbladder** where it is stored between meals, but once you eat, the body sends a series of hormonal and nerve cell signals to this organ to tell it to contract and empty bile salts into the small intestine where it mixes with food.

Bile has two important jobs. It helps the body digest fats and also helps eliminate certain waste products, including iron-rich haemoglobin from destroyed red blood cells and excess cholesterol. Bile salts also stimulate the secretion of water by the cells lining the intestinal tract to keep waste fluid and moving along.

If you know you have a toxic lifestyle – smoking, drinking, poor quality foods – then the production and flow of bile is even more relevant since drugs and other harmful wastes are excreted in bile and later eliminated from the body.

Bile salts are reabsorbed into the small intestine, extracted by the liver and resecreted into the bile – a process known as enterohepatic circulation. In fact, all the bile salts in your body circulate between ten and twelve times a day.

Gallstones form when bile becomes too 'dense' to remain soluble in the gallbladder. The solubility of this digestive fluid depends on the relative concentrations of cholesterol, bile acids, phosphatidycholine and water in the mix so, again, you can see that to take a holistic approach you need to think more about what happens to food when it enters the body. A simple **gallbladder flush** combines a tablespoon of **olive oil** and the juice of half a **lemon,** which you simply mix and drink, to help keep bile soluble and prevent the formation of stones, a problem that is the most common reason for the surgical removal of the gallbladder.

Globe artichokes work well to support the liver and gallbladder but, as is common in natural health, the name of the supplement I am going to recommend – **cynara** – has no obvious link with the plant. This is because it is named after the active agent, cynarin, which is extracted from the leaves. Cynara works to increase the secretion of bile, which helps enzymes in the gut break down fats and other foods, but it also helps slow the production of cholesterol by the liver.

In test-tube trials on cultured liver cells, artichoke extract not only provided significant antioxidant protection from a toxic, chemically induced assault but also showed a diminished loss of cellular glutathione reserves. (Glutathione is the body's own major mine-sweeping antioxidant which works to clear out toxins, especially from environmental and dietary pollutants such as excess alcohol and cigarette smoking.) For more details on how cynara works, contact the UK herbal makers Lichtwer Pharma (01803 528668).

Going Out – the Large Intestine or Colon

The large intestine secretes mucus and is largely responsible for the absorption of water and electrolytes from the faeces. This is where the so-called 'friendly' or good bacteria can aid digestion and the absorption of nutrients, but only when they outnumber the less friendly or pathogenic ones.

Sickness and antibiotics can both disrupt this balance, making probiotic supplementation (see Chapter 1, page 9, and Chapter 2, page 65) crucial, especially if you already suffer from any form of digestive disorder.

Glutamine is the single most abundant amino acid in the bloodstream. It is produced by the body, primarily in the skeletal system, but is also present in high levels in cabbage and beets. This nutrient plays a key role in detoxification processes in the gut and is critical to healthy digestion. It helps prevent the passage of bacteria and toxins across the intestinal wall and into the bloodstream and is also used as a food source by the intestinal immune cells (see page 64 for how digestion and immunity are interlinked). It also provides antioxidant protection to the intestinal cells and is needed to eliminate toxins from the intestinal tissues.

A struggling digestive system, trauma, infection, starvation and chemotherapy treatments can all take their toll on glutamine levels, which will then need to be rebuilt via supplementation.

Tried and Applied

Allergy Research Group's Permavite combines L-glutamine with N-acetyl-D-glucosamine and slippery elm in powder form. Practitioners love it and I cannot think of a better supplement to support the digestive–immune relationship. Mail order from the NutriCentre (0800 587 2290; www.NutriCentre.com) and take 1–3 tablespoons a day.

Getting Naturopathic – Colon Cleansing

There is only one place any self-respecting naturopath will begin a treatment regimen and that is with a congested gut, which they believe lies at the root of more than 70 per cent of all ailments. In fact, anything else you do to try to tackle health problems is a waste of time if the digestive tract is overburdened and struggling to do its job.

The simplest way to cleanse the colon is to fast, but since this is also the quickest way to trigger what natural therapists call a 'healing crisis', which can include blinding migraines, nausea and cramping, I would not embark on a serious fast or one lasting more than a day without supervision by a naturopath or other qualified practitioner with expertise in this field.

Complementary health practitioners at the Organic Pharmacy (020 7351 2232; www.TheOrganicPharmacy.com) in London, for example, have developed an ingenious pre-detox programme that works to strengthen the organs of the digestive tract before embarking on any cleansing or detoxification programme. This is an excellent example of adopting a truly holistic approach to health and well-being and will help to avoid triggering the uncomfortable signs of a healing crisis, which can include stomach cramping, headaches, nausea, rashes and flu-like symptoms.

The second worse thing you can do (aside from starve yourself for three days and still expect to function as normal) is to fast and then tuck into a roast dinner when you decide to eat again. Again, if you have no experience of fasting, ask for help from someone such as a qualified herbalist, nutritionist or naturopath who knows what they are doing, who can tailor a programme to help you through the detox and who can support you through the sometimes dramatic adjustments your body will have to make.

If fasting is not your thing, you can use herbal supplements to cleanse the colon. The most important one is **psyllium husks**, which absorb moisture in the body and swell to bulk faeces and keep the colon clean. They also stimulate peristalsis, the wave-like contractions of the gut that keep waste moving through. If you can bear to swallow something that tastes and smells like sawdust, use **Lepicol**, which combines psyllium husks with both pre- and probiotics. (Call 0121 779 6619, or sales@leppin-health.com, for more details.)

Cornflakes and Colonic Irrigation

Although the ancient Egyptians regularly used enemas, irrigation of the entire colon did not start in the west until the 1800s. In the US, this method of relieving gastrointestinal problems was popularized by Dr John Harvey Kellogg – the natural health zealot and Seventh Day Adventist, and one of two brothers who also brought cornflakes to our breakfast tables.

There is almost no real research proving the effects of colonic irrigation one way or the other, but according to a new trial by the Meridian Institute in Virginia, the infusion of warm, filtered water into the rectum to cleanse the large intestine and encourage peristalsis (the wave-like action that moves waste through the gut) can be helpful for people with indigestion, gas, headaches, joint problems, allergies, asthma and skin disorders, but should *NOT* be used on anyone who has Crohn's disease, ulcerative colitis, severe haemorrhoids, diverticulitis, blood in the stool, heart problems or colorectal cancers. This is worth reporting since it is the only piece of research, as opposed to anecdotal evidence, that I have encountered on the subject.

What I would also say is that with the guidance of a qualified herbalist, you can cleanse the colon just as effectively using herbs, especially the Ayurvedic cleanser **Triphala** (see page 83), and you might take the view that if you were supposed to sluice water up your bottom, the Creator would have installed a tap!

Tried and Applied

Get a meditation stool. This will not only come in handy for your yoga classes and meditation sessions, but also for sitting on the loo. The human body was never designed for the modern toilet. When sitting, you can facilitate the elimination process by raising both feet on a small stool. If your budget is tight, use a child's step and keep it in the bathroom.

Immune System

Although they appear to have nothing in common, you cannot separate the body's own natural defences in the form of its immune system from the digestive tract and its related organs. Think of both systems as close work colleagues, partners if you like, and be aware that the healthy functioning of one will have a direct impact on the health and well-being of the other.

What you eat can affect your immune system and your immune system will affect how your digestive tract can absorb or eliminate what you eat. In addition, both systems also work together to protect your body from invasion by bacteria, viruses and other harmful pathogens.

As we have seen, the gut is where you really interface with the outside world, and so your primary defences are the B and T immune system cells, which form part of what is called gut-associated lymphoid tissue (GALT). The B cells, for instance, produce antigens against toxins and pathogens, making them a kind of front-line defence troop.

In laboratory studies, researchers have shown that something as simple as feeding cabbage juice to rats stimulates the immune system, thanks to the presence of an unidentified compound, believed to be glutamine (see page 61) since cabbage is such a rich source of this protective amino acid. So if you do nothing else to support the link between your immune system and your digestive tract, fill your shopping trolley with organic cabbage and get juicing.

Tried and Applied

Superjuice: To boost the link between digestion and immunity, juice glutamine-rich cabbage and beetroot with carrots, celery and apples. Add a probiotic acidophilus powder to further boost levels of good gut bacteria.

The Better Bug Debate – Pre- and Probiotics

Because digestion is so crucial to well-being and vitality, and is often at the root of sickness and chronic ailments, you will be told in this book, again and again, if you do nothing else for your health, take a good quality **probiotic**.

You may already know that probiotics are the supplements that rebuild good gut health by replenishing levels of the so-called 'friendly' bacteria in the gut, but the smart thing is to take a combined pre- and probiotic which will selectively 'feed up' these bacteria to the detriment of the other, less helpful micro-organisms present in the gut. The best known pre-biotic is still the plant sugar known as **fructo-oligosaccharides (FOS)**.

One of the best prebiotic powders I have found comes from a wonderful New Zealand company called Annie's which, primarily, produces pure, unadulterated 'fruit waves' for kids to replace those disgusting artificial fruit-winders which, sadly, have become a staple in most school lunchboxes, despite the fact they have more in common with a chemical air freshener than any real live piece of fruit. Visit Annie's website (www.annies.co.nz) to find local stockists. Mail order Nutrition Now's Acidophilus with FOS, an excellent combined pre- and probiotic supplement in capsule form from Victoria Health (0800 389 8195; www.victoriahealth.com).

Why 'good quality probiotic'? Are some better than others? The simple answer is that in independent testing, scientists have confirmed what I have long suspected – that many of the probiotics on sale contain nothing like the number of replacement bacteria promised on the label or even the best strains.

In other words, *not all probiotics are equal* and not everyone agrees on which is the best form to take – a powder you must keep in the fridge, or an enteric-coated capsule to protect the bacteria on their journey through the gut to reach the place they are needed: the colon.

See Chapter 1 (pages 9–10) for a discussion on the two key strains of bacteria that we know are safe for human consumption and that you should be looking for when you select a probiotic brand, and then ask yourself why, if these strains are supposed to be in the colon naturally, they need an expensive coating process to get there?

Health stores and supplement makers may tell you that enteric-coated capsules are the only way to get these bacteria to survive their journey through the acidic environment of the stomach, but some insiders would argue that this process is a poor substitute for using strains that are already acid resistant. There is a very real risk the process of enteric coating may kill off live bacteria or reduce their viability and, as far as I am aware, there are no convincing studies showing that enteric-coated probiotics really do outperform those that are not coated.

The question I would keep asking is why do they need a protective coat when they do not come that way naturally?

The One to Watch – Artemisia

You can also use herbs to rebalance the gut flora of the digestive tract, but only if you know what you are doing. The herb I am going to recommend grows vigorously in my own herb garden, but is too foul-tasting for its medicinal properties to be harnessed by most of us in a tincture or tea.

The herb is Artemisia annua or sweet wormwood, a traditional anti-malarial agent which has also been used by Chinese physicians to treat ulcerative colitis (see page 103). The active agent is artemisinin or qinghaosu, which has now been encapsulated in tablet form by US market leaders the Allergy Research Group, as part of its Nutricology range. To find out more about this range, which is targeted at doctors and other health professionals in the

US, visit my website and check out Allergy Research Group on the links page.

The plant itself contains around 0.3–0.5 per cent artemisinin, so this new supplement provides a therapeutic dosage hundreds of times higher than you would get if you harvested your own plants. The way it works is that unlike probiotics, which rebuild levels of the good gut bacteria (see pages 9 and 65), artemisinin has an antiparasitic and antipathogen action, and so kills off the bad bacteria that would otherwise compete with the good ones, allowing the latter to flourish.

Clever or what?

Tried and Applied

Whatever else you are doing to tackle digestive disorders, make silica an adjunct, since this trace mineral works to support the lining of the digestive tract. You can take it in the form of biochemic tissue salts, which, like homeopathic pills, pass straight into the bloodstream and bypass the stomach, or in liquid form, which you dilute in water or fruit juice and take before a meal. Look for Huber's Original Silicea, which is now on sale in good health stores.

Feeding Your Digestive System – which type of fibre?

When most people think of fibre they think of bran, but there are, essentially, five different types of fibre, which work in different ways in the body.

Hemicellulose fibres, found in bran and other cereals, Brussels sprouts and beetroot, absorb water to bulk and soften waste as it moves through the colon, making them very effective in preventing constipation and treating problems such as irritable bowel syndrome (IBS).

Cellulose fibres, found in beans, broccoli, peppers, apples and carrots, work in the same way as the hemicellulose, above.

Lignin is found in breakfast cereals and, more interestingly, older vegetables, which have a higher lignin content than fresh produce. Lignin reduces the digestibility of other fibres in the food you have been eating (ensuring more useful bulk in the stools) and binds with bile acids to lower cholesterol and speed the passage of food through the gut.

Gums, found in oatmeal and dried beans, are another type of fibre. These bind with bile acids to decrease fat absorption and delay stomach-emptying by coating the lining of the gut.

Pectin, found in apples, citrus fruits, carrots, cabbage, cauliflower, green beans, potatoes and strawberries, is the last type. This agent is often used in natural slimming aids.

Some foods, such as bran, contain more than one type of fibre. To work out which fibre you need most, do your homework. Read more about your problem, what causes it, why you have it and which of the above will best help. For example, if you suffer from constipation, you need one of the bulking (hemicellulose) fibres, which will help move waste out of the body. If you want to prevent bloating and lose some weight, increase your intake of the gum fibres in foods such as oats.

Tried and Applied

I dislike the dry, often bland taste of lots of ready-made mueslis and so always make my own breakfast cereal by mixing jumbo-sized organic oats with linseeds, sunflower seeds, pumpkin seeds, sesame seeds, raisins, dried apricots, chopped pecan and brazil nuts, bran flakes and millet. This is not a precise science: use oats as your base and add the other ingredients to taste. Tip your serving into a bowl and soak with hot water for 20 minutes to help the body better absorb the grains. Add a teaspoon of flaxseed oil and use oat milk instead of dairy. The oats in this recipe help maintain blood-sugar levels throughout the morning (which means you won't be craving a mid-morning snack). This breakfast will help keep many of the more common digestive complaints at bay.

Living Foods and Simple Sprouting

The very term 'living foods' suggests there must be other foods that are nutritionally 'dead'. What living foods provide, gram for gram, and thanks to their dense chlorophyll content, are more nutrients than any other natural food. In health stores you can buy ready-made powders and even grain snack bars made from these 'living foods', but if you grew mustard & cress as a child, you've already grown your own and taken your first step towards sprouting, which means you can easily harvest your own living foods at home. (And if you never did grow mustard & cress, I can assure you it's easy.)

And while you can buy starter kits, all you really need to get started at home is an old jam jar, a muslin or mesh sieve to cover the top, some water and some seeds. If you are not sure what to sprout, then start with organic alfalfa, sunflower, peas or mung bean seeds.

How to Sprout: Soak your chosen seeds overnight, then put them into the jar with three times as much water (i.e. one cup of seeds, three cups of water) and cover the top with your muslin sieve. Leave to soak again overnight. In the morning, drain the water off but keep it – this liquid is now an enzyme-rich solution known as rejuvenac. Sip throughout the day to boost digestive health and pour any that is left over on your houseplants.

Leave your drained seeds alone for 12 hours, then rinse in fresh, lukewarm water and drain again. Repeat this rinsing and leaving process over the next three to five days until your sprouting seeds start to form little green leaves. Harvest and toss into salads.

Once you get the hang of sprouting, you can start to get more technical about your yield. Different seeds, for instance, need a different number of rinses. Alfalfa, for example, needs only two rinses and should be harvested when the sprouts are 2.5–5 cm/1–2in high. This should take four days. Chickpeas need five rinses, also take four days to yield, and you eat them when the shoots reach 1–2.5cm/½–1in high.

Green Superfoods

Spirulina* is rich in vitamin B5, which helps support healthy digestion. A blue-green micro-algae that thrives in hot climates, it produces twenty times more protein than soybeans growing on the same size patch of land, and is probably the most nutrient-dense superfood known to humankind.

It is a superb adjunct for anyone considering fasting since it works in the body to cleanse and heal, at the same time curbing appetite. It is also excellent for diabetics, since the high-protein content means it can help stabilize blood-sugar levels between meals. Test-tube studies show it has a liver-protecting role, making it a useful addition to any regimen designed to clear heavy-metal pollutants out of the body.

Natural healers often link heavy-metal contamination to a range of chronic conditions, from digestive disorders to chronic fatigue. When you think about all the chemicals in your daily life, you realize they may have a point. Heavy-metal pollutants are stored in the body but you can use chlorophyll-rich foods including spirulina and wheatgrass to leach these toxins from the body.

* Spirulina is safe to take during pregnancy.

If you want to introduce any of the Green Superfoods into your diet (you can find out about them from many different sources), start slowly with a small dosage and build up to around 40g a day. Also, make sure you source these supplements from specialist companies who ensure their supplies of spirulina, for example, come from non-contaminated sources and so have not built up their own load of lead, cadmium and mercury. I use the UK specialist Xynergy (08456 585858; www.xynergy.co.uk).

Forget Seafood – It's Sea Vegetables You Need

Brown seaweeds such as **kombu** and **wakame** provide a bounty of minerals, vitamins, protein and fibre to support the digestive system and good gut flora. They are an excellent source of gut-protecting super-nutrition because they themselves absorb minerals from seawater. They are also a good source of iodine, which supports the thymus gland, which, in turn, regulates the body's metabolism.

The problem is that outside Japan, where sea vegetables make up 10 per cent of the normal diet, they are definitely an acquired taste and most of us don't know how to use them.

The trick if you are new to these foods is to toast them first and then crumble them over rice, baked potatoes, casserole dishes or even popcorn, or add them as a thickening agent to spaghetti sauces or quiches, use in soup stock, beans, soups and stews, or even learn to make your own sushi (which is easier than you might think).

Instead of using gelatin, which is a by-product of the slaughterhouse made from the bones, cartilages and hides of horses, pigs and cattle, use the sea vegetable **agar agar**, which is a natural gelling agent and one that is very soothing to the digestive tract.

You can now buy these foods in most independent health

stores; if you prefer the convenience of mail order, the UK specialist Clearspring has an extensive list of sea greens (0871 871 6611; www.clearspring.co.uk).

Six of the Best – Sea Greens

Agar Agar Produced from the mucilage of several species of sea greens and usually sold as a powder or as flakes, this is a good substitute for animal gelatin to make summer fruit jellies. Rich in nutrients, plus iodine, it adds bulk to meals without increasing calories and so is excellent for curbing appetite.

Arame Brown and stringy but high in iron and calcium and good for the thyroid and digestion. Soak for 5 minutes before cooking. It supports the thyroid and is good for high blood pressure, bones and teeth.

Dulse Red and blue pigmentation, it has a salty flavour and is rich in iodine and manganese. It also has the highest iron content of any food and so is excellent for those with anaemia. Prevents seasickness, inhibits the herpes virus and is a good salt substitute.

Kombu Unlocks the nutritional value of foods prepared with it. Used to treat arthritis, rheumatism, high blood pressure, thrush, prostate and ovarian problems, lymphatic swellings and water retention. Good for weight loss and can help reduce cancer tumours. Soak for 20–30 minutes or allow an hour's cooking time. Use one or two strips to tenderize beans. (It will also reduce the resulting flatulence.)

Nori Rich in fibre and low in fat, use in salads, soups and for making sushi. It contains more vitamin C than oranges and is delicious roasted. No need to soak. Very cooling and rich in vitamin A to maintain skin and membranes. It can reduce phlegm, lower cholesterol and is the most easily digested of all the sea greens. Known as 'sloke' in Ireland, and 'laver' in Scotland and Wales.

Wakame Olive-coloured wakame should be soaked for 5 minutes, and cooked for 45. It has anti-cancer properties and is higher in calcium than most other sea greens. Promotes healthy hair, nails and skin. Traditionally used in Japan to purify the blood after childbirth; it supports the liver and has a sweet flavour.

Mud, Mud, Glorious Mud

No, I'm not kidding.

Your body is programmed to heal itself but you do not live in a vacuum and nature has very cleverly provided not only plants, but also the beneficial bacteria that help develop an immune system, and which work with and not against your digestive tract.

Both chronic digestive disorders and malabsorption syndromes have been shown to improve dramatically in clinical trials where sufferers were given a supplement containing precision-bred homeostatic soil organisms (HSO). This is a fancy term for the micro-organisms that live in untreated soil.

People who have retained the ability to think for themselves (no mean feat in itself) have long expressed concern about the over-clean and oversterilized environments most of us in the west live in. These people are not nutters with nothing better to think about. They know, thanks to new research, that the micro-organisms found in dirt influence the maturation of the immune system and can help determine whether it becomes functional or dysfunctional in later life.

They know, too, that when children are exposed to adequate levels of viruses, bacteria and micro-organisms – i.e. when you allow them to play in mud and put dirty fingers into their mouths – the T-helper cells of their immune system mature properly, but that without this internal exposure to soil microbes, immune cells can become hypersensitized and tend to overreact.

Think about it. Unless you are a keen and gloveless gardener, when did you last get your hands really dirty?

You can now buy HSO formulations such as Primal Defense that has a very specialized delivery mechanism to get the microbes through the acidic environment of the stomach and into the gut. This range is produced by American manufacturer Garden of Life. For more information, visit www.gardenoflifeusa.com.

Tried and Applied

Rezonate is a natural digestive tonic made from organic apple cider vinegar and native New Zealand manuka and tamari honeys. The latter are rich in fructo-oligosaccharide prebiotic plant sugars (see page 65), and this tonic will also aid the absorption of other nutrients. To mail order from the UK, call 01730 813642.

Food Allergies and Intolerance

The UK government might believe food intolerances are all in the mind* and simply a way of getting more attention at the

---

* UK government scientists have stipulated that, while the idea of food intolerances has become so fashionable that a third of the adult population believes themselves to be affected, only about 2 per cent of us genuinely do suffer from them. Rubbish!

dinner table, but if you are a sufferer, pay no heed, since you will discover for yourself that eliminating foods your body has become intolerant to can really boost your overall vitality and health, and, especially, the working of your digestive system.

Natural healers would argue that food intolerances are the new silent epidemic of the 21st century, and while doctors are quick to diagnose allergies, they remain largely uninformed about intolerances to everyday foods such as wheat and dairy products.

According to Paleolithic nutrition experts, our ancestors survived on a diet of mostly fruits, vegetables and lean game meats. The agriculture of cereal grains first started some 10,000 years ago but did not spread to Europe until 5000 years ago. Over that period of time, changes in our genetic make-up are negligible, which is why some anthropological nutritionists will argue that human beings are still best suited to a grain-free diet.

While our genetic make-up has changed little, what has changed drastically is our consumption of wheat, thanks to the technical and production revolutions that have given us supermarket shelves heaving with packaged and processed 'unnatural' foods containing wheat that has been altered by technology to increase its gluten content. Today, 50 per cent of the protein in wheat is gluten – a component that facilitates baking and adapts this grain well to cultivation and harvesting.

If you suffer from coeliac disease (CD) then you already know about allergy to gluten, and that when you eat foods containing it the immune system produces antibodies that damage the lining of the intestinal tract. The only way to cope with this is to avoid gluten in the diet, which, when you consider how often it crops up as a hidden binder, filler and starch in foods and even in some vitamins and medications, is easier said than done.

Doctors are taught that one in 5000 suffer from CD, but according to researchers at the University of Maryland medical school, the true figure is closer to one in 150. What is even more alarming is that the majority who do suffer may not even know because it is commonly misdiagnosed and confused with other conditions including irritable bowel syndrome (IBS), anaemia, stress, colitis, diabetes, depression, joint pain, lactose intolerance, viral gastroenteritis, ulcers and gallbladder problems. If you have even half a hunch you may be a sufferer, go back to your doctor and ask to be tested for the antibodies the immune system is producing in response to a food the body cannot tolerate.

Researchers have now identified a connection between gluten intolerance and other, seemingly unrelated problems, which they now label 'overlapping syndromes'. The link is that these conditions – including chronic fatigue, fibromyalgia, autism in children and rheumatic joint problems (see Chapter 4, page 177) – display the very same abnormal biochemical, neurological and immune responses as intolerance to gluten.

Common food allergens besides wheat include: rye, barley, oats, dairy foods and citrus fruits. Remember, too, when shopping, that a 'wheat-free' label does not necessarily mean gluten-free as well.

If you think you may have a food intolerance, consult a practitioner who can arrange screening and testing procedures to confirm your hunch and then prescribe a tailor-made treatment programme. There are also health centres, such as the Diagnostic Clinic (020 7009 4650) in London, where you can, in effect, walk in off the street, and where the treatment options include a medically supervised integrated approach combining complementary and conventional medicine. The problem is that none of these tests come cheap and you can pay up to £800 for an integrated health MOT, which is too expensive for most normal family budgets.

You know your body better than anyone else and remember, the only language it has to make itself heard is sickness, so start listening to it before it has to shout at you symptoms you cannot ignore.

A–Z of Gut-Nourishing Foods

A is for asparagus, which can help prevent constipation and bloating, plus artichokes which are rich in magnesium to help relieve indigestion. The French eat artichokes the day after indulging in a heavy meal.

B is for bananas, the best natural probiotic, and broccoli, a vegetable rich in glutamine, a crucial amino acid that can detoxify carcinogens in the digestive tract and thus help protect the colon from cancer.

C is for cider vinegar, which helps strengthen digestion and prevent diarrhoea; chicken, which is a good source of gut-protecting B vitamins, and cabbage, which stimulates the immune system to further protect the digestive tract. Cabbage juice will also soothe inflammation and stomach ulcers.

D is for dill, a member of the parsley family with a potent antidiarrhoea action in the body. Use dill oil to stop hiccups and flatulence. Dates, which are high in vitamin B6, will help the body properly assimilate proteins and fats, and work as a natural diuretic to stop bloating from water retention.

E is for elderberries, which provide folic acid to help the body metabolize protein and protect against intestinal parasites and food poisoning. This important nutrient is also present in egg yolks.

F is for fennel, which is widely used in Ayurvedic medicine as a natural laxative to help relieve everyday digestive problems, especially gas and constipation.

G is for ginger – one of the all-time best digestive tonics. Make your own Ayurvedic pre-dinner digestive aid by mixing a little grated ginger with fresh lemon juice, honey and warm water. Drink half an hour before you eat to stimulate the gastric juices.

H is for horseradish, a digestive stimulant which can break down the protein fibres in meat – which is why your granny serves horseradish sauce with her Sunday roast beef.

I is for ice cream of the oat variety from a company called First Foods (01494 431355; www.first-foods.com). Oats contain gum fibres that bind with bile acids to decrease fat absorption and delay stomach emptying by coating the lining of the gut. This slows down sugar absorption after a meal and means you will not suffer the blood-sugar highs that trigger sweet food cravings.

J is for juniper berries, first used in the 1500s to make an inexpensive diuretic and digestive tonic known as gin ... These berries, which are used to flavour sauerkraut, can help eliminate wind and cramps.

K is for kale, another bowel-cancer-protecting cruciferous vegetable which provides colon-protecting glutamine; plus kidney beans, another diuretic which can help prevent bloating.

L is for liver and lentils, both good sources of cancer-protecting glutamine (see broccoli and kale); lentils are also simple to sprout for extra nutrients and intestinal protection. Also linseeds (psyllium) which help bulk waste for easier transit through the digestive tract (see the breakfast recipe on page 68).

M is for millet, a sacred, ceremonial grain in China where it was eaten as a niacin-rich (vitamin B3) porridge to support healthy digestion; plus malt, which is a good source of other B vitamins that aid digestion, and which, in 1800s Britain, was known as a restorative food for invalids and sickly children. Use malt extract from the health store to make a nourishing malted drink.

N is for nori, the Japanese seaweed used in its dried form to make the outside skin of a Californian sushi roll. In Wales and Scotland, this same seaweed is known as laver and used to make traditional laver bread. Nori can help the body better digest fried foods.

O is for onions which, when cooked, can help relieve indigestion and wind. They are also a good source of folic acid to help with digestion and protect the gastrointestinal tract.

P is for prunes, a natural laxative; parsley, a plant that is not only nutritious in its own right but can also aid the digestive process, plus potatoes, which provide gut-protecting silicon. Peppermint can help ease digestive spasms; grow your own and make fresh peppermint tea.

Q is for quinoa, rich in the digestion-supporting B vitamins, with the highest protein content of any of the natural grains. Use as a substitute for rice or in soups or as a side dish.

R is for rye, another good food source of silicon and nutrients that support other organs linked with digestion, especially the pancreas, liver and gallbladder. Eat rye bread, sprout rye seeds or use rye flakes in cereals. Drink rooibos (red bush) tea to counter stomach spasms caused by IBS.

S is for sprouting (see page 69). It's also for spinach, which has a cleansing action in the intestinal tract and is also rich in antioxidant nutrients to counter the otherwise harmful effects of environmental and dietary pollutants.

T **is for** tahini and turmeric, both foods that work to support healthy digestion. Tahini is a magnesium-rich paste made from ground sesame seeds which retain all their nutrients intact. It can help counter indigestion. Turmeric acts as an intestinal antiseptic, making it a powerful cleansing agent for the digestive system.

U **is for** unsulphured dried fruits. Sulphur is used to preserve the drying fruits and make sure they retain a more appealing light colour. Without this agent, dried fruits turn an unappetizing dark brown or black after drying (but don't be put off by the dark colour – they taste just as good and are much better for you).

V **is for** vitamin B5 (pantethine), which is found in wholegrains and plays a role in converting fats, proteins and carbohydrates in food into energy. Also vitamin B3 (niacin), which promotes healthy digestion and is found in fish, eggs, poultry, avocados, dates and prunes.

W **is for** wheat (one to avoid if you have digestive problems) and wheatgrass juice, which is a potent detoxifying agent but also an acquired taste, so build up your tolerance by adding a small amount to your superjuices.

Y **is for** bioactive yoghurts which provide probiotic bacteria (see page 9) to help rebuild a healthy digestion. The trouble is that you do not always know what strain of bacteria you are ingesting or whether you will get a therapeutic dosage.

Z **is for** zinc, the nutrient that plays a key role in your sense of taste and smell. If you've lost either, take a zinc supplement and eat more zinc-rich seafoods, nuts and seeds.

What is a Legume?

You read about the health properties of legumes in health books all the time but do you really know what they are? Quiz your friends and see how many of them know they include the following foods: peas, lentils, carob, peanuts and beans, plus soybeans and soybean products such as tofu, soy milk and tempeh.

Legumes grow in pods on vines and contain even more protein than eggs or many meats (namely 25 to 38 per cent) but have the advantage of no cholesterol or saturated-fat content.

They also contain complex carbohydrates that have a low glycaemic index (GI), which means they raise blood sugar levels more slowly than refined, sugary foods, and they are high in the omega-3 essential fatty acid that is difficult to source in the diet.

Finally, legumes contain phytochemicals that have anti-cancer properties and reduce cholesterol levels, making them beneficial for almost all the body's organs and the intestinal tract.

Tried and Applied

You can travel throughout India and not fall prey to a gippy tummy if you start the day the same way as Indian families do with a lassi. I have had delicious lassi drinks combining papaya, pineapple, banana and mango with fermented live yoghurt, which acts as a natural gut-protecting probiotic. To make your own, blend one glass of live yoghurt with two tablespoons of coconut milk, one dessertspoon of honey and a pinch of ground cardamom. Add the fruit of your choice, blend again and drink straight away.

Ancient Wisdom, 21st-century Healing

Traditional Chinese Medicine (TCM)

I really like the word 'tonic'. It makes me think of rose-covered idyllic cottages, a warm, soft grandmother baking scones, and some homemade delicious liquor to strengthen your constitution and fortify you for the real world.

Tonics play an important role in TCM and those formulated for the digestive system almost always include warming ginger and liquorice to support all its related organs. Making your own tonic remedies is too much of a faff for most people. The Chinese Herbasway range does the same job with an energizing digestive tonic that combines liquorice with immune-supporting astragalus, ginger, bitter orange, Chinese blackberry and vitality-boosting schisandra. Since this formulation includes stevia, a natural sweetener that is, in my opinion, suspiciously banned in the UK, you will have to get this tonic from the internet. (I say suspiciously because the evidence that suggests it may do more harm than good is pathetically weak, unlike the might of the companies that make billions producing synthetic artificial sweeteners such as aspartame, which really do raise health concerns.) For maximum therapeutic benefits, though, you should find an accredited practitioner in your area. To do this, contact the Register of Chinese Herbalists on page 448.

If you want an all-natural sweetener which contains no stevia or aspartame, use TriMedica's SlimSweet from Rio Trading (01273 570987; www.riohealth.com).

Ayurvedic (Indian) Remedies

The Ayurvedic supplement I am going to recommend is a

traditional mix of three herbs that has been used for over 2000 years in India to help relieve chronic constipation and to detoxify and cleanse the colon.

In fact, it works so fast, you're going to think it's nothing short of miraculous.

Triphala tablets combine Terminalia chebula, Terminalia belerica and Phyllanthus embilica to help restore healthy peristalsis (which is, you'll remember, the wave-like action that moves waste through the digestive tract). Buy the Maharishi Ayur-Veda brand from the NutriCentre (0800 587 2290; www.NutriCentre.com) and take two tablets at bedtime with warm water. The following night, take three tablets, and the night after, take four. After two or three days at this maximum dosage, you can then cut back to three and two tablets, eventually weaning yourself off them unless or until the problem returns. Alternatively, use a Triphala tincture from Pukka Herbs (08456 585858; www.pukkaherbs.com).

Native American Remedies

We have seen in this chapter how you cannot separate the gut from its related organs and one of the best herbs you can use to support the digestive tract holistically, from the mouth to the anus, is **yarrow**.

Native American healers rate this plant so highly, it is one of their key cancer-preventing agents. It has anti-inflammatory, antibiotic and detoxifying properties. It will help regulate and improve liver function, prevent abdominal bloating and cramping and tone the mucous membranes of the stomach and bowels. Rich in vitamin A, it works to support the immune system. It can prevent diarrhoea, flatulence and ulcers and has a potent blood-cleansing action in the body.

You can now buy yarrow tea bags in health stores (the active part of the plant is the flower) but, if you have a garden, this attractive plant with its soft, feathery leaves thrives in a temperate climate, so you can easily grow it and make your own brew. For convenience, the Eclectic range includes an organic yarrow tincture, which you mix in warm water to make a quick tea (for stockists, visit www.eclecticherb.com).

Native New Zealand Remedies

Kawakawa – which you must not confuse with the now and again suspiciously* banned Kava Kava – was traditionally used by Maori healers as a digestive tonic. Commonly known as the New Zealand Peppertree, the indigenous population would chew the leaves to settle stomach upsets and help prevent indigestion.

It has a mildly bitter taste so can help stimulate appetite, and the root of the plant was chewed to treat both dysentery and diarrhoea.

Thankfully, today you do not have to chew on leaves or chomp on roots to get the same health benefits. Kiwiherb has harnessed the digestive healing properties of kawakawa in a new organic herbal tonic that combines it with soothing ginger. This is a great remedy for anyone convalescing from sickness; visit www.kiwiherb.com or mail order from Xynergy (08456 585858; www.xynergy.co.uk), which now imports this range.

---

* Suspiciously this time because the ban followed reports of possible liver toxicity in 29 German users. What those reports did not admit was that 28 of these 29 people were using other medications at the time that could equally have been responsible for these side effects. The question I would want answering is why, with a supplement as popular worldwide as Kava Kava, did all these cases come from just one country?

Still Using Laxatives? What You Need is a Walk in the Park

Believe it or not . . . **exercise** is one of the best ways to keep your gastrointestinal tract healthy and you don't have to spend all week in the gym to benefit. In one study, scientists found men who burned just 500 calories a week through exercise were 20 per cent less likely to get bowel cancer than men who did not exercise. Just **four hours of walking each week** will give you the same benefits so if you don't already have one, get a dog, and if you do, thank it for making you walk every day.

Commercial laxatives only serve to make the colon lazy so while you might be using them for expediency, when you stop the problem will be worse. Senna is a popular (and natural) alternative but even this is too aggressive, in my opinion.

My breakfast recipe (see page 68) includes a teaspoon of **flaxseed oil** a day which will help keep food moving through the digestive tract, but if you are in dire need of a laxative, then use **psyllium husks** (see Lepicol, page 62), which swell with moisture in the gut to gently bulk faeces and kick-start the peristaltic wave-like action.

Top Three Products For Healthy Digestion

Digestive disorders are distressing because you cannot help but try to hide them from the world. If you simply don't have time for a long and involved detox diet, here are my three best nutraceutical solutions.

Digestive enzymes

These are now widely on sale in good health stores but make sure you buy a brand that contains all three of the major enzyme groups – amylase, protease and lipase – to break down all food groups. If you cannot source one locally, mail order Source Natural's supplement from Revital (0800 252875; www.revital.com).

Alternatively, make your own digestive enzymes by drying papaya seeds and grinding them into a pepper to sprinkle on food.

Aloe vera juice

Make space in the fridge for this soothing remedy which can help relieve inflammation of the digestive tract. To take internally, look for products that are 98–99 per cent pure and thus higher in the protective mucopolysaccharides that have a healing effect on the digestive tract. I recommend the Living Nature brand, which is hard to beat for purity. Whether you suffer from constipation or diarrhoea, aloe vera can help return stools to normal, and one of the best natural colon cleansers (if you want a simple alternative to colonic irrigation) is a combination of aloe vera juice with psyllium husks. Add one generous teaspoon of husks to a quarter of a glass of aloe vera juice and drink in the morning.

Ultimate Cleanse

Nature's Secret do an amazing dual-pack super colon cleanse which provides colon cleansing herbs in one capsule, and fibre plus probiotic in the other. You take one tablet from each pack in the morning and again at night and increase this dosage until you achieve three bowel movements a day. Since the Ultimate Cleanse formulation includes psyllium husks that swell to bulk stools and kick-start peristalsis, you must make sure you drink enough water too (8–10 glasses a day). For more on how this works, visit www.naturessecret.com.

Weight Loss and the Magic Pill We're All Waiting For

Currently, the most talked about (and controversial) natural appetite-suppressant is **Hoodia gordonii**, a cactus plant traditionally used by the desperately poor San tribespeople of the Kalahari desert to stave off hunger pangs during long hunting expeditions.

Scientists in Cambridge have isolated and patented the single plant molecule they believe is responsible for this action, and drugs giant, Pfizer, which paid £30 million for a licence to use this discovery, started to develop a miracle slimming pill, but then abandoned the project amid controversy over who owns the 'rights' to this traditional knowledge.

It all sounded too good to be true and it was. The bio-piracy issues surrounding the exploitation of this plant remain largely unresolved. While you can patent a molecule, you cannot patent a natural substance like a whole plant, which is why supplement makers have been able to jump on the bandwagon to make slimming formulations that include the hoodia plant.

The issue here is that if the hoodia is not coming from authorized suppliers in South Africa, then it is being either grown or harvested illegally. And even if it is being farmed with the blessing of the South African government, you might still want to ask what those farmers and the retailers selling the finished product are doing to compensate the indigenous tribes for their discovery of the plant.

If you can find the answer to this, you are a better reporter than me, since my researches appear to falter at the point where I am told that Thermokinetix, a hoodia-containing supplement that is now available in the UK, for instance, comes via Bulgarian suppliers who sell the raw ingredients to the American manufacturer but who are not able to explain where in South Africa they source the hoodia from, or how they resolve the bio-piracy concerns.

Furthermore, some of the American supplements you can currently buy over the internet have been found to contain no hoodia whatsoever.

You can, of course, choose to ignore these issues because these supplements are available now but if you prefer to take a more moral stand – which is that the people profiting from the enormous potential of this plant should compensate the San tribespeople who first discovered its appetite-suppressing properties – I suggest you use an 'alternative' alternative and wait for the issues to be fairly resolved.

Top Three Natural Slimming Aids

The brutal truth, if you want to lose weight and keep it off, is that you have to eat less of the wrong foods, eat more of the right kinds of foods and exercise more. Exercise is especially important if you are over the age of thirty-five when, unless you take hold of yourself, you will find you can be eating the same amount but still spreading round the middle.

Yoga, for instance, is great for flexibility, which is important to maintain and will help develop core strength and stability (which is more important than looking good in a swimsuit), but unless you are doing one of the more dynamic and vigorous forms, such as Astanga yoga, you are not going to increase muscle mass in any way.

Why should you care? Because muscle burns fat at a faster rate, so the more toned you are, the more likely it is that you can eat a sensible diet and still stay in good shape.

If you can afford it, get a personal trainer who can work with your body and at your pace, not least because hurling yourself into the gym without proper supervision can do more harm, in the long term, than good. Unless you are already steeped in the fitness culture, you cannot expect to maintain proper alignment when you exercise without assistance. You may build muscle and tone by going to the gym, but you will also, inadvertently, be exacerbating the underlying structural imbalances that we all have and that will cause you problems in later life.

Health stores, of course, sell plenty of natural weight-loss products but many of the agents that work to suppress the appetite are sold in combination formulas with **chromium,** which has been shown to be helpful in weight management but may soon disappear from sale following a recent report by the **Food Standards Agency (FSA)** calling for a ban.

There's money in them there pills and so supplement makers will never give up trying to find the magic weight-loss cure that will make them millions. There are literally hundreds to choose from; here are my top three that will help support a weight-loss programme which includes moderating your diet and doing more exercise, and will still allow you to sleep with an easy conscience at night.

Green Tea

This may be making its UK TV debut as an additive being used in fabric conditioners for your clothes, but green tea can do a lot more than make your clothes feel soft – it can make them hang off you more attractively too. This is because green tea extract, which is also now available in capsule form, has similar fat-burning properties to hoodia. In university trials carried out in Geneva, scientists reporting their findings in the *American Journal of Clinical Nutrition* confirmed that taking green tea extract over ten weeks prompted significant and dramatic weight loss among those taking part in the trials. There are lots of makes around but I like Metasys Green Tea Extract. Mail order from Victoria Health (0800 389 8195; www.victoriahealth.com).

Slim-Mist

Cravings are usually a sign that you are trying to lose weight via the deprivation route, and if that is the case, you will eventually succumb and grab that packet of crisps. Since your body is programmed to lay down fat stores just in case you run into a famine, you need to cheat it into thinking it has already eaten plenty of calories, and one of the newer ways to do this is to use Slim-Mist, an oral spray that will make you feel you have eaten more than you actually have. The good news is you can still have your chocolate ... because one of the flavours is Choco-Lite. The sprays include L-carnitine, a nutrient that encourages the body to satisfy cravings from fat reserves, rather than glucose from yet another snack. You can mail order the mists from Indigo Health (0871 871 8192). There are four flavours, which cost £24 each.

Conjugaic Linoleic Acid

It may not sound as sexy as a spray mist, but I still rate conjugaic linoleic acid (CLA), which has been shown in trials to promote an average 20 per cent reduction in body fat if taken for at least three months. In studies concentrating on body builders, researchers at Kent State University in Ohio showed that taking regular supplements of CLA increased arm girth, boosted lean muscle mass and enhanced overall muscle strength. First of all, CLA regulates several of the enzymes involved in fat metabolism, including one called lipoprotein lipase, which works to break down fat globules in the blood. It increases the activity of this enzyme, and at the same time reduces the action of a second enzyme, called heparin-releasable lipoprotein lipase, which works to increase the uptake of fats into the fat cells. In other words, it speeds up fat breakdown and blocks fat uptake.

Secondly, it acts on the way the body uses its fat stores for the production of energy. This process relies on a key vitamin-like nutrient called carnitine and, again, CLA works on a related enzyme, carnitine-palmityl transferase, which controls how quickly muscles can burn off fat.

CLA is one of the active agents in SlenderDay & SlenderNight, weight-loss supplements from Lifes2Good, the company whose founder, James Murphy, first introduced the Slendertone slimming system to the UK. For more information, visit www.lifes2good.com.

Metabolic Typing . . .

. . . or why you may be wasting your time on that best-selling diet book that worked for your best friend.

Everyone knows that to lose weight and keep it off, you need to eat less and exercise more, but that does not explain why some of the best-selling diet books can recommend eating plans that completely contradict each other and yet still work.

For example, in his best-selling book *Eat More, Weigh Less*, American doctor Dean Ornish recommends a high-carbohydrate, low-protein and low-fat diet, while in his book, *Diet Revolution*, the late Dr Robert Atkins recommended a high-protein, moderate-fat and low-carbohydrate diet.

The reason both work – but not for everyone – is that some people are better at metabolizing carbohydrates, while others are better at metabolizing protein. In other words, if you are serious about weight loss and keeping the weight off, you should find out more about your metabolic type by visiting www.metabolictesting.com.

Diabetes

There are two forms of diabetes: type I (insulin-dependent) and type II (non-insulin dependent). Type II is more common but can be very effectively controlled by changing the diet and using natural remedies.

Most people understand that with diabetes the body is not able to control blood sugar (glucose) levels. The difference between type I and type II is that with the former, the pancreas is not making enough of the hormone, insulin, which controls glucose metabolism, whereas with type II, enough insulin is produced but the body is not able to use it effectively. This is known as 'insulin resistance' and results in a more gradual change in blood sugar levels; hence the more insidious onset of type II diabetes, which is more likely to affect anyone over thirty, and which becomes more common with increasing age.

Symptoms include tiredness, repeated infections (including recurrent boils), excessive thirst and excessive urination. Although nobody knows what triggers type II diabetes, you are more at risk if there is a family history of this condition, if you are of Indian or African descent, and if you are obese – since obesity and diabetes are linked in 90 per cent of cases. That said, there may be very few symptoms in the early stages, and since only a third of sufferers show any symptoms at all, the majority of people with this condition do not know they have it until complications develop. Lots of integrated health clinics now offer screening and testing for this condition (see Chapter 4, page 205) so if you are not sure whether you suffer from it, get tested.

There is some evidence that chromium can moderately help control both type I and type II forms of diabetes if you stick to a safe dosage of 200mcg (micrograms) a day. However, chromium is a heavy metal so there is always a risk that levels can build up and cause problems in the future. In the UK, chromium has had such negative press that at the time of writing the Food Standards Agency (FSA) was considering calling for a total ban on its inclusion in supplements.

Certainly there have been reports of kidney damage in people taking a high dose of 1,200mcg or more for several months, and since the most effective dosage for type II individuals appears to be 1000mcg daily, I think you need to consider these risks.

A better solution is the Indian Ayurvedic herb, **gymnema sylvestre**. The part of the plant used to control diabetes is the leaf, which contains gymnemic acids that have been shown to reduce the rate of intestinal absorption of glucose and to stimulate the pancreas to increase insulin production. Gymnemic acid also has the ability to inhibit the taste of sweetness. If you chew the leaf and then eat sugar, it will taste of grit or sandpaper with no sweet flavour at all.

In trials on gymnema, no adverse side effects have been reported to date although some preparations can decrease the absorption of iron in the body. That said, the extract used in clinical studies is known as GS4, which does not include the constituents that can cause this problem. The daily dose you need to be taking is 400mg. Mail order from the NutriCentre (0800 587 2290; www.NutriCentre.com).

For type I sufferers, gymnema can enhance the blood glucose-lowering effects of insulin but you should not self-medicate or take the herb without medical supervision and medical monitoring of your blood glucose levels.

Tried and Applied

B-complex combines all the B vitamins, which work best when taken together, and which are known as 'nature's stress-busters'. They also improve the absorption of all the other nutrients you eat so make sure you are taking a B-complex supplement to supply them in the correct ratios.

What Really Works for Digestive Complaints

As I explained in the previous chapter, I could recommend some thirty different remedies for almost any chronic condition you care to suggest, but what good is that? You need to know what really works and which of these thirty to try, so here are my 1, 2, 3 . . . Easy Steps for everyday chronic digestive complaints.

Bloating

Bloating is often a sign of a hidden wheat or dairy intolerance caused by Irritable Bowel Syndrome or IBS (see page 99). To relieve it, eliminate these foods from the diet and try a simple herbal remedy called **gentian**. This works to stop bloating by stimulating the release of gastric juices, including bile, which helps break down fats for digestion. It can also help prevent a build-up of abdominal discomfort and wind.

According to practitioners, the best way to take this herb is to brew the dried form of the root into a tea. This could not be simpler. Just add half a teaspoon of the herbal powder to half a cup of water and boil for five minutes. Strain and drink the liquid half an hour before you plan to eat.

1, 2, 3 . . . Easy Steps to Help Prevent Bloating

Take a probiotic (see page 65).

Drink peppermint tea; you can grow peppermint in a window-pot and use the leaves to brew a fresh tea.

Use gentian; you can mail order this herb in powder form from Napiers (0131 553 3500); if you don't have time to brew a tea or find the taste too bitter, use a tincture instead and sweeten it with manuka honey, which has an additional probiotic action in the gut.

Candida

I could write an entire book about tackling this everyday complaint, but to keep it simple, while we all have this organism in our bodies, a healthy immune system will keep it in check, so if it is running riot, your first step should be to support the gut–immune relationship with a glutamine supplement (see page 61).

There are over 150 different strains of candidiasis; eight are pathogenic to humans and all of them thrive on refined sugar, so cut this and alcohol from your diet too.

Horopito is one of New Zealand's 2000 or so little-known

native plants, and it has performed well in small-scale preliminary trials there, where it was used to treat vaginal thrush. Over the course of two months, none of the 22 female volunteers in the trial suffered a relapse of infection.

1, 2, 3 . . . Easy Steps to Help Tackle Candida

Take Solgar's L-glutamine supplement, 2 x 500mg once a day. Call 01442 890355 for stockists.

Use a probiotic (see pages 9–10) that includes the strain Lactobacillus acidophilus, especially if infection follows a course of antibiotic treatment (which is not uncommon), and take it with Candiclear tincture from the Organic Pharmacy (020 7351 2232; www.TheOrganicPharmacy.com) – this combines the anti-candida herb pau d'arco with immune-boosting echinacea and goldenseal.

Use the New Zealand herb horopito both internally and, if you have a vaginal infection, as a topical cream. (To use internally, apply the cream to a cotton tampon.) To source it, visit www.kolorex.com.

Constipation

I once heard a woman in my local health store tell the sales assistant she had suffered from constipation for twenty years before finding out that something as simple as sprinkling linseeds on her breakfast cereal could help.

This discovery, she said, had changed her whole life . . . for the better – but it made me sad to think she had suffered for so long before finding a relatively simple and inexpensive solution. If you do use linseeds, you can sprinkle them on your breakfast cereal or over salads, or you may prefer to take the same remedy in liquid form, as flaxseed oil, which is what I use. Add a spoonful to your morning cereal or blend it into a smoothie to disguise the distinctive taste.

Refer to the section on Irritable Bowel Syndrome (IBS) on page 99, since constipation is an early sign of this condition, and, if the situation is dire, use the Ayurvedic herbal formulation Triphala (see page 83) to clear your system out or look out for Nature's Secret's Ultimate Cleanse (see page 86).

1, 2, 3 . . . Easy Steps to Help Prevent Constipation

Once you have cleansed the colon, use psyllium husks to bulk waste and stimulate wave-like peristalsis (which keeps faecal matter moving through the colon). Use Lepicol (0121 779 6619), which combines the husks with a prebiotic and a probiotic.

Take up some form of exercise, even if it is only brisk walking for 20 minutes a day. Scientists have shown that men who burn up just 500 calories a week through exercise are 20 per cent less likely to get bowel cancer than couch potatoes who do no exercise at all.

Drink gut-healing aloe vera juice: a quarter of a glass in the morning and again at night. I use Aloe Pura's cranberry-flavoured aloe vera juice, which disguises the otherwise distinctive taste of this important digestive remedy.

Crohn's Disease

Crohn's disease is an autoimmune disease and inflammatory condition that affects the intestinal lining, causing severe problems including pain, diarrhoea and rectal bleeding.

There is definitely a link with food allergies and intolerances that have given rise to a pre-condition known as 'leaky gut' (see page 101), where damaged cells in the wall of the intestinal lining leave 'gaps' which larger proteins can pass through, triggering an abnormal immune response and inflammation in the gut mucosa.

Typical allergens include chocolate, dairy products, yeast, cereal grains, fats and artificial sweeteners, and elimination diets excluding these foods have been shown to effect a remission twice as long as that gained from using the conventional corticosteroid treatments.

Zinc is a commonly-identified deficiency among sufferers so make sure you are taking a good multisupplement that provides the equivalent of 30mg a day, and while the clinical evidence remains scant, there is lots of good anecdotal evidence for increasing your intake of antioxidants, especially vitamin E, to help alleviate the symptoms.

1, 2, 3 . . . Easy Steps to Help Manage Crohn's Disease
Take L-glutamine (see above), 2 x 500mg once a day.

Avoid milk. Researchers believe there may be a link between a bacteria called Mycobacterium paratuberculosis (Para-T) which causes diarrhoea in cows – and which, since it is not destroyed by pasteurization, passes on to humans in milk – and Crohn's disease. Start your day with half a glass of anti-inflammatory aloe vera juice instead.

Olive-leaf extract can also help. Use Allergy Research Group's Prolive supplement (www.allergyresearchgroup.com).

Diarrhoea

This can be a sign of Irritable Bowel Syndrome (IBS) or may be triggered by an intestinal infection. Repeated bouts of diarrhoea may also be a sign of lactose intolerance – an underlying inability to digest the milk sugar lactose. This is not the same as a milk allergy, but is due to a lack or deficiency in the specific enzyme lactase, which is manufactured in the small intestine, where it splits lactose into glucose and galactose.

The symptoms, which usually start up to two hours after the consumption of dairy foods, include gas, diarrhoea and stomach cramping, and are the result of undigested lactose fermenting in the colon. This intolerance has become so widespread that for many adults in the west it's become a fact of everyday life.

Whatever the underlying cause of your diarrhoea, you will need to make sure you rehydrate and support the body's tissues after a bout by drinking plenty of water and taking a good quality multi-supplement such as Sage Organics Healthy Woman or Healthy Man formulation (www.sageorganic.com; helpline on 0870 4412 9599).

1, 2, 3 . . . Easy Steps to Stop Diarrhoea

Start the day with a quarter of a glass of aloe vera juice, and also drink Rezonate (01730 813642), a nutrient-rich tonic with pro-biotic New Zealand natural honeys, which will help the digestive tract settle down again.

If you suspect an underlying lactose intolerance, use Nutrition Now's Lacto Safe, which can help the body better digest dairy products including milk (www.nutritionnow.com).

IDS (intestinal digestive support) supplement combines L-glutamine, fructo-oligosaccharides (FOS), slippery elm and the anti-inflammatory herb Boswellia serrata. Again, from Nutrition Now, as above.

Diverticulitis

Diverticulitis is the inflammation of 'out-pouches' or diverticular sacs, which form along the linings of the small and large intestinal tracts. If left untreated, an inflamed pouch can become a small, hard mass known as a fecalth, caused by the combination of undi-gested food residues and bacterial infection.

More common in men than women, this condition is almost inevitable in later life. Some 50 per cent of the population aged between sixty and eighty and almost everyone over the age of eighty will be a sufferer.

Switching to a diet that is high in the right kind of fibre (see page 67) will help prevent the onset of this condition, or its deteri-oration if you already have it. It is often linked with a history of irritable bowel syndrome (IBS) and can cause similar bloating, stomach pains, cramping and constipation followed by diarrhoea, so check my recommendations for these problems too.

Anthropological studies show, again and again, that the best way to prevent these digestive conditions is to adopt a diet that is rich in wholegrains, vegetables, legumes (see page 81) and sprouts, all of which pass more easily through the gastrointestinal tract. For details on simple sprouting, see page 69.

1, 2, 3 . . . Easy Steps to Help Manage Diverticulitis

Olive-leaf extract can kill off the bacteria causing the inflammation around the sacs. Take Allergy Research Group's Prolive (www.allergyresearchgroup.com).

As with almost all these digestive disorders, aloe vera juice can help heal an inflamed gut lining and a good quality probiotic will rebuild levels of the good bacteria that aid digestion.

Bowel hygiene and a healthy balance of good gut bacteria are crucial to digestive health. If the flora are out of balance (a condition known as dysbiosis) then toxic metabolites and mutagenic compounds may be produced, giving rise to damaged tissues and poor assimilation of nutrients. The underrated rainforest herb cat's claw can help redress this since it works not only to soothe irritated tissues but also to eliminate pathogens from the gastrointestinal tract. Take a therapeutic dose of 500mg, three times a day.

Irritable Bowel Syndrome (IBS)

This is probably the most common of all the gastrointestinal disorders and is now so widespread that it has become the second most common reason for days off work after the common cold. Put simply, what is happening is that the large intestine or colon (see page 60) is not functioning properly. Typical symptoms include constipation or diarrhoea, excessive production of mucus in the colon, indigestion, flatulence and cramping, and can be so severe that sufferers will stay at home rather than risk the embarrassment of dealing with these symptoms in public.

Food intolerances (see page 74) can exacerbate the symptoms so, if you are a sufferer, eliminate troublesome foods from the diet and take a good quality probiotic (see page 65) every day. Dandelion (taraxacum) root is a traditional and very effective IBS remedy, and in recent trials researchers discovered that one of its active agents, a substance called inulin, is a preferred food of the good gut bacteria that aid digestion. In one small trial, IBS patients given a dandelion root supplement showed a 10 per cent increase in levels of Lactobacillus bifidobacteria in the gut (see Chapter 1, pages 9–10 for an explanation of the best probiotic strains), and a decrease in the pathogenic gut flora responsible for disease.

1, 2, 3 ... Easy Steps to Help Prevent IBS

Fennel and peppermint oils have both been shown to help relax the smooth muscle in the colon, helping prevent intestinal spasms. Biocare has formulated an excellent new internal digestive-support supplement that combines fennel and peppermint with cardamom oils. The latter also works to soothe mucous membranes. Call 0121 433 3727 for details.

Almost all the natural regimens for digestive health start with aloe vera juice: drink a quarter of a glass at breakfast and again at night. Take L-glutamine to help rebuild the damaged intestinal tissues.

Dandelion will selectively 'feed up' the good bacteria already present in the gut and those in the probiotic you are taking. There are lots of good dandelion supplements on sale, and make sure you use one made from the root, not the leaves. Take a therapeutic dosage of 250–500mg, three times a day.

Leaky Gut Syndrome

This is often a root cause of many of the more common digestive disorders covered in this chapter, including IBS, Crohn's disease and ulcerative colitis. What is happening is that the intestinal mucosa cells have become damaged, resulting in a dramatic increase in their permeability, and so instead of screening out large molecules that can trigger an abnormal immune response and an inflammatory reaction, they allow these substances to pass into the bloodstream.

How has this happened? It is usually the result of impaired digestion leading to the production of intestinal endotoxins – i.e. the toxic by-products of the fermentation of poorly digested foods. These toxins, which include putrescine, methane and cadaverine, then attack the intestinal mucosa, thus compromising the integrity of the intestinal tract. They will also, thanks to the damage they have caused and the increased permeability of the gastrointestinal lining, pass into the bloodstream to cause what naturopaths describe as a generalized toxaemia.

1, 2, 3 . . . Easy Steps to Help Heal Leaky Gut

Drink aloe vera juice, which can help soothe inflammation of the gut lining and which will encourage the repair of the mucosa cells.

Support the compromised immune–gut relationship by taking L-glutamine.

Take a good quality probiotic to rebuild levels of good bacteria that aid proper digestion, and help improve digestion by taking digestive enzymes (see page 85).

Parasites

Whether it's the children coming home from school with an infestation of threadworms, or picking up a tropical infection when travelling, parasites, however much we don't like to think about them, are part of the risks of everyday life.

I never travel to India or the Amazon without a combination antiparasitic formulation of artemisia (known as wormwood), tansy and quassia, made up for me by the UK company Herbs of Grace (www.herbsofgrace.com).

Citricidal tastes vile but will prevent parasites. Again, I never travel without it. Hold your nose while you dose yourself with five drops of this purple tincture added to water or juice in the morning, and take another five drops in the same way at night. Mail order from Revital (0800 252875; www.revital.com).

Colostrum – the fluid that new mothers produce during the first few days after birth to provide infants with a rich mix of antibodies and growth factors – is now widely on sale in health stores as an immune stimulant, and studies have shown that it can also help protect against parasitic infection and relieve diarrhoea too. The colostrum you can now buy is collected from cows, and whether cow antibodies can do the same for the human immune system remains unproven. What has been shown is that patients deliberately infected with bacteria who took colostrums as well were more protected than a control group, members of which suffered more diarrhoea and more fever symptoms. To learn more, see Chapter 5, Stress and Immunity, page 295.

Stomach Ulcers

Most stomach ulcers are not caused by stress or bad diets but by a bacterium called Helicobacter pylori, which causes inflammation and pain when it burrows into the lining of the stomach and small intestine. This organism survives the stomach's strong acid secretions by producing a compound called urase that neutralizes these acids and then causes symptoms ranging from a blunt, gnawing or sharp stomach pain to lower backache and discomfort when passing stools. (A bleeding ulcer occurs only when the ulcer has penetrated a blood vessel; this then requires medical intervention.)

The best natural remedy for stomach and duodenal ulcers is mastic gum, produced from the resin of the Mediterranean Pistacia lentiscus tree. Laboratory tests show it has the potency to kill off seven different strains of this bacteria, and in addition, in 70 per cent of ulcer sufferers using this remedy, the damaged tissue repairs itself so well it is as if there never was an ulceration. New generation formulations of this active agent combine it with liquorice (see below).

1, 2, 3 . . . Easy Steps to Help Prevent or Relieve Stomach Ulcers

Ceasefire . . . this is a new supplement that combines mastic gum with DGL, a form of liquorice where those agents that would otherwise increase blood pressure and cause water retention have been removed from the root of the herb (the part of the plant used). Liquorice root has long been used to soothe the irritated and injured mucous lining of the digestive tract. It works by increasing the body's production of mucin, the substance that naturally protects the body against stomach acid and other harmful agents. DGL stands for deglycyrrhizinated, and this form of liquorice has been shown to be more effective than standard anti-ulcer drugs. Ceasefire is made by Allergy Research Group, a US company that specializes in making supplements for doctors and health practitioners (www.allergyresearchgroup.com).

Take 1 tablespoon of flaxseed oil daily (see breakfast recipe, page 68, and increase the amount of flaxseed oil).

Preliminary studies now suggest plant bioflavonoids can help inhibit the growth of Helicobacter pylori. Take 500mg of a quercetin (bioflavonoid) supplement, three times a day.

Ulcerative Colitis

Confined, usually, to the colon and rectum, this is another inflammatory disease that may also be triggering an abnormal immune response. It is most common in people aged fifteen to forty and occurs equally in men and women. It can run in families, and, since about five per cent of sufferers do go on to develop cancer of the colon, it should never be ignored.

Symptoms, generally, include bloody diarrhoea and abdominal pain, and the condition is usually graded as mild, moderate or severe. With moderate UC, a low-grade fever may be present too. Smokers who suffer from UC and who quit the habit may experience a flare-up as nicotine leaves the body, and should consider asking the doctor for a nicotine patch to improve symptoms during this time.

1, 2, 3 . . . Easy Steps to Help Manage Ulcerative Colitis
Take a glutamine powder supplement, 20g a day.

Use anti-inflammatory bromelain. The daily therapeutic dose is 320mg, three times a day.

Use psyllium husks (see Lepicol, page 62) to bulk stools and keep waste moving; make sure you take a good quality probiotic (see page 65), and, if you are taking anti-inflammatory drugs to control the symptoms, make sure you take a supplement of folic acid too, since low levels are common among those following a conventional treatment route. Folic acid may also play an important role in protecting against colon cancer, so take a supplement and step up your intake of folate-rich foods (see A–Z, pages 77–80), including liver and lentils.

Roll Out Your Yoga Mat

A serious yoga practitioner will use kryias (see page 168) or cleansing practices to keep the digestive system working optimally, but since these practices can include drinking gallons of salt water to induce vomiting and swallowing yards of soft cloth to regurgitate, they are too extreme for most of us. As well as bringing physical cleansing benefits, kryias are also meant to get the yoga student to overcome any sense of repulsion about the internal workings of their body. Again, this is sound in theory, but difficult to put into practice, since most of us do not want to think about slippery entrails and excretions.

Thankfully, many of the estimated 840,000 different yoga postures or asanas work to tone and stimulate the digestive system. Here are my **1, 2, 3 best yoga asanas** for doing just that.

Ustrasana (Camel Pose)

This is one of my all-time favourite yoga poses. If you are new to yoga, you will need to work on stretching and warming the spine before attempting the backwards bend this posture calls for. Keeping on the tip of your toes will also reduce the stretch to the spine and intestinal organs, although it is this stretch that you are, ultimately, aiming for.

Begin by kneeling on your mat with your bottom tucked over your heels. Lift your torso into a high kneeling position and reach back with both hands to clasp the ankles. If you do not feel bendy, make sure you are kneeling with your feet balancing on the tips of the toes. If you are comfortable stretching the front of the body, let the tops of the feet remain flat on the mat.

It is important not to strain to get into this posture. Just allow your whole body to stretch backwards until your head is hanging back, with the throat stretching. Close your eyes as you lean back and enjoy this deep stretch to the stomach and intestines. Stay in the posture for as long as you are comfortable and take care, when you come out of it, to move in a slow and controlled way: lifting the head back up first, keeping the arms strong and straight as you raise and return them to the front of the body, and keeping the high kneeling position.

If you have never done this posture before, position your mat up against a wall, which you can use as support as you roll the body back down. As you begin to arch the body backwards, use your hands against the wall for support.

Counter this posture by folding the body forward into the pose of the child (see page 50) for five minutes.

Meru Wakrasana (Spinal Twist)

This posture, as you concentrate on twisting the spine round first to the right and then to the left, helps massage the liver and pancreas. All the spinal twists encourage the flow of prana – the invisible and re-energizing lifeforce – to the naval region to nourish the organs of the digestive system. Because you practise in first one and then the other direction, you alternately contract and stretch these organs, which will help improve their tone. And this posture could not be more easy to do.

Simply sit on your yoga mat, with both legs stretched out in front of you. Turn your trunk slightly to the right and place the right hand behind the body, close to your bottom with the fingers pointing backwards.

Now place the left hand behind you, slightly to the side of the right buttock and as close as possible to the right hand. Again, make sure the fingers are pointing backwards.

Bend the left knee and place the left foot along the outside of the right leg, close to the knee. Keep your bottom on the floor and slowly twist the head and torso as far to the right as you can, using the arms as levers but keeping the spine upright and straight. Look over your right shoulder as far as you can and hold this position for as long as you feel comfortable.

Now do the same thing twisting to the left.

You will twist further and more easily if you breathe in and hold the breath as you twist, and exhale as you let the body recentre and settle after each twist.

Halasana (Plough)

If you are not familiar with this posture or your body is stiff, make sure that you warm up, and that you use a stable chair or the wall to lower the feet onto or against instead of the floor. Do not strain to get your feet to the floor if this is too advanced for you. It will come with gentle practice.

Lie on your back on your yoga mat with your arms stretched along the sides of your body, palms facing down on the mat. Raise the body into the shoulderstand (see page 50), making sure you support the back with your hands, keeping your elbows tucked in to the sides.

Now, slowly lower your feet, keeping your legs straight, over your head and down onto the chair if you are using one, against the wall if that is your preference, or onto the floor if you are comfortable with this posture.

Breathe slowly and deeply and hold the pose for as long as you can without straining. You can feel how this position massages all the internal organs, including and especially the digestive tract.

Take as much care moving the body out of halasana as you have taken moving into it. Support the middle of the back with both hands, raise the feet up from the floor or chair, and fold the knees down into the chest. Allow the spine to 'unroll' back down onto the mat, lifting the head as you release from the asana.

Counter the pose by massaging the lower back into the

floor. To do this, keep the knees bent in towards the chest, place one hand on each knee and make circular motions with the knees which, in turn, will rotate the hips and sacrum and release the lower back into the floor.

Tried and Applied

If you are already a serious practitioner, please remember these postures are for beginners. If you would like to know more about advanced postures that do the same job, I suggest you add a copy of Swami Satyananada Saraswati's excellent book, *Asana Pranayama Mudra Bandha* (ISBN: 81-86336-14-1) to your library, since it documents the physical as well as the spiritual benefits of all the postures you will have been taught.

CHAPTER THREE

Heart, Blood and Lungs

If it inflates, deflates, pumps, circulates, flows, filters, screens, transports or clots, then it is part of the body that will be included in this chapter, which is loosely called Heart, Blood and Lungs. The exception is the lymphatic system, which I will examine in more depth in Chapter 5.

This is the chapter that gets down to the nitty-gritty of the unsexy but important hidden body bits that need to function optimally to keep us in good health, but which, unlike the skin and digestion, often get overlooked. It is about the body's transportation systems, breathing mechanisms and storage facilities – all systems that are equally prone to the oxidative damage that is the underlying cause of most chronic cardiovascular and respiratory diseases.

The Heart

Cutting to the chase, heart failure is the term medics use to describe not a heart that has stopped working altogether but a heart that is struggling to do its job of contracting and pumping blood around the body. Any disease that adversely affects the heart and disrupts circulation can lead to heart failure, and while it is a frightening diagnosis to contemplate, it is not an automatic death sentence. True, it is likely to worsen over time, but lots of people with heart failure live for many years following the diagnosis.

The single most common cause of heart failure is coronary artery disease, which limits blood flow to the heart muscle and can lead to a heart attack. Other factors that can damage the heart muscle itself include a bacterial infection or myocarditis (see page 117), diabetes (see page 91), obesity (see page 123) and an overactive thyroid gland (see Chapter 8, page 394).

Problems with the valves that regulate blood flow between the heart's four distinct chambers can obstruct circulation and cause problems, and, in effect, anything that increases the workload of this muscle will eventually weaken the force of its contractions. There are, of course, other diseases that affect the electrical conduction system that determines heartbeat, and since slow, fast or irregular beats cannot pump blood as effectively, again the heart muscle will end up overworked.

If you are concerned about heart disease, ask your doctor to give you a check-up. He or she will look for a positive response to some of the following symptoms to make a diagnosis that can easily and quickly be confirmed by a chest X-ray.

- You feel weak and tired when you have to perform physical activities (this symptom is a sign that the muscles are not getting enough blood).
- You have a rapid and weak pulse rate.
- You have reduced blood pressure.

- You have swollen neck veins.
- You are short of breath (this symptom is a sign of fluid on the lungs and is almost always worse when you lie down and better if you sit up).
- You report rapid weight gain (a rapid increase of more than 2lb (about a kilogram) a day can be a sign of worsening heart failure).
- The liver has become enlarged and the abdomen swollen.
- You complain of water retention in the legs.

I do not for one moment recommend you embark on a DIY programme of natural remedies if you know you have underlying cardiovascular disease. Rather, this section is to encourage those who are still unaware of any cardio- or pulmonary problems to take extra care of this aspect of their health. It is also an encouragement to those who are seeking more natural solutions to existing problems, such as high cholesterol levels or insulin resistance (see page 91), to talk to their health advisors about the role of some of the remedies I am going to be recommending either as an adjunct or an alternative to current medication.

You must not treat any of the information in this book as a substitute for excellent and supervised medical care. See it more as a way of doing your homework before talking to your advisors so that you are better informed if you have to make health choices about prevention or cure.

The Blood

You might find the sight of your own blood too alarming to contemplate but the biology of blood is fascinating enough to fill a book in its own right. In essence, your blood is a combination of liquid (plasma) which is made up mostly of water, containing proteins and dissolved salts, plus red and white blood cells, platelets and other particles that flow through the arteries and veins, delivering oxygen and essential nutrients to the body's organs and tissues and taking waste, including carbon dioxide, away.

Fats (which we also call lipids) are energy-rich substances that provide the body with a source of fuel for its metabolic processes. There are two types of fats in the blood – cholesterol and triglyceride – both of which travel round the bloodstream by attaching themselves to proteins, at which point they become known as lipoproteins. For more on lowering blood-fat levels, see page 118.

As we get older, our blood vessels become less elastic, more rigid and more stiff. As a result, blood starts to flow more slowly through the capillaries and this, in turn, increases its tendency to coagulate and the risk of a clot forming. Exercise helps maintain stretchy blood vessels but if your lifestyle is, mostly, sedentary, that all-important elasticity will go. If you are over thirty and have any of the risk factors outlined in this chapter (see page 115), do yourself a huge favour and find a way to incorporate supervised exercise into your life. You should also consider those natural remedies that have been shown to support circulation and help strengthen and maintain the integrity of blood vessels. These include: **vitamin C** (see page 129), **horse chestnut** (see page 169), **ginkgo biloba** (see page 317), **rutin** and **bilberry.** Rutin is often included in haemorrhoid creams, for example, but newer research suggests bilberry, more traditionally used to support eyesight, may perform even better since it has a two-pronged advantage over other vascular treatments. First, because it encourages the production of collagen, it works to strengthen the connective tissue that surrounds the veins, and, secondly, it also improves the endothelium, the layer of cells that lines the blood vessels, the heart and the lymphatic vessels.

The recommended dose of bilberry extract (providing 25 per cent anthocyanidin content) is 80–160mg a day. **Remember, though, that herbs can be as powerful as prescription drugs and** can affect any medication you are already taking. Do not, for example, self-dose if you are already taking heart or blood-pressure medicine. Instead, consult a qualified medical herbalist (see Useful Contacts, page 447).

Live Blood Analysis – No Place to Hide

I have been prodded and poked and manhandled and massaged, measured and monitored (inside and out) and scanned, all in the name of reporting on natural health. But I had never felt more 'exposed' than when I agreed to provide a blood sample to enable New Zealand-based holistic physician Dr Tim Ewer to demonstrate the workings of darkfield microscopy and a relatively little-used and still controversial* diagnostic tool called Live Blood Analysis.

I cannot think of a single experience that compares with facing a TV screen displaying for all to see what is usually the secret workings of your circulatory system. I cannot say I relished the experience but I also cannot deny that it was fascinating to see for myself the then 'sticky' state of my red blood cells, along with circulating fat globules, unexpectedly large numbers of white blood cells (antibodies that had been produced in response to an infection I was not aware I had – though I was feeling tired and run down), plus strands of a protein called fibrin.

The strands of fibrin, when activated, form fibrinogen, a

---

* Live Blood Analysis has not been accepted as a useful diagnostic tool by main-stream medicine and so is still not widely available. Critics argue that pill pushers can use it to dupe vulnerable patients into buying expensive supplements they may not need but that does not mean, of course, the technique does not work or is not a useful diagnostic tool – in the right hands. You can now make your own mind up. In the UK, you can book a Live Blood Analysis test with holistic doctors at the Diagnostic Clinic (020 7009 4651). It will cost between £75 and £150.

substance that then plays a key role in blood clotting – this is an important protective mechanism which stops us from bleeding to death when we cut ourselves, but which can, commonly, get stuck revved up in top gear. (To tackle this, see nattokinase, page 147.)

The bad news was that it was clear from this somewhat alarming analysis of my live blood that I was not, at that time, as healthy as I would have liked to be, and it was also clear that a lot of inflammation was present in my body. The good news was that I could work out precisely what my system needed to give my overall health and vitality a much-needed boost, to springclean the blood (see Chapter 1, page 29) and to reduce the strain of inflammation on my system.

In other words, this was no guessing game. I could see for myself what was wrong and take holistic health advice on what to do about it – and you cannot get a more motivating start to deciding the time has come to do something positive about your health, instead of just talking or thinking about it.

The Spleen

If you consult with a Traditional Chinese Medicine practitioner, you will soon hear mention of the spleen, a key organ that is otherwise primarily overlooked and ignored by a more conventional medical approach.

Your medical dictionary will tell you the soft, spongy and purplish-coloured spleen – which is about the size of a bunched adult fist and which is tucked up under the ribcage on the left-hand side of the body – is responsible for the production, monitoring, storage and destruction of blood cells, and I will talk about this organ in more detail in Chapter 5 (Stress and Immunity).

The point I want to make here is that in TCM the role of organs is not limited to their anatomical functions but is widened to include their bio-energetic roles in the body, and in this context the spleen has two important jobs: (1) to help transform food into energy, and (2) to make sure that food is used to make healthy blood which can then transport vital qi (chi) energy around the body.

Atherosclerosis and Coronary Heart Disease

Coronary heart disease (CHD) is still the No.1 killer in both men and women living in the west. Between the ages of thirty-five and fifty-five, the death rate is higher for men than women. After fifty-five, the rate for men starts to decline while the rate for women continues to climb. Among heart attack survivors, women are also more likely to suffer a second heart attack than men.

According to mainstream medical thinking, you are most at risk of developing atheroma – i.e. plaque deposits that can block blood vessels, which is still the primary risk factor for heart failure – if:

- you smoke cigarettes and drink too much alcohol (see page 139 for help on stopping smoking);
- you have high blood pressure and eat a lot of salt (see Syndrome X, page 122, for natural remedies that can re-regulate this);
- you have diabetes (see Syndrome X, page 122, and Chapter 2, page 91);
- you are obese and eat a high-fat diet (see Syndrome X, page 122, and weight loss recommendations, Chapter 2, page 88);
- you do no real physical exercise (see Chapter 4 for a discussion of the importance of targeted training to build strength and core stability, especially as you age);
- you have a low ratio of 'good' cholesterol to total cholesterol (see Syndrome X, page 122, and cholesterol levels, below);

- you have high homocysteine and low potassium levels (see homocysteine, below);
- you are getting older and heavier (increase in blood pressure with age is always a result of creeping atherosclerosis, or hardening of the arteries, and increasing body weight; see Chapter 7 for a discussion on ageing).

So how come someone who never smokes or gets fat, who spends half the week in the gym and who has no history of heart disease, can have a heart attack?

While the first signs of heart disease – arterial plaque and fatty deposits – have been noted in kids as young as twelve, the fact is that half of all those who die from a heart attack have none of the risk factors (see above) that have long been identified.

For many years, calcified fatty deposits (plaque) that restrict blood flow in the coronary arteries have been seen as the primary cause of heart attacks. Yet studies involving autopsies of heart-attack victims failed to find significant plaque deposits at the site of the occlusion in over two-thirds of victims.

What these findings suggest is that alongside those well-documented risk factors for CHD that we all know about, something else must be going on.

That something else is now thought likely to be: (a) bacterial infection, which has been identified in the 50 per cent of cases who had no other risk factor for a heart attack (see page 117), and/or (b) the formation of something called 'vulnerable plaque', which builds up inside, not along, the arterial wall and which cannot be detected by a standard angiogram.

Clinical trials by cardiologists have shown that statin drugs, which work to lower 'bad' (LDL) cholesterol to levels around 90mg per decilitre (mg/dL) of blood, can help shrink vulnerable plaque. Natural remedies that can achieve the same results without the risk of side effects include red yeast (see page 119), which works in the same way as the statin drugs.

The Role of Infection in Cardiovascular Disease

Researchers are now looking carefully at the role of infectious agents in heart disease, especially a bacterium called Chlamydia pneumoniae which, as the name suggests, causes pneumonia but which has now also been linked with cardiovascular problems.

In animal trials, rabbits fed a high fat and cholesterol diet that were then infected with Chlamydia pneumoniae developed plaque more rapidly than the control group of animals fed the diet only. We also know that, statistically, a higher use of antibiotics in humans correlates to a lower risk of heart disease, and that patients with acute myocardial infarction have a high blood plasma concentration of those markers of inflammation such as fibrinogen or white blood cells (see Live Blood Analysis, page 113).

Research alert: New research published in the *European Heart Journal* turns conventional thinking on its head by suggesting that men with lower levels of testosterone have a higher risk of developing coronary heart disease (CHD) or atherosclerosis. Since, traditionally, men have higher rates of heart disease than women, it had always been assumed that testosterone and other androgens increased the risk. You can increase levels of the male hormones naturally by taking the aptly named supplement Manpower, which provides a daily dose of 250mg of the hormone-boosting adaptogenic east-European herb, **tribulus terrestris**. This is part of the American Lifetime range, available in the UK from Victoria Health (0800 389 8195; www.victoriahealth.com).

Cholesterol Levels

The health risks of high cholesterol levels have been hammered home so effectively that we now all (mistakenly) believe that the lower our cholesterol levels, the better. Nothing could be further from the truth since there are also health risks – including mood disorders, depression, feelings of violence and a higher risk of stroke – when cholesterol levels are too low.

The real predictor of your risk of heart disease, if you are sticking with cholesterol monitoring, is the ratio of so-called 'good' high density lipid (HDL) cholesterol to total cholesterol, and so this is the test you should ask for. Medics deem an ideal cholesterol level to be between 140 and 200 milligrams per decilitre (mg/dL) of blood and it is true that at levels higher than 300mg/dL, the risk of a heart attack appears to double.

The preferred levels of good cholesterol (HDL) to bad (low density lipid or LDL) are as follows: LDL should be below 130mg/dL and HDL should be above 40mg/dL. In addition, HDL should account for more than 25 per cent of the total cholesterol. *Remember, the total cholesterol level is less important as a reliable predictor of the risk of heart disease than the ratio of HDL to total cholesterol.*

The good news about natural remedies for lowering cholesterol levels is that (a) they really do work and (b) they work as effectively as the conventional medications without the additional risk of side effects that, according to new reports, can include an increased risk of cancer.

Both classes of the two most popular cholesterol-controlling prescription drugs – the fibrates and the statins – have been shown to cause cancer in rodents, often at levels close to the dosages prescribed for humans. I know you can argue that a risk in rats cannot be extrapolated to a risk in humans but I would argue back that until we have longer-term clinical trials and surveillance of the use of these drugs, they should be reserved for the short-term use of patients known to be at high risk of a heart attack, especially when we have risk-free alternatives, such as red yeast (also known as red rice; see below), which we know work.

This is important because health experts predict that, in the future, 50 per cent of the population will be taking these cholesterol-lowering drugs, and if they are right, that means either you or someone very close to you will be affected.

The One to Watch – Red Yeast

Most of the cholesterol in your body – over 80 per cent – is not from the diet but is produced by your own liver, so you need an agent that will reduce this production without damaging that organ. The herb that does this is a Chinese plant called **red yeast** (**hong qu**) or **red rice**. This is the substance that gives the popular Chinese dish Peking Duck its distinctive colouring, but red yeast supplements are not the same as the red yeast rice sold in Chinese supermarkets. Instead, they are made by fermenting rice with a yeast called Monascus purpureus in a carefully controlled environment.

In clinical trials, patients taking red yeast for just eight weeks reduced cholesterol levels by 23 per cent. Most studies were using 2.4g a day but researchers have recorded benefits with a lower dose of 1.2g a day and, in one trial, red yeast was found to be as effective as the cholesterol-lowering statin prescription drug, Zocor (simvastatin).

You can mail order Nature's Plus Pure Red Rice Yeast from Revital (0800 252875; www.revital.com).

Tried and Applied

Take a leaf from Madonna's book and order real ale next time you are in the pub ... agricultural chemists at the University of Oregon have found that hops contain active agents which help prevent the tissue-damaging oxidation of 'bad' cholesterol (LDL), and German research confirms that the odds of developing a heart attack are 45 per cent lower in moderate beer drinkers than non-drinkers. The researchers on this occasion confined their studies to beer and did not investigate the health benefits of drinking wine or other types of alcohol.

H is for Homocysteine

I first wrote about homocysteine as a better indicator of your risk of heart problems than cholesterol five or six years ago. At that time, I received angry letters from both doctors and nurses, specializing in cardiovascular health, accusing me of peddling nonsense, and I wonder if these same highly opinionated correspondents are sending similar letters of complaint to their own medical journals, which have now started reporting the usefulness of measuring homocysteine levels. Probably not, is my guess.

Homocysteine, in case you haven't heard about it, is an amino acid and a normal by-product of the metabolism of protein, which is now reckoned to be about 40 times more accurate as a tool for predicting your risk of heart problems than cholesterol levels.

Raised homocysteine levels have been found in the blood of 40 per cent of patients suffering from heart disease, and we know that around 80 per cent of all fatal heart attacks, for example, occur in men who do not have high cholesterol levels. One possible explanation is that homocysteine in some way promotes atherosclerosis – the life-threatening hardening of the arteries – and the formation of plaque deposits made up of cholesterol and calcium, which can trigger a heart attack by restricting blood and oxygen flow to the heart.

Both cigarette smoking and high coffee consumption are known to be linked with an increased risk of heart disease. What is less well known is that they have also been associated with high levels of homocysteine.

If the body makes it naturally, why is homocysteine a problem?

In good health, the body not only makes but then detoxifies homocysteine by converting it back to methionine, from which it was produced in the first place, or by breaking it down even further to form a more harmless substance called cystathionine. Factors that can interfere with this process include either (a) a genetic fault in one of the enzymes responsible for this chemical breakdown, or (b) a deficiency in any one of the nutrients needed to activate these enzymes in the first place.

What we also know is that several of the B vitamins, including folic acid (which is more usually taken by women wanting to conceive and by mothers-to-be in the first trimester of pregnancy to protect against neural tube defects), can also lower levels of homocysteine. The two important vitamins to take if you have high homocysteine are B6 and B12, both of which act as cofactors for the enzymes that keep levels low. Where there has been an increase in homocysteine levels as a result of a nutritional deficiency, you need only take 400mcg of folic acid, 10mg of vitamin B6 and 50mcg of vitamin B12 every day.

The point about taking all three of these nutrients is that they are synergistic (i.e. one does not work as well without the other). And if you are still not convinced, you should know that tests on men with high levels of homocysteine revealed sub-optimal levels of all three of these nutrients.

Since homocysteine is made from methionine, if you know you have high levels there seems to be some sense in avoiding those foods that are a natural source of this substance. These include meat, fish, chicken and eggs. Foods that can help keep homocysteine levels lower include beans and dark leafy greens such as spinach.

You can ask your GP to test your homocysteine levels. If they are too high, discuss supplementation with your health practitioner. Solgar's Homocysteine Modulators provide folic acid and vitamins B6 and B12 to lower blood levels of homocysteine. To find a local stockist, call 01442 890355.

Cholesterol vs Homocysteine – Why You Need to Monitor Both

The simple answer is that although homocysteine is now accepted by mainstream medicine as a 40-times-more-accurate predictor of the risk of heart disease than cholesterol levels, what we also know is that while high cholesterol levels will give rise, more frequently, to plaque deposits in the coronary arteries servicing the heart, high homocysteine levels will give rise, more frequently, to plaque deposits in blood vessels other than the coronary arteries. In other words, while one can increase the risk of heart attack, the other can increase the risk of blood clots and related coronary disease.

Syndrome X . . .

. . . how high blood-sugar levels, high cholesterol and high blood pressure can add up to heart disease.

In 1988, US endocrinologist Gerald Reaven – who had studied insulin resistance for some twenty years – made an important connection. He realized that sometimes this disorder was part of a group of related symptoms which had the worrying effect of increasing a person's risk of both diabetes and heart disease.

He coined the term 'Syndrome X' to describe this cluster of symptoms which includes:

- insulin resistance,
- glucose intolerance,
- obesity,
- blood-fat abnormalities, and
- hypertension.

At the moment, all the above conditions are treated by allopathic medicine with aggressive drugs that come with significant adverse side effects, when the solution could be as simple as changing your diet.

What causes Syndrome X is an excess of sugar in the blood, and where has this sugar come from? A diet that is rich in refined sugars and refined, highly processed, rapidly digested carbohydrate convenience foods. (See The GI Index; What Not To Eat, page 124.)

When we eat this type of typical western diet, the pancreas responds by releasing large amounts of insulin (see Chapter 2, page 58) to reduce high glucose levels and, over time, it is as if the cells become deaf to this chemical messenger, so that more and more insulin has to be released to get the same effect. This is known as insulin resistance, and the upshot will be glucose intolerance; in other words, two of the symptoms already listed as related under the umbrella term Syndrome X.

Just to worsen the picture, insulin also promotes the formation of fat, and so the more insulin a person makes, the more likely he or she is to gain weight, which, if not addressed, will result in yet another of the Syndrome X symptoms: obesity.

If you have even a hint of this insulin resistance/glucose intolerance – which is now thought to affect almost half the adult population in the west – you need to switch to a more natural diet rich in the complex carbohydrates that are present in fruits and vegetables, and eliminate refined sugars.

The **Glycaemic Index (GI)**: This is a ranking of hundreds of everyday carbohydrate foods (starches and sugars) showing how quickly they affect blood-sugar levels after ingestion. Most studies use pure glucose as the reference food, giving it a GI of 100. The idea then is to eat more low GI foods (low = below 55) and fewer high GI foods, and what is shocking about using this index to support your diet is that foods you might have thought of as healthy can have a high ranking (e.g. pumpkin is 75) while those you would have avoided as being a health hazard have a lower one (e.g. a Snickers bar, which is ranked at 41). Carrots, for instance, have a stonking ranking of 90, while chocolate is 49 and rice cakes, which health gurus love, are an alarming 82.

Here's what not to eat: white flour products, colas and pops, hydrogenated oils in margarines and cooking oils, and processed convenience foods, including commercial breakfast cereals.

My Top Twenty Low-GI Foods You Should Try to Eat More Often

In alphabetical order:
 Apple (GI=36)
 Baked beans (GI = 48)
 Barley (GI = 25)
 Cherries (GI = 22)
 Dried apricots (GI = 29)
 Grapefruit (GI = 25)
 Green peas (GI = 49)
 Kidney beans (GI = 27)

Lentils (GI = 29)

Non-fat yoghurt (GI = 14)

Peanuts (GI = 14)

Pears (GI = 38)

Potato chips (GI = 54)

Rice bran (GI = 19)

Soybeans (GI = 17)

Split peas (GI = 32)

Strawberry jam (GI = 51)

Watermelon (GI = 7)

Whole milk (GI = 23)

Wholewheat spaghetti (GI = 37)

Visit www.glycemicindex.com and use the search facility to find the GI ranking of your favourite foods.

Potato chips, for example, have a surprisingly low GI (lower than baked potatoes, which most people would consider healthier) because fat takes the stomach longer to digest. Combining high and low GI foods in the same meal will also help moderate blood sugar levels and is a smart way to vary your diet and better avoid the slippery slope of insulin resistance and Syndrome X.

If you start your day with a low GI food, such as grapefruit or stewed apples, you will not be reaching for the biscuits by mid-morning to stave off hunger pangs. Try it; it really works.

Can You Really Reverse Heart Disease?

Coronary calcifications or arterial deposits grow at the rate of 44 per cent, i.e. almost half again, each year, according to some reports, but there is a single nutrient that might not only slow down this growth rate but also work to reverse plaque deposits and heart disease.

In a report, published in the *Journal of Applied Nutrition*,

American researcher, doctor and champion of vitamin C Dr Mattias Rath reported that when 55 patients went on a specially devised vitamin programme, including up to 3g of vitamin C*, for six months, this trend was reversed and the calcium deposits in some patients actually disappeared.

Humans, unlike animals, cannot make vitamin C in their bodies and so must get it from their diet. For more about Dr Rath's theories on reversing heart disease, read his thought-provoking book, *Why Animals Don't Get Heart Attacks . . . But People Do!*, in which he argues that heart attacks and strokes are not diseases but signs of a deficiency in vitamin C and other important vitamins.

The Kidneys

The kidneys remove waste products from the body, regulate chemical levels, maintain the water balance and work to normalize blood pressure and red-blood-cell production. Each kidney contains about a million minuscule filtering units (nephrons) and these organs, along with the heart and brain, boast the body's highest levels of mitochondria – the cells' own energy-production units that are most dense in the hardest working of the body's organs.

Hormones, the body's own chemical messengers, control kidney function, and the concentration of urine is determined by the body's need for water. Most adults pass around three cups of urine a day, and most people urinate four to six times in 24 hours, mostly in the daytime. Increased urination and excessive thirst can both be signs of type II diabetes (see Chapter 2, page 91) so do not ignore either.

---

* Doses of vitamin C over 2g a day are likely to cause stomach upset, including diarrhoea.

I know just how nasty **kidney stones** can be since for some extraordinary reason, I had a small one in my late twenties – followed by a kidney infection – both of which were sheer agony. Vitamin C, in large doses, is often implicated in the formation of kidney stones. This was certainly not the case for me, but to be safe, split your daily vitamin C dose into no more than 250mg per hit. In other words, if you are taking 1g of vitamin C, divide your supplement into four 250mg doses, which is the level at which tissues become saturated, and take them at four evenly spaced intervals (e.g. one every four hours) throughout the day.

My health books tell me that testing the kind of stone that is passed will give a clue to what foods need to be eliminated from the diet to prevent the formation of these hardened, crystallized deposits of excess minerals and oxalates, but this didn't happen in my case and I never suffered again.

Do not think you must stop calcium supplementation to prevent kidney stones (you might think this on the grounds that the stones are made up in part from calcium deposits) – ironically, lower calcium levels could *increase* your risk, since this mineral binds with oxalates in the gut to prevent their absorption and thus help prevent the formation of kidney stones.

Magnesium (see page 136) can help lower the risk of kidney stones if you are prone. You need 200–400mg a day in the form of magnesium citrate. Avoid oxalate-rich foods, the eclectic list of which includes: chocolate, spinach, rhubarb, beetroot, tea, wheat bran, nuts, almonds, peanuts and strawberries.

Research alert: New studies show that the antihangover, antioxidant amino acid N-acetyl cysteine (NAC) can also help protect the kidneys from damage caused by the radio-opaque dyes doctors use in imaging tests in patients who have kidney problems or diabetes. Ironically, NAC, which is also used to treat lung disease, is so effective that many patients and reporters now think it is a drug and not simply a nutrient you can buy in your local health store. It is also one of the active agents in the SinuFix formula (see page 144).

Urinary Tract Infections (UTIs)

I often get asked whether commercial cranberry juice really can, despite its high sugar content, help banish urinary tract infections, and the answer is that, although supplementation would be better, yes, commercial juices do work.

The reason **cranberry** works is that it makes the urine more acidic, creating a more hostile environment for bacteria such as E. coli, which are usually causing the problem. It also stops these bacteria from establishing themselves on the bladder wall, and if they cannot get a 'foothold' they are then flushed out of the bladder along with the stream of urine.

What cranberry can do is help tackle chronic infections and halt the cycle of repeated infections. In trials, women taking even a supermarket cocktail of cranberry plus another juice had 58 per cent less bacteria in their urine than those given a placebo pill.

If you prefer a supplement, use Planetary Formula's Cranberry Concentrate; it provides the equivalent of 200ml/7fl oz of cranberry juice in each 500mg tablet. If not available at your local UK health store, mail order from the NutriCentre on 0800 587 2290; www.NutriCentre.com.

The other herb that is useful for milder urinary tract infections is **uva ursi** (or bearberry), which can help stop the bacteria that are causing the infection from multiplying. Uva ursi works best when the urine is alkaline. What this then means is that you need to avoid taking it with a more acidic remedy, such as cranberry juice. In other words, don't be tempted to think you'll get double the results by doubling up the remedies.

Top Ten Natural Agents to Help Protect Against Heart and Lung Disease

Ask your health practitioner about these.

Vitamin C

Reports that suggest vitamin C may do more harm to arteries than good were widely discredited when researchers admitted that the techniques they had been using to assess the impact of this nutrient on healthy cells in test-tube studies had caused damage to the DNA of those cells. In other words, it was the science, not the nutrient, causing the problem. Study after study has shown how taking a daily dose of vitamin C (1g a day) really can lower your risk of cardiovascular disease. This nutrient also protects the lungs, especially in smokers. (Smoking increases your need for vitamin C and smokers are recommended to take an extra 35mg a day to compensate.) Taking the contraceptive pill can also affect levels of vitamin C, since oestrogens work to increase elimination of this nutrient. The richest food source of vitamin C is acerola berries, and Viridian (www.viridian.com) has launched a new vitamin C made from these fruits.

Therapeutic dose

1g a day, split into 4 doses taken throughout the day.

Contraindications

Do not take vitamin C alongside antacid prescription drugs, aspirin or warfarin. The body cannot store vitamin C and so will flush out any excess, which means you need to replenish levels every day.

Hawthorn

Roman physicians used hawthorn as a cardio tonic in the first century AD, and clinical studies now show that its healing action is thanks to the presence of **proanthocyanidins** – red and purple pigments (sometimes called anthocyanins) found in plants which help prevent degenerative diseases of the heart, blood vessels and lungs, and are thought to help reverse artherosclerotic plaque deposits.

Cleverly, hawthorn can re-regulate both high and low blood pressure (see pages 164 and 165), and works to dilate both peripheral and coronary blood vessels, making it a useful aid in the management of angina.

Therapeutic dose

250mg, 3 times a day. Use a supplement that is a mix of the leaf and flowers.

Contraindications

Do not use this herb without medical supervision if you are already taking drugs for cardiovascular problems, if you are pregnant, or if you are taking antidepressants. Remember, all herbal remedies will take a month or so to kick in and you need to take them for at least three months to get the maximum therapeutic benefits.

Garlic

With the advent of more cutting-edge remedies, such as red yeast (see page 119), it seems almost old-fashioned now to recommend garlic as a cardiovascular tonic, but it does still merit a mention as a broad-spectrum treatment for arterial disease.

The active agent is an odourless chemical called alliin. When you cut or crush raw garlic, this is immediately converted to allicin, which is the substance that gives garlic its powerful smell. Allicin then rapidly breaks down into various components, and unless herbal remedy manufacturers, who want to offer odourless capsules, find a way to stop this process, no active agents will be left. This is the reason there is so much controversy about the different brands and forms of garlic.

Therapeutic dose

To be safe, either stick with the traditional dosage of two raw cloves a day, or take odourless Allicin capsules from Health Perception (www.health-perception.co.uk).

Contraindications

Do not combine garlic with blood-thinning medications such as warfarin or aspirin, or other herbal remedies that have the same action, including high-dose vitamin E or ginkgo biloba. Do not use raw garlic topically, since it can blister the skin.

Apples

An apple a day may help keep lung cancer at bay, according to preliminary evidence that suggests a very positive relationship between eating five or more apples a week and healthy lung function. Researchers admit they cannot explain why eating apples can offset normal age-related deterioration in lung functioning but suggest it may be thanks to the presence of two active agents – **quercetin** and **pectin**.

Quercetin (see pages 153 and 163) is a natural antioxidant and anti-inflammatory agent, and pectin has been shown in animal studies to help boost the immune system to protect cells from mutagenic toxins. It can also help reduce high cholesterol and triglyceride levels (see page 118).

Therapeutic dose

One organic apple (with the skin) a day or, if you prefer supplementation, 1 x 500mg apple pectin capsule taken daily.

Contraindications

Do not use pectin supplements if you are taking medications for cardiovascular problems or antibiotics, since pectin supplements can interfere with the absorption of these prescription drugs.

Dandelion

This humble backyard weed is a powerhouse of nutrients that work together to promote healthy heart and lung functioning. Although better known as a digestive tonic (when the remedy has been made from root extracts of the plant), it can also work to promote good cholesterol (HDL) and has a diuretic effect in the body, which then works to regulate blood pressure, when you use the leaves.

Dandelion provides more membrane and lung-supporting vitamin A than carrots, is an excellent source of heart-protecting potassium, and can help maintain good iron levels to prevent anaemia. The young leaves are delicious tossed into a summer salad.

Therapeutic dose

1 x 500mg capsule made from standardized leaf extract taken 3 times a day, with food.

Do not use dandelion if you have gallstones or if you have diabetes, since it can interfere with blood glucose levels, or if you are taking lithium.

Guggul

This is a mixture of gum resin substances taken from the plant Commiphora mukul, which is approved for use as a cholesterol-lowering agent in India. In one small-scale trial, serum cholesterol levels dropped by 17.5 per cent, and in studies combining this natural remedy with the drug chlofibrate, levels of good HDL cholesterol rose by 60 per cent in the group taking the two combined, but remained the same in the control group taking chlofibrate alone.

Guggul, which can also play a role in the treatment of acne (see Chapter 1, page 31), has also been shown to exert protective properties against drug-induced myocardial necrosis and is thought to have useful anti-inflammatory properties.

Therapeutic dose

25mg, taken 3 times a day. You need to persist for at least 12 weeks before evaluating the effects of this herb.

Contraindications

Stop if you get stomach upsets, headaches or mild nausea. Do not take this herb with thyroid medication.

Taurine

A sulphur-containing amino acid present in high levels in meats and fish, taurine, taken as a supplement, has been shown to lower blood pressure and plasma epinephrine (adrenaline) levels. People with high blood pressure and heart problems have higher levels of this hormone circulating in the blood – since it helps the heart work harder to increase its output of blood and thus compensate for any pumping problems – but lower levels in the heart muscle itself, which usually has more taurine present than any other amino acid.

Taurine, which can also help relax blood vessels, is present in human breast milk and it works to lower bad cholesterol levels (see page 118), regulate heart rhythm, maintain cardiac contraction, maintain normal blood pressure and help blood clot when it needs to.

Therapeutic dose

Sold as L-taurine in health stores, clinical trials investigating its use for congestive heart failure used 2–4g a day. Normal maintenance dose is 1.5g a day.

Contraindications

None documented.

Arginine

Sold in supplement form as L-arginine, the body uses this amino acid as a precursor to nitric oxide, which, in turn, dilates blood vessels and lowers blood pressure. It has been successfully used to help support stable angina patients and, in clinical trials, high dosages (17g a day) have been shown to lower 'bad' cholesterol (LDL) without affecting levels of 'good' cholesterol (HDL). (At these high doses, you run the risk of side effects including digestive disturbances and watery diarrhoea.)

Arginine is found naturally in meats, dairy products, poultry and fish, and has been found to be a useful adjunct to treatments for people suffering from intermittent claudication. This is the name given to a condition where, thanks to advanced atherosclerosis, the arteries supplying the legs with blood have become hardened. This makes walking painful because the muscles in the legs are starved of oxygen, and the intensity of this condition is often measured by how far a patient can walk before severe, cramping pains set in.

In one study, where patients were given a daily dose of 6g of arginine split into two equal dosages, after just two weeks all participants were able to walk 66 per cent further than when they started the study.

Therapeutic dose

Sold as L-arginine in health stores, take 3g twice a day on an empty stomach.

Contraindications

Do not use this supplement if you suffer from herpes (see page 44) since it can trigger the usually dormant virus to replicate, and avoid if you have liver or kidney disease.

Homocysteine Modulators

For the full story on homocysteine, which is a 40-times more accurate predictor of the risk of heart disease than cholesterol levels, see page 120. Homocysteine itself is not a natural protector against heart disease, but the agents used to regulate its levels are.

Therapeutic dose

Solgar's Homocysteine Modulators supplement combines Folic acid (400ug) with vitamins B12 (500ug) and B6 (50mg). Call 01442 890355 for UK stockists.

Contraindications

Do not self-diagnose or self-treat high homocysteine levels, but work with a qualified health practitioner who can monitor your progress. See page 447 for a list of referral organizations in the UK.

Magnesium and Potassium

Many unexpected adult deaths are thought to occur as a result of fatal heart rhythm disturbances. We know that magnesium deficiency, which is common in men and women, predisposes to higher risks of these kinds of disturbance, so taking a therapeutic daily dose of a magnesium supplement would seem sensible, along with increasing your dietary intake of this nutrient (see M is for Magnesium, page 152).

We know that potassium works with sodium to regulate the body's water balance and normalize heart rhythms (potassium works inside the cells; sodium works outside them) and documented research proves that a low-potassium, high-sodium (salt) diet is linked with high blood pressure.

Therapeutic dose

Look for a good multimineral supplement that provides both magnesium and potassium. I like New Chapter's MultiMineral (www.new-chapter.com); take 4 a day to boost your intake of magnesium by 200mg. No dietary allowance has been set for potassium but a daily intake of 900mg a day is considered optimum for maintaining good health.

Contraindications

Taking a good general multi mineral-and-vitamin supplement is sensible, but since boosting levels of one mineral can adversely affect another, do not try to self-dose minerals without medical supervision.

Watch the Hype

Co-enzyme Q10 is much mooted as an important nutrient to help prevent heart disease, but in clinical trials it does not always perform as well as the marketing hype would have you believe.

What is known is that one in 500 high-cholesterol patients also have what is called impaired LDL receptors (which is a genetic complaint) and if you are one of these patients you do need CoQ10 because your cholesterol-lowering prescription drugs will block this important nutrient.

If this is the case, take a supplement called Carni Q-Gel Forte, which combines co-enzyme Q10 with L-carnitine (see Chapter 7, Energy and Fatigue) for maximum effectiveness.

Tried and Applied

Invest in a clever little pill-splitter, especially if, like me, you have trouble swallowing tablets the size of horse pills. This little splitter and crusher may not be the best-looking gadget on your shelf but it takes the hard work out of supplementation. You can either split or grind your pills into a fine powder you can then sprinkle over food. For mail order details, call 01273 558112, or visit UK suppliers www.lemonburst.co.uk.

The Breath and the Lungs

In yoga, we say the breath is the bridge to the divine, and one of my favourite yogic references to the importance of the life force – the breath plus that magic ingredient known as 'prana' or 'chi' – comes from the *Brihadaranyaka Upanishad*, which explains how we are all linked by the breath: '. . . verily, by air, as by a thread, this world, the other world and all beings are held together . . .'

If you practise yoga but your teacher has not yet introduced you to the study of pranayama (the science and control of the breath), then ask them why not, or find a teacher who has a special interest in this fascinating topic. For my part, I enjoyed the study and practice of pranayama far more than the practice of asana (postures), and if you think this is a lot of spiritual nonsense, consider this: a third of the air in your lungs at any one time is stale. In yoga, we seek to reduce this and to increase both the amount of oxygen getting into the body and the amount of noxious carbon dioxide waste gas we exhale. We achieve this through the practice of selected asanas and pranayama (see my top three yoga practices for this chapter, page 172) and for confirmation that it really does work, turn to page 172 now.

In yoga, we also recognize that the primary mechanism we must use to improve lung capacity (and thus enhance breathing and the transportation of richly oxygenated blood to the body's tissues) is the diaphragm and its associated musculature. Believe it or not, the diaphragm is responsible for 75 per cent of all respiratory efforts, making it three times more important than the action of the intercostal muscles that expand the ribcage and which, in fact, most people rely on, because instead of breathing deep from the diaphragm they shallow-breathe from the top of the lungs.

Fitness trainer Ann Thompson*, with whom I train (and who is, coincidentally, a specialist in cardiovascular fitness and recovery), gets driven to distraction by what she calls my 'slow yoga breathing'. Rather than sit and twiddle her thumbs while I breathe out, she now asks me to quicken my breath to do an exercise at what she calls 'normal', not yoga, pace. It is something we have agreed to disagree about, but it is highly novel to be working out to a pattern of pranayama.

* For specialist advice on fitness for cardiovascular health and for training regimens to aid recovery from cardiac events, contact Ann Thompson at www.info@fitness.co.uk.

Coughs, Colds and Flu? Think Black Elderberry

Healthy adults should succumb to no more than two common colds a year. If you are prone to repeated infections, you need to build up the body's natural defences by supporting your immune system. For a more detailed programme showing how to do this, see Chapter 5. In the meantime, take **black elderberry** (Sambucus nigra), which has been shown in clinical trials in Israel not only to reduce your risk of developing colds and flu, but also to lessen their severity and shorten the duration of an attack.

Researchers at the Department of Virology at the Hebrew University Hadassah Medical School in Jerusalem discovered that flu patients taking this herb recovered twice as quickly as those taking a placebo pill, and concluded that the active agents could shorten the duration of a flu attack, for example, to just four days.

Smoking and Quitting the Evil Weed

I know it is boring to bang on about it but one of the reasons cigarette smoking is so harmful is that it actually *decreases* levels of the high density lipoprotein (HDL) 'good' cholesterol and *increases* levels of the low density lipoprotein (LDL) 'bad' cholesterol. It also raises the level of carbon monoxide in the blood, and raised levels of this can damage the lining of the arterial walls and, worse, constrict arteries already narrowed by atherosclerosis, further decreasing the amount of blood reaching the tissues. Smoking also increases blood's tendency to clot (see nattokinase, page 147).

That said, it is also bloody hard to stop, and I know this because I have smoked, stopped for years, lapsed when I was feeling under pressure, started again and stopped again, which means

I now know I will always be a smoker who is simply not having a cigarette, and I will always be in danger of caving in. I also know nicotine is probably the most addictive substance known to man and so I forgive myself for being human.

One of the reasons many women are scared to stop smoking is fear of weight gain and, sadly, it is true, you can stop smoking, eat no more than you were eating before and still put on weight. The reason this happens is that the very act of smoking accelerates all the body's systems, including the metabolic rate, which also determines how quickly you burn up calories from food and metabolize fat stores.

A single cigarette has been shown to increase blood pressure by 15mm and pulse rate by 15 beats per minute, so the only way to keep your weight the same if you do quit smoking is to exercise more, and to eat less of the wrong foods and more of the right, health-promoting ones.

Since over the years I have had my own struggles with the weed, what I can tell you is that there is only one way to stop smoking and here is how you do it.

1 Throw out anything in the house that has an association with smoking, including lighters, ashtrays and secret duty-free hoards. If there is anything to smoke in the house, you will cave in at the first craving and use this 'failure' as an excuse to carry on smoking.

2 Stop doing the things you always associate with having a cigarette. For example, if you have one first thing in the morning with coffee, stop drinking coffee first thing in the morning and drink something else instead.

3 Do not tell anyone you are stopping. If family or friends ask, say you have a sore throat and so are trying not to smoke. Say you are on a short detox. The reason for this is that anyone who is still smoking will want you to carry on and will feel threatened by your decision to stop – so don't tell them.

4 Do not allow anyone else to smoke in your house or car. If you have stopped and are enjoying the benefits of a sweet-smelling home, do not let anyone else come in and foul it up again.

5 Take yourself in hand and spend the money you were wasting on cigarettes on working out instead. If you are new to training, get a personal trainer who will make sure you work out safely at the beginning. This will pay dividends in the long run and will also help you stay stopped because you will soon start to look and feel so much better.

6 Do not tell yourself, or anyone else, that you have stopped for ever. In fact, don't think about tomorrow, let alone for ever. Take it one day at a time. What you are trying to do is break a horribly addictive habit, so simply tell yourself: I will not smoke today. If you feel you have lost your best friend, get another – replace this habit with a more healthy one: go line dancing, drink peppermint tea every time you want to smoke, get addicted to something else.

7 Focus on the benefits of stopping. Notice how you and your clothes smell so much better. Notice how everyone has an opinion about smokers but nothing to say about people who do not smoke. Notice how, within days, you are no longer clearing your throat or coughing your way through every conversation.

8 Use nicotine patches to help break the physical habit of smoking, and investigate how natural remedies (see page 143) can help steady nerves and steel willpower to help you through the first few weeks. Take comfort from knowing that it takes three months for all traces of nicotine to leave the body. After that period, any cravings are purely psychological and will pass.

9 Remember that most of us who have stopped did not do so overnight. It took me four years to stop completely and another year to stop again after I had lapsed. It's not easy and you should reward yourself for trying and trying again.

10 Copy this out, and also What Happens When You Stop Smoking? (see below). Pin these around the house to remind you of why you have stopped.

People who stop smoking have only half the risk of coronary heart disease of those who continue to smoke – regardless of how long they smoked before quitting. It is never too late to stop, and always, always, worth it for the real health benefits, which are as follows:

What Happens When You Stop Smoking?*

- 20 minutes after the last cigarette, blood pressure returns to normal.
- 8 hours after the last cigarette, blood oxygen levels return to normal, and nicotine and carbon monoxide levels reduce by half.
- 24 hours after the last cigarette, there will be no more carbon monoxide in the body, and the lungs start to clear out mucus and other smoking debris.
- 48 hours after the last cigarette, your senses of taste and smell start to improve.
- 72 hours after the last cigarette, breathing becomes easier; bronchial tubes begin to relax and energy levels increase.
- 2–12 weeks after the last cigarette, circulation improves.
- 3–9 months after the last cigarette, coughs, wheezing and breathing problems all improve as lung function increases by up to 10 per cent.
- 1 year after the last cigarette, your risk of a heart attack has dropped to about half that of a smoker.

* Taken from *The Health Benefits of Smoking Cessation: A Report of the Surgeon General*, US DHHS, 1990

- 10 years after the last cigarette, your risk of lung cancer has dropped to half that of a smoker.
- 15 years after the last cigarette, your risk of heart attack has dropped to the same risk as someone who has never smoked a single cigarette.

Tried and Applied

Vega's Nico-Quit herbal capsules can help you stop smoking. They combine calming oats with St John's wort. The latter has been shown in trials to maintain mood so that smokers who want to quit do not lapse because they feel depressed.

Why, If You Plan to Carry On Smoking, You Need to Eat Fiery Chillies

Hispanic populations living in the Los Angeles area who smoke but who eat lots of chillies in their everyday diet have a surprisingly low incidence of respiratory problems, according to Dr Irwin Ziment, a professor at the University of California, who, based on these findings, now prescribes **chillies** to patients with lung-related problems.

Chillies, which are native to America, work to open up the body's airways, including sinuses. They break down mucus in the lungs, help prevent blood clots and can also help alleviate both bronchitis and emphysema. The pharmacological agent is capsaicin, a compound that gives chillies their fiery taste. Green chillies are also rich in rutin, a bioflavonoid that works to support and maintain the integrity of blood vessels.

See page 129 for why **vitamin C** is a crucial nutrient for smokers too.

Other Open Spaces — Nose, Ears, Sinus Passages

The sinuses are, in effect, open spaces in the skull whose job is to warm, moisten and filter the air coming from outside and going into the lungs. The trouble with spaces in the body is that they are the first places to become congested when any kind of infection takes hold. When the sinuses are congested, blocked, irritated or inflamed, they can trigger a whole range of secondary symptoms, including earache, headache, toothache, pain in the face, loss of the sense of smell, bad breath and tenderness in those affected areas.

Chronic sinusitis is often linked to asthma and the result of an allergic reaction. That means it won't go away until you identify the food or environmental triggers and remove them. Dairy products and milk are not helpful since they trigger the production of even more and thicker mucus, which will be harder to drain – so be strict and try cutting down on both these in your diet.

Look for a supplement that combines **quercetin**, which works to reduce the body's inflammatory response to allergens and other irritants, and **nettle** which, far from being another annoying weed, is a hotbed of herbal pharmacological activity and one of the most effective remedies for hay fever and other allergic reactions. Nettles contain, for example, vitamins C and K, as well as immune-boosting proteins and an anti-inflammatory agent called scopoletin that will counter the action of the body's histamine discharge causing your blocked sinuses. Check out SinuFix from NaturalCare (www.enaturalcare.com), which also provides mucus-busting turmeric to keep sinus passages clear.

Ringing in the Ears?

Tackle tinnitus by taking a high daily dose of vitamin B12. You need 2000mcg (micrograms) a day; which everyone will tell you is too high and could be dangerous. It is not. There are no reported side effects with this nutrient, but make sure you avoid synthetic brands.

Why should it work?

Because vitamin B12 plays a key role in neurological functioning, and in trials 47 per cent of patients with both tinnitus and noise-induced loss of hearing were shown to be deficient in this nutrient, which the body also uses to make myelin, the protein sheath that covers nerve fibres. Researchers therefore concluded that, in some cases, there is definitely a link between B12 deficiency and auditory dysfunction, and you just might be one of those cases.

Some studies have shown that tinnitus patients who switch to a low-fat, low-cholesterol diet also experience a significant reduction in symptoms, and in further trials investigating the usefulness of the circulation-boosting Chinese herb ginkgo biloba, 12 of the 33 patients participating in the study recovered completely. If you take this route, you will need to be patient, since it can take a month for the effect of the herb to kick in, and you will also find that the longer you take it, the greater the benefits.

I have upset the 'establishment' over and over again with these recommendations. One correspondent, the chairman of a tinnitus support group, was furious that I had ignored the results of the largest-ever trial conducted into the usefulness of ginkgo in the management of this condition. This particular study had recruited over 1000 sufferers and been reported in the *British Medical Journal*. Its researchers were forced to conclude ginkgo biloba was ineffective as a remedy for tinnitus, but what sufferers were not told was that this so-called study simply involved sending a questionnaire and supplements out to the volunteers. In other words, there was no doctor–patient contact.

Such studies are often criticized because patient compliance is always an issue. People lie about taking their tablets and researchers know that. In other words, and in my opinion of course, the 'establishment' is relying on pretty shaky ground which it perceives as solid, simply because it has been reported in a prestigious mainstream medical journal.

I am not in the business of giving false hope, but we know that both ginkgo and vitamin B12 really can help with this distressing condition and I believe sufferers have a right to know that and do not deserve, because of some other agenda, to be kept in the dark with blinkers on.

Solgar vitamins make a single B12 supplement in 1000mcg (microgram) tablets. Call 01442 890355 for local stockists and take two a day.

Tried and Applied

Nourish the lungs and other airways with a minty-flavoured respiratory tonic taken from the Ayurvedic healing system: mix a teaspoon of mint juice with two teaspoons of malt vinegar, two teaspoons of a locally harvested honey and 120ml carrot juice. Drink this three times a day to keep the breath fresh and reduce congestion in all the body's air passages.

The Other One to Watch – Natto

Natto is a traditional Japanese fermented food, made by adding the spores of the Bacillus natto bacterium (hence its name) to boiled soybeans. It is also known, thanks to its taste, as vegetable cheese.

In 1980, Japanese researchers investigating the blood-clot-busting properties of almost 200 natural foods discovered that natto exhibited the strongest thombocytic activity, thanks to the presence of a potent enzyme that could not only help prevent the formation of life-threatening blood clots but could also dissolve fibrous blood clots that had already formed. This enzyme is called nattokinase, and further research confirms that 100g of natto has the same clot-preventing action as a therapeutic dose of the anti-coagulant prescription drug urokinase. Even more promising, while an injection of urokinase is effective for between just four and twenty minutes, nattokinase remains active for between four and eight hours and has no recorded side effects.

In fact, natto is so effective that lots of natural health experts are now describing it as the poor man's way of cleaning out the arteries. You can, if you get hold of the fresh microbe spores from specialist suppliers, make your own vegetable cheese (natto), but since this book is all about convenience, check out the **nattokinase supplement** from US specialists Allergy Research Group (www.allergyresearchgroup.com) and take one tablet in the morning and two at bedtime.

Feeding Your Cardiovascular System

Since most degenerative and chronic health problems are the result of oxidative tissue damage, there is nothing more important than antioxidant protection. The most important antioxidant that the body produces naturally is glutathione, which has a mine-sweeping action, clearing out toxins from both dietary and environmental pollutants. There is some concern that glutathione supplements are not readily absorbed by the body so a better way to boost levels, especially if you either drink or smoke heavily, is to take a supplement of **N-acetyl cysteine (NAC)**, which the body uses to make glutathione.

To remember the three most important antioxidants, simply start at the beginning of the alphabet with the letter A. The three big hitters are: ACE (vitamins A, C and E), astaxanthin (which is even more potent when combined with the bioflavonoid, Pycnogenol) and alpha linoleic acid (ALA), which can help halve your risk of a heart attack.

Top Three Over-the-Counter Antioxidant Remedies

If you cannot find these on sale in your local UK health store, you can mail order all three from Revital (0800 252875; www.revital.com).

ACE

Super10 antioxidant from the Country Life range will provide 10,000 IUs of vitamin A, 1g of vitamin C and 400 IUs of vitamin E per two capsules.

Astaxanthin and Pycnogenol

You need to take these individually. HealthPlus Inc make 1mg capsules of astaxanthin and Solgar makes a 30mg Pycnogenol, both of which you take twice a day.

ALA

Fresh linseed oil by Solgar (1200mg) will provide a therapeutic dose. Alternatively, if you can tolerate the taste, add two table-spoons of flaxseed oil to your food each day. (See my breakfast cereal, Chapter 2, page 68, and increase the dose.)

The Dollar-a-Day Indo-Mediterranean Diet

Researchers are reporting near epidemic levels of heart disease among people of South Asian origin (mainly Indian and Pakistani) who live in developed countries. The risk is greatest among affluent, urban city dwellers, but cannot be explained by the usual cardiac risk factors, including a high-fat diet and high cholesterol levels (see page 115), since most of those being monitored are vegetarians.

In a recent study, reported in the British medical journal *The Lancet*, one thousand South Asians deemed at high risk of heart disease were put on one of two diets. Diet 1 was an Indian version of the 'prudent' diet recommended by the American Heart Association. Diet 2 was the same but enhanced by elements of the Mediterranean diet to create a new hybrid called the Indo-Mediterranean diet, which promoted a higher consumption of fish, wholegrains, fruits, vegetables, almonds, walnuts and other sources of **alpha linoleic acid (ALA)**. Those patients following diet 2 cooked with olive oil. Everyone followed their diet for two years.

The difference in cardiovascular risks between the two groups at the end of the two years was astonishing. In those patients following the antioxidant-rich Indo-Med diet, the intake of ALA doubled, while the incidence of heart disease halved. The risk of stroke and the number of cardiovascular problems all fell accordingly and, even better, this hybrid diet appeared to work for those who had already suffered a heart attack, suggesting it could help prevent a second attack or strokes.

According to American health experts, the cost of producing the foods incorporated in the Indo-Med diet by US farmers would be around one US dollar a day, giving rise to the name, the Dollar-a-Day Diet.

If the idea of a hybrid diet is too way out for you, make sure that at the very least you start your day with a bowl of cereal (see my breakfast muesli, Chapter 2, page 68), since research has also shown that people who consumed cereal on a regular basis had a significantly lower risk of coronary heart disease, thanks to the presence of both soluble fibre and antioxidant nutrients in this healthy breakfast dish.

> ### Tried and Applied
> When making your own health-promoting fresh juices, use high water content vegetables, such as carrots, apples, grapes and cabbage, as your base, and only small quantities of stronger-tasting plants such as onions or celery. Never juice rhubarb greens or carrot tops, which would be toxic.

A–Z of Heart and Lung Nourishing Foods

A is for antioxidant-rich avocado, asparagus and apricots, plus organic apples which may help keep lung cancer at bay (see page 131). Almonds can help lower bad cholesterol and acerola berries are a brilliant source of lung- and heart-protecting vitamin C.

B is for chromium-rich brewer's yeast that can help normalize blood-sugar levels, and broccoli that contains anti-cancer agents plus vitamin K, which will help keep legs free from unsightly spider and varicose veins. Also bananas, which are an excellent source of heart-protecting potassium.

C is for chocolate and cocoa powder; not a food you would expect to find in a health book, but one that is so rich in tissue-protecting antioxidants, it may help prevent the oxidation of bad cholesterol (LDL) and lower your risk of heart disease. We are not talking Mars Bars here, but the darker the chocolate and the higher the cocoa content, the better it is for you. Milk chocolate, for instance, has twice as many antioxidants as blueberries, and plain chocolate has five times as many. Cocoa powder, which is devoid of fat, is best of all, and boasts twice as many antioxidants as dark varieties of chocolate. Also see lung-protecting chillies (page 143).

D is for iron-rich dried fruits and magnesium-rich dark green leafy vegetables (see Magnesium, page 152); also arginine-rich dairy foods (see page 134) and the potassium-rich seaweed dulse (see Sea Vegetables, page 71).

E is for vitamin E that can help protect against heart disease; you'll find this nutrient in eggs, avocado, legumes, nuts and seeds, wholegrains, organ meats, vegetable oils and molasses. Also eggs, which far from being unhealthy, are a rich source of lecithin, a nutrient that can help lower bad cholesterol. The important thing is to avoid unhealthy frying and restrict your intake to just three eggs a week.

F is for fenugreek, a member of the bean family that works in the body to reduce mucus in both sinusitis and asthmatic conditions. Newer research suggests it can also help lower bad cholesterol. Gargle a warm tea made from the seeds to soothe a sore throat; to make this, simmer two tablespoons of seeds in 1 litre of water for half an hour, cool a little and then strain.

G is for garlic (see page 131), a plant that has both anticoagulant and cholesterol-lowering properties. It is also an effective expectorant and so can expel mucus from the bronchial tubes. Also vitamin C-rich guava, sprouted grains (see page 69) and cholesterol-lowering grapefruit. In animal trials, green tea has been shown to inhibit cancer of the lungs.

H is for horseradish sauce which, like garlic, onions and chilli peppers, can open air passages by thinning mucus, and prevent congestion. Also the hemicellulose fibres (see page 67) found in apples, beets, wholegrain cereals, cabbage, broccoli, green beans, bananas and pears, which will help maintain optimum weight levels and reduce the risk of cardiovascular disease due to excess weight.

I is for iron which you can get from fresh leafy vegetables, meat, poultry, fish, eggs, fortified breads, potatoes, figs, milk, raisins, asparagus and soybeans. Both protein and vitamin C help the body to better absorb iron from the diet by a process called chelation, whereby they attach themselves to the iron molecule to carry it across the intestinal wall.

J is for juicing, the fastest way to get live enzymes into your system. Papaya juice is good for heartburn, grape juice can help reduce water retention, beetroot juice is a brilliant blood tonic and apple juice will help lower cholesterol levels.

K is for vitamin K, which can help prevent the deterioration of blood vessels that causes spider and later varicose veins. Foods that are a good natural source of this nutrient include eggs, soybeans, oats, broccoli, cabbage, liver, rye, cauliflower, whole wheat and the seaweed kelp (see pages 220 and 384), which can also protect against heart disease.

L is for lignan, one of the fibres found in cabbage, beans, cauliflower, carrots, peas, tomatoes, strawberries, wholegrains, brazil nuts, peaches and potatoes. It works to lower cholesterol levels, regulate blood pressure and help reduce the risk of heart disease.

M is for magnesium, which is crucial for cardiovascular health (see page 136). Eat more nuts, wholegrains, beans, dark leafy greens, fish, meats, kiwi fruits and dairy produce, and make your own magnesium- and potassium-rich hummus by blending raw garlic (four juicy cloves), 150ml olive oil and 50g of toasted sesame seeds.

N is for nuts: almonds, cashews, chestnuts, pistachios, hazelnuts, peanuts (these are actually legumes, see page 81), pecans, pine nuts, walnuts and brazil nuts – all of which are good sources of heart- and lung-protecting nutrients including potassium and vitamin A. Add pine nuts to fruits and salads for variety, but limit your intake of cashews since the good nutrients are offset by a high and bad-for-you fat content.

O is for onions, a vegetable that stimulates the production of IgA, an immune-response antibody that coats potential allergens to prevent their absorption. Onions, both raw and cooked, also reduce platelet-clumping by decreasing levels of fibrinogen, the basic clot-promoting substance. Increase your intake if you suffer from hay fever, asthma, sinusitis or any of the allergy-related respiratory complaints. O is also for vitamin-K-rich oats and iron-rich oysters.

P is for potassium, a mineral that crops up again and again in this list of heart-nourishing foods because, together with sodium, it maintains the water balance of the body, which, in turn, affects cardiovascular functioning. Legumes, fish, fruits and poultry are among the healthier, low-fat potassium-rich foods you should be stepping up in your diet.

Q is for quercetin, a bioflavonoid and one of the active agents believed to give apples their lung-protecting and cancer-fighting properties. Found in shallots, onions, summer squash, broccoli and grapefruit, it is also present in many red wines – a presence many believe explains why indigenous populations living in the South of France, for example, can eat a high-fat diet but, thanks to their consumption of red wine, still suffer lower than expected rates of heart disease.

R is for rye, a complex carbohydrate that helps stabilize blood sugars and a plant now providing the active agents in one of the more exciting natural remedies for asthma and respiratory problems, especially in children (see page 160). Also for raspberries, which contain folic acid to help regulate homocysteine levels (see page 120), and iron-rich raisins, which I gently warm in oil until they begin to swell and then toss into a spinach leaf salad with toasted pine nuts. Serve this topped with grilled goat's cheese. Simple, chic and nutritious.

S is for spinach, a good natural source of cardiovascular-protecting co-enzyme Q10 (see page 136) and other blood-cleansing nutrients, plus salmon, which is rich in the omega-3 fatty acids (see page 314) that are important to good health. Also sage, which is fantastic for healing sore throats, tonsillitis, mouth and throat ulcers, and for supporting the lungs.

T is for taurine, found in meat, fish and human breast milk; this is the most abundant amino acid present in a healthy heart (see page 133). T is also for tuna, which is rich in the tissue-protecting antioxidant selenium, and black tea, a good source of health-promoting bioflavonoids. For more on the health-promoting properties of teas, see page 384.

U is for umeboshi plum, a fermented pickle my Irish husband reintroduced me to when he opened a sushi bar and began catering Japanese food! The first bite flashed me back to my teens when my parents often hosted overseas students, including Japanese girls, who would live with us for months on end and then thank us by cooking up a feast of their traditional dishes. Fermented foods support a healthy balance of good gut flora (see page 71) and help the body produce its own anti-cancer compounds.

V is for vegetable oils, which are a good source of vitamin E (see page 151), and magnesium- and fibre-rich vegetables. Also herb vinegars, a more creative way to benefit from the health properties of everyday herbs. Use raw apple cider, rice or malt vinegar as your base, add the fresh or dried herbs of your choice e.g. sage (see above), bottle and cap and leave for two months, unopened, to allow flavours to fully develop before use.

W is for wheatgrass, the king of juices and nature's most potent blood purifier – once you get used to the taste, which can be over-powering, and even make you feel nauseous if you are not careful to build slowly to a daily dose of a teaspoon a day. Experiment with wheatgrass and if you are stuck for ideas, order a copy of *The Little Sweet Wheat Recipe Book* from UK suppliers Xynergy (08456 585858; www.xynergy.co.uk). Watercress is another high-chlorophyll-content plant that is rich in potassium and magnesium to help protect the cardiovascular system. Walnuts are an excellent source of the heart-protecting omega-3 fatty acids, which can help reduce blood-vessel constriction, prevent blood clots and lower homocysteine levels (see page 120).

Y is for yams or sweet potatoes which, according to studies, can both help protect against lung cancer and lower blood cholesterol levels. These delicious but often underused vegetables are rich in substances called protease inhibitors, which have been found in animal studies to help prevent cancer and to protect the body against infection by bacteria and viruses. If you live in a polluted city, with a smoker or smoke yourself, try to eat at least one por-tion of yams, carrots or squash each day. I use yams in my Chillit pie; for the recipe, see Chapter 6, page 340.

Z is for zinc, a nutrient that is so important it is involved in some 200 different processes in the body, including helping to decrease cholesterol deposits. Most zinc in food is stripped out by food processing techniques, or was lacking in the first place thanks to nutrient-poor soil. When food shopping, don't be taken in by a label that says 'enriched'. 'Partially restored' would be a more honest claim. Natural sources of zinc include shellfish, especially oysters, and eggs, black-eyed beans, poultry, pumpkin seeds and sardines.

Ancient Wisdom, 21st-century Healing

Traditional Chinese Medicine (TCM)

Ginkgo biloba is probably the best-known (in the west) cardiovascular tonic (see DVT, page 157) but the one I really rate is a mushroom called **cordyceps**, which works to support the lungs and the kidneys, and which has impressive anti-asthmatic properties (see asthma, page 161).

Cordyceps (dong chong xia cao) was first harvested over 1000 years ago by Tibetan monks who, so the story goes, noticed that yaks would happily graze on this fungus and then 'frolic with great passion and energy'. A potent antioxidant, cordyceps also works to boost stamina and strengthen the immune system, protect the lungs and increase circulating oxygen levels.

If you plan to use the fresh mushroom, its potency, apparently, increases when cooked with duck.

If you want a supplement, check out the New Chapter range (www.newchapter.com), which includes a single cordyceps supplement, and Host Defence, a powerful formulation that combines cordyceps with reishi, shiitake and maitake mushrooms. You can mail order both these in the UK from Victoria Health (0800 389 8195; www.victoriahealth.com).

For maximum therapeutic benefits with TCM, find an accredited practitioner in your area. To do this, contact the Register of Chinese Herbalists (see Useful Contacts on page 448).

Ayurvedic (Indian) Remedies

Water retention can also be a sign of a struggling cardiovascular system, as can spider or varicose veins. There are lots of good natural diuretics, but one of the very best, **gotu kola**, remains little known outside India, where it is known, in Hindi, as Brahmi-manduki. In Ayurvedic medicine, this is treated as the most sattwic herb (see Chapter 6 for more on the sattwic properties of plants, people, and the foods we eat).

This herb works to support both the circulatory and respiratory systems and, despite only limited western clinical evidence to prove its efficacy, is the herb I use when I travel long-haul to help prevent water retention and reduce the risk of deep vein thrombosis (DVT).

Gotu kola (Centella asiatica) will support microcirculation in the peripheral blood vessels, and also works to strengthen the connective tissue of the circulatory system. It can help prevent oxidative damage, and has been shown to reduce the risk of DVT by stabilizing plaque in the femoral arteries of the legs, and lower the risk of stroke by acting in the same way on carotoid plaque that has formed in the arteries supplying the brain.

If you want to use gotu kola, get it from Pukka Herbs (08456 585858; www.pukkaherbs.com).

Native American Remedies

Native American tribes used a plant called **horsetail** or shavegrass as a diuretic and a tonic to boost blood flow to the body's tissues and organs. The Hopi tribe of New Mexico, for example, mixed this plant with corn meal to make a spreadable mush to eat with bread.

Horsetail is rich in the trace mineral **silica**, which we now know works in the body to strengthen the connective tissues of the circulatory system. It also has cleansing properties, which herbalists believe help keep both the blood and its vessels free from toxins and deposits. Horsetail tinctures are widely on sale in good independent health stores. Take as directed on the bottle.

Finally, horsetail is also a good source of heart-protecting vitamin E, which is stored in the heart and blood and which works as both a vasodilator and anticoagulant. Lots of people now take vitamin E to protect their cardiovascular system – the typical therapeutic daily dose is 60–75 IUs of natural (not synthetic) vitamin E – but you should not use this nutrient if you are already taking blood-thinning or blood-pressure medications.

Native New Zealand Remedies

In the early 1900s, almost half of the Maori patients being treated by allopathic doctors were suffering from respiratory, especially bronchial, problems. At that time, two indigenous herbs were successfully used to help alleviate these complaints: kawakawa, which I first introduced as a digestive tonic in Chapter 2 (page 84), and a second herb called kumarahou, which was also known as gumdigger's soap, since you can crush the flowerheads in your hands, mix them with a little water and create a soapy lather.

To treat coughs and colds and chest complaints, including

asthma, the Maori would boil kumarahou leaves in hot water to make a medicinal tea. I have not to date found anyone making commercial remedies from this plant*, and so if you want a New Zealand remedy for chest disorders, you will have to use kawakawa, which is now incorporated in the new Kiwiherb range, available from the NutriCentre (0800 587 2290; www.NutriCentre.com).

Tried and Applied

If you frequently travel long-haul, invest in a Deep Vein Exerciser (DVE), an ingenious little foot pedal you keep on the floor to exercise your legs and keep blood flowing to the extremities. Mail order from JJ Orthopaedic Development Ltd on 020 8786 7039. Both gotu kola and ginkgo biloba also help boost microcirculation to reduce the risk of DVT.

✼

What Really Works for Heart and Lungs

As before, I could recommend some thirty different remedies for almost any chronic condition you care to suggest, but what good is that? You need to know what really works and which of these thirty to try, so here are my 1, 2, 3 . . . Easy Steps to help prevent or manage chronic health complaints that involve the circulatory system, blood and breath. **Do not treat this advice as a substitute for medical supervision. Instead, and for best long-term results, find a qualified health practitioner who specializes in integrated medicine. (See Useful Contacts, page 447.)**

---

* If anyone does know about remedies made from kumarahou (Pomaderris kumerahou) please contact me: susan@thenaturalhealthclub.com.

Anaemia/Iron deficiency

Anaemias – and it is plural because there are several different types and causes – are those conditions in which the number of red blood cells or the amount of haemoglobin in them is below normal.

The average human body contains about 4g of iron, approximately two-thirds of which is in the form of haemoglobin. If you think you might be anaemic, get checked by your GP or another qualified health specialist, and do not simply try to self-treat by taking iron supplements, which could do more harm than good since inorganic iron is actually quite toxic.

1, 2, 3 ... Easy Steps to Help Prevent Anaemia

The Ayurvedic herb ashwagandha* is an excellent natural source of iron. Mail order from Pukka Herbs (08456 585858; www.pukkaherbs.com) and take as directed on the bottle.

Levels of hydrochloric acid in the stomach affect iron absorption. Patients with low levels have reduced iron absorption and increased intestinal bacterial overgrowth, so take betaine hydrochloride (see Chapter 2, page 55) and a good quality probiotic (see Chapter 2, page 65).

Take vitamin A (10,000–25,000 IUs) with your iron supplements. Some 50 per cent of pregnant women in developing countries suffer iron-deficiency anaemia and studies show that giving them vitamin A, along with iron supplements in the form of ferrous sulphate, improved iron take-up levels.

Asthma

Defined by the American Thoracic Society as a disease characterized by increased responsiveness of the trachea and bronchi to a

* Males with known cardiovascular problems should avoid this herb because it has the potential to accelerate the risk.

number of stimuli, and manifested by a widespread narrowing of the airways, there are two types of asthma: intrinsic and extrinsic.

Intrinsic asthma usually develops in adulthood and may be the result of cold air, exercise or emotional trauma. Extrinsic, or atopic, asthma is considered an immunologically mediated condition that is accompanied by a rise in blood serum antibody levels.

The telltale signs are wheezing, coughing and shortness of breath, the severity and duration of which will vary. The key triggers include viral or bacterial upper-respiratory-tract infections, exercise, exposure to allergens or irritants, psychological problems or climate.

1, 2, 3 . . . Easy Steps to Help Prevent Asthma

Take cordyceps (see page 156) which, as well as improving cardiopulmonary function, can modulate the immune system and help increase energy levels.

Studies show a strong relationship between magnesium levels and bronchial reactivity. Take a therapeutic dose of 250mg a day of food-state magnesium from the Nature's Plus range.

Food intolerances are often a common trigger for many asthmatics (see Chapter 2) so supporting the digestive system will also help. Take a lactobacillus acidophilus probiotic and add L-glutamine to your supplement regimen. See pages 95 and 98 for sourcing details.

Bronchitis

More people consult the doctor about respiratory-tract infections than any other condition, and while the body's own defences can usually protect the lungs and airways from invaders, when the immune system and normal defences are compromised, especially by an assault such as heavy cigarette smoking, infection is almost inevitable.

Although quite common, bronchitis – which is an inflammation of the bronchial tube lining – places high levels of stress on the body, and while antibiotics work for most people, they take their toll too. You can counter the side effects by taking a good quality probiotic to rebuild levels of the good bacteria that live in the gut where they keep digestion healthy and, by association, support the immune system, which has taken quite a battering.

To treat any lingering respiratory infection, take a multi-supplement that combines three of the most powerful medicinal mushrooms known to man. **Triton** is made up of **cordyceps** (Cordyceps sinensis), **reishi** (Ganoderma lucidum) and **shiitake** (Lentinula edodes) mushrooms. These will work collectively to boost the immune system, increase aerobic performance and counter infection.

1, 2, 3 . . . Easy Steps to Help Prevent Bronchitis

Take Triton: mail order from Lemonburst on 01273 558112. This supplement contains 166mg of each mushroom and is sold in pots of 90 x 500mg tablets to last for six weeks.

N-acetyl cysteine (NAC) is a mucolytic agent that has been shown to help reduce the number of acute attacks and lower the rate of hospitalizations among sufferers taking 400mg a day for at least six months. This agent is now widely on sale in supplements in health stores.

If you have been taking antiobiotics, take a probiotic to rebuild good bacteria in the gut; mail order Biocare's lactobacillus acidophilus powder on 0121 433 3727.

Hay Fever

Hay fever – or allergic rhinitis – is a reaction of the mucous membranes of the eyes, nose and airways to seasonal pollens and other everyday allergens, including dust, feathers, animal hairs and environmental pollutants. When this happens, the body releases large numbers of antibodies to fight the perceived allergen, but these antibodies also produce the histamine that causes swelling and irritation to the body's own tissues.

Vitamin C not only supports the immune system, but also helps the body defend itself against the consequences of having too much histamine released. Ironically, the same stress that triggers the release of histamine in the first place also increases the body's need for more vitamin C.

In one study by scientists at the Arizona State University, researchers gave allergy sufferers, including patients with hay fever, increasing doses of vitamin C, starting with 500mg daily and increasing to 2g* per day over a period of six weeks. They found that by the time the higher levels of vitamin C were reached, volunteers' histamine levels had dropped by 40 per cent.

Quercetin, an anti-inflammatory bioflavonoid, will also help since it works to stabilize the cell membranes of those cells that would otherwise discharge their supply of histamine into the surrounding blood and tissue when there is an allergic attack.

If you spend half the year dreading the arrival of spring because you know you will suffer, then you should be taking **Alleraide**: a German homeopathic formulation that cleverly combines three herbs which work specifically to stop all the hay fever symptoms that can make life a misery. The first of this trio is cardiospermum, a tropical vine from India, which will help to prevent inflammation of the nasal and sinus passages, and thus stop sneezing. The second herb, galphimia, comes from Mexico, where it is used to prevent the sensation of burning eyes that accompanies this condition. The third, luffa, works to desensitize the nasal

---

* Remember, taking more than 1g of vitamin C daily can cause stomach upset. It is important to build up to higher dosages. You cannot overdose on this nutrient since it is water-soluble and the body will flush out any excess. Split the daily dosage into three or four equal amounts to take throughout the day or opt for timed-release capsules.

membranes, and since this is a homeopathic preparation, it is 100 per cent safe to take continuously and alongside conventional medicines and to give to children.

1, 2, 3 . . . Easy Steps to Help Prevent Hay Fever

Alleraide is available from Victoria Health (0800 389 8195; www.victoriahealth.com); take one tablet every hour for acute symptoms, and one tablet, three times a day, for prevention.

Start the day with a teaspoon of locally produced honey in warm water to help build resistance to local pollens.

Take a combined vitamin C with rosehip or vitamin C with quercetin formulation to reduce inflammation and the body's production of histamine. If you take more than 2g of vitamin C, expect side effects including stomach upsets and diarrhoea.

High Blood Pressure (Hypertension)

Blood pressure is, of course, the amount of force required for the heart to pump blood round the body. Under normal conditions, and while it may peak during physical or emotional stress and drop during sleep, blood pressure stays within a narrow range of normal limits.

Hypertension or high blood pressure is a cardiovascular disease characterized by the elevation of blood pressure above arbitrary values considered normal for people of the same sex, and similar age, racial and environmental background.

In the vast majority of people with hypertension, no single cause is identified, however, and around a third of sufferers have high blood pressure without knowing it. The good news is that it is a condition that is not only easy to detect, it is not too difficult to manage and bring back under control.

1, 2, 3 . . . Easy Steps to Help Prevent Hypertension

Take the Chinese herbal remedy Lifeflower (see Stroke, page 170) and take Drs A–Z diuretic water pills alongside. You can mail order both from Victoria Health (0800 389 8195; www.victoriahealth.com). Take Lifeflower as directed on the box, and take one water pill tablet up to three times a day.

Vitamin C will help lower blood pressure. Take 1g a day.

Co-enzyme Q10 can help but only if you take a high dose (225mg a day), which works out as expensive. That said, in trials on over one hundred hypertensive patients, adding this high dose CoQ10 to their regular blood pressure medication paved the way for a significant reduction* in the use of antihypertensive drugs over six months.

Low Blood Pressure (Hypotension)

Low blood pressure (hypotension) can cause fainting spells, dizziness, lightheadedness, dimming vision, paleness and general weakness.

Siberian ginseng is one of the adaptogenic herbs (see Chapter 5, page 252) that help normalize the body's various systems, including blood pressure. The best way to benefit, according to patient trials, is to take a therapeutic daily dose for two months, take a break of two or three weeks and then start again. This is known as a multiple treatment regimen.

Siberian ginseng also has an oestrogenic effect in the body; this means women with hormone-sensitive conditions, such as breast or ovarian cancers, endometriosis and fibroids, and anyone taking HRT should not use it. You should also avoid coffee, alcohol and spicy foods if you plan to take it since all three increase the risk of side effects.

1, 2, 3 . . . Easy Steps to Help Prevent Hypotension

Take Siberian ginseng (2500mg a day) but do not confuse it with the more expensive energy-boosting American or panax ginseng.

---

* Do not reduce or stop prescription medicines for hypertension without seeking qualified medical advice.

Take a silica supplement or use silica-rich horsetail tincture (see pages 158 and 181) to further support blood vessels that have lost their elasticity.

The adrenal glands secrete hormones that help regulate blood pressure. They contain more vitamin C than any other organ in the human body so supplement the diet with vitamin C too (see Chapter 5, Stress and Immunity, Top Ten Natural Remedies, page 277).

Raynaud's Disease

Raynaud's disease, which affects an estimated 10 million Britons, is the result of the constriction of the small arteries (arterioles) in the fingers and toes which can go into spasm, causing the skin to turn pale or blue and the fingers and toes to go numb. It can also affect the nose, cheeks and tips of the ears, which will all throb, tingle and even swell when the circulation returns to normal. Most common in younger women, it usually happens after exposure to the cold and so is usually only a problem in winter.

Evening primrose oil can help because it inhibits the action of substances called prostaglandins, which are found naturally in the body and which can otherwise promote the constriction of blood vessels. A deficiency in magnesium (see pages 136 and 152), which can also result in spasms of the blood vessels, can also cause similar symptoms to Raynaud's disease, which is why, although there are no clinical trials to support the theory, some nutritionists will recommend a daily dose of between 200–600mg of this mineral.

Another less well-known supplement that has been shown to make a real difference to sufferers is **L-carnitine**. In a small, twenty-day pilot study, where twelve sufferers were given 1g of this vitamin-like nutrient three times a day, all those taking part reported fewer blood vessel spasms in their fingertips after being in the cold.

Ginkgo biloba – take the equivalent of 40mg, three times a day, or use Seredrin, from Health Perceptions (www.health-perception.co.uk), the ready-made supplement that has been tested with Raynaud's patients in UK clinical trials.

Use evening primrose oil. In research trials, daily doses of between 3g and 6g were used to help reduce both the number and the severity of attacks.

Take 1g daily of L-carnitine in supplement form.

Sarcoidosis

This is a disease that tends to develop in young adults. It happens when abnormal collections of inflammatory cells called granulomas form in the body's different organs, especially the lungs. Some doctors believe it is the legacy of an infection; others suggest it is an abnormal immune system response.

Many sufferers have no symptoms at all and the problem is only discovered by accident when it shows up on a chest X-ray taken for other reasons. Fever, weight loss and aching joints are all likely symptoms. It is seldom fatal and usually burns itself out within two years. In fact, more than two-thirds of those diagnosed with lung sarcoidosis will have no symptoms at all nine years later.

Most natural healers give this condition a wide berth but some doctors with an interest in complementary medicine report excellent results when the patient adopts a 'mucus-less' diet. Mucus-forming foods are those high in protein, and so cutting out meat and dairy products could help keep you off the steroids. Because it is still such a mysterious condition, I would also consult a homeopath, who will give you what is called a constitutional diagnosis and remedy (see page 448), which will then underpin any other treatment you receive.

If you have this condition, you should not take vitamin D or calcium supplements without consulting a qualified health practitioner.

1, 2, 3 . . . *Easy Steps to Help Prevent Sarcoidosis*

Adopt a mucus-less diet under the supervision of a qualified naturopath. (For a referral in your area, see Useful Contacts, page 448.)

Take bromelain (500mg a day), an anti-inflammatory agent made from the stems of fresh pineapple, which helps heal connective tissues and hence the inflammation that accompanies this condition.

Think about a liver-cleansing programme (see page 58) and use the Ayurvedic herb gotu kola, which can support the lymphatic system that will also be affected.

Sinusitis

Jala neti is one of the cleansing yoga practices that are known collectively as the kryias, and if you study the yoga texts, you will learn that the primary purpose of the kryias is to cleanse the mind and body, to clear the nadis (energy channels in the body), increase vitality and help develop greater awareness of the functioning of the chakra energy centres.

The jala neti pot looks like a small spouted jug which you fill with water that you have boiled, dissolved salt into and allowed to cool to room temperature. You then hang over the sink to tip this saline solution through one nostril, tilting your head to allow it to emerge from the other nostril. Keep a box of tissues nearby to blow your nose; you will need to do this in between cleansing each nostril.

Not only is jala neti simple to do, it is perfectly safe and 100 per cent effective. The sensation of the fluid passing into your nostrils does take some getting used to but I cannot think of a better way of keeping the nasal passages clear of infection, and there really is no need to be apprehensive.

Practise jala neti; you can get a jala neti pot from the Sivananda Yoga Centre in Putney, London (020 8780 0160).

Take SinuFix (see page 144). Mail order from Victoria Health (0800 389 8195; www.victoriahealth.com).

Take a good quality probiotic (see Chapter 2), since a large number of cases of sinusitis have now been linked with a hidden fungal infection.

Spider/Varicose Veins

Varicose veins, which are the result of blood pooling and stretching the vein wall causing damage to the lining, are three times more common in women than men. Pregnancy exacerbates the problem because the growing foetus puts increasing pressure on the abdomen, which makes it more difficult for the blood vessels in the leg to pump the blood back up the body.

The good news is that there has been more extensive scientific research into the use of herbs for this condition than any other (aside from prostate problems), and although it is not yet proven, the general consensus is that regular use of these herbs can help prevent existing varicose veins deteriorating and new ones developing.

Currently the most widely documented herbal remedy is **horse chestnut**. Research, which started in the 1960s, culminated in Germany's Commission E health watchdog body approving this herb for venous diseases of the legs and in that country it is now the third most commonly prescribed herb.

The active agents are a complex group of related chemicals known, collectively, as aescin, which is often the name you will see on the box when you buy this remedy. These chemicals help reduce the rate of leakage from damaged blood vessels and, while nobody really knows how, the theory is they somehow plug the leaking capillaries and inhibit the enzymes which would otherwise break down collagen causing open holes in the blood vessels.

1, 2, 3 . . . Easy Steps to Help Prevent Spider/Varicose Veins

Bioforce (01294 277344; www.bioforce.co.uk) make a good aesculus (horse chestnut) tincture and topical gel.

Derma E Clear Vein Creme combines horse chestnut with both antioxidant grapeskin extract and pycnogenol (see pages 25 and 148) and is brilliant for both spider veins and skin bruising. Only available in the UK from Victoria Health (0800 389 8195; www.victoriahealth.com).

Gotu kola (see page 157) will also provide good phytonutrient support for damaged blood vessels.

Stroke

A stroke – which is also called a cerebrovascular accident – is the death of brain tissue following a lack of blood flow and thus insufficient oxygen to the brain. There are generally two underlying causes. With the more common ischemic stroke (85–90 per cent of all cases), the blood supply has been cut off because either atherosclerosis (see page 115) or a blood clot (see nattokinase, page 147) has blocked a blood vessel. In a haemorrhagic stroke, a blood vessel has burst, preventing the normal flow and allowing blood to seep into part of the brain and destroy it.

A stroke usually damages only one side of the brain but it will be the opposite side of the body that is affected (because nerves in the brain cross over: nerves in the right-hand side of the brain affect the left-hand side of the body, and vice versa). Individuals with cardiac disease have twice the risk of a stroke, compared with healthier 'matched' individuals (that is, as similar as possible in age, weight, height, lifestyle, sex, and so on). High levels of homocysteine (see page 120) have also been linked with a higher risk of stroke.

Formulated from the Chinese herb erigeron breviscapinus and sold as Breviscapini, **Lifeflower** is new to the west but now available in the UK. In clinical trials in China, where it was administered intravenously to stroke patients, over 80 per cent of participants under investigation reported improved brain function.

The reason it is so effective is that as well as having an 85 per cent bioavailability, Lifeflower can cross the blood–brain barrier to boost supplies of oxygen and glucose to the brain. There are no known contraindications for this herb but it would be wise to consult with your current health advisors before taking it.

1, 2, 3 . . . Easy Steps To Help Prevent or Recover From A Stroke

Lifeflower is only available from Victoria Health (0800 389 8195; www.victoriahealth.com). Take as directed on the bottle.

Nattokinase works better than any other natural agent to prevent blood clots. (See page 147.)

Acupuncture treatments carried out in those first crucial few days after a stroke can dramatically help improve recovery, and thus the patient's quality of life thereafter. The trouble is, who is going to tell you this, or be brave enough to insist the doctors and nurses allow an acupuncturist onto the hospital ward? If this were me or a relative of mine, I would take the view this is a fight worth having. To find an acupuncturist with experience of treating stroke patients, contact the Register of Chinese Herbalists (see Useful Contacts, page 448).

Roll Out Your Yoga Mat

In March 2000, a groundbreaking study conducted for the Center for Natural Medicine and Prevention in America was published in the American Heart Association journal *Stroke*, which showed, *conclusively*, that meditation really could reduce the thickness of arterial walls to lower blood pressure and reduce any associated risk of heart attack and stroke.

As well as teaching meditation techniques, yoga should also include pranayama (the science of 'proper breathing') because western science can now tell us what the yogis have known all along: that breath-control exercises, coupled with active asanas, really can improve the vital capacity and functioning of the respiratory mechanisms, including the lungs.

In one trial, researchers compared the effects of virasana (the warrior pose) and simply sitting in a chair on lung function in ten healthy males, aged twenty-five to thirty-seven. They found that heart rate and oxygen consumption increased among the volunteers in the more active pose (as you would expect) but, interestingly, further studies showed that a combination of active postures and relaxation improved cardiopulmonary status greater than either active postures or relaxation alone. In other words, you need to do both – and please remember that this is active yoga relaxation, not slobbing out on the couch.

So here are my **1, 2, 3 best yoga practices** for improving cardiopulmonary function.

Virasana (Warrior Pose)

'Vir' means hero, warrior or champion, and this is a deceptively simple-looking posture that is harder to master than it might first appear, not least because you need to keep the body 'soft' to release enough to kneel, keep the bottom on the floor and allow each leg to rest by the side of the hips.

To start, kneel on the floor, keeping the knees together and the feet about 18 inches apart.

Now rest the bottom on the floor, but keep the body off the feet. This will take some getting used to. The idea is that the feet stay alongside the thighs and each inner calf muscle rests alongside each outer thigh.

Keep the spine erect and place the wrists on the knees, palms facing upwards, and bring the thumb and index fingers on each hand together to form a mudra, which helps to open the lungs. Keep all the other fingers extended. (See Chapter 6, page 352, for the healing powers of yoga mudras.)

Close your eyes, and concentrate on slowing down your breath. Stay in this asana only for as long as you feel comfortable. If your ankles hurt, soften the surface they are resting on by placing a blanket over your yoga mat.

Nadi Shodhana (Calming Alternate-nostril Breathing)

This is so calming that by the end of your practice you will feel you have entered a different way of being. You need to remember just three things:

You must close the nostrils very gently – we do nothing in yoga with force.

A round counts as one inhalation through the left nostril, one exhalation through the right nostril, one inhalation through the right nostril and one exhalation through the left nostril.

You must always start your 'round' by closing the right nostril and breathing in through the left. You always complete a round by breathing out through the left nostril.

Again, you need to find a comfortable sitting position where you can keep your spine straight and your head upright.

Raise your right hand towards your nose and close the right nostril by gently placing your thumb against the side of the nose. Keep the index and second fingers pointing down and the third finger raised since this is the digit you will use to close the left-hand nostril. It is important to maintain this hand position – this is what is known as a mudra (see Chapter 6 for more on yogic mudras).

To start nadi shodhana, gently close the right nostril and breathe in through the left nostril to a slow count of four. Now, carefully close the left nostril with the third digit of the right hand, and slowly exhale through the right nostril to a slow and controlled count of eight. Keep the left nostril closed and slowly inhale through the right, to a slow count of four. Now close the right nostril with the thumb and open the left nostril to slowly exhale to a count of eight.

This counts as one complete round.

Practise this pranayama until you can comfortably do twelve rounds. Make sure you keep the body, including the hands, relaxed, and ensure that both your breathing and your hand movements are slow, gentle and controlled.

The benefits of nadi shodhana are amazing. It works to ensure the whole body is better oxygenated and to help expel carbon dioxide from the body and toxins from the blood supply. It increases vitality, lowers stress levels and generates feelings of tranquillity and calm. You will not believe any of this until you try it for yourself so I am saying no more. It can take time to master but it really is worth every minute you invest in getting used to it.

Trataka (Easy Candle Meditation for Beginners)

This is probably my all-time favourite meditation. The beauty of this exercise lies in its sheer simplicity and I cannot think of a better introduction to the art of sitting still and clearing the constant chatter from your mind.

Simply light a candle and place it on a stable surface so that the flame is around your eye level when you are sitting.

Choose any comfortable sitting position, as long as it

maintains a straight spine and upright head, and sit yourself one arm's length away from your candle.

Close your eyes for a moment, relax the body and become aware of simply sitting still. Try to keep that stillness throughout this practice.

Now, open your eyes and gaze steadily at the wick of the candle. Try not to blink or allow your gaze to wander away from this focal point.

Keep gazing at the flame until your eyes start to water. When this happens, close your eyes and concentrate on the after-image of the candle flame that you can now see inside your head.

Try to hold this image in your 'mind's eye' for as long as you can. Once it has faded away, repeat the exercise again, two or three times, and then stop.

This is a brilliant technique for helping relieve anxiety and tension that's causing insomnia; practise it last thing at night.

CHAPTER FOUR

The Spine and Joints

The skeleton, muscles, tendons, ligaments and other components of the joints together make up the musculo-skeletal system. Western populations may be living longer, but they are living longer with more chronic health complaints, most of which relate to this all-important system. In fact, musculo-skeletal disorders are the single biggest cause of pain and disability, because although these body parts thrive on use, the wrong kind of use – e.g. sitting for long hours, from the age of five, on hard chairs at desks that are too high or too low – will generate imbalances that will have more serious repercussions later on in life.

Since I have reached that forty-something age where these imbalances are now too glaring for me to ignore (knees that sometimes hurt just walking upstairs in winter; a shoulder injury that prevented me from practising yoga for several months), I know that I too have to do something about them. That said, what I have discovered is that in any search for the right natural remedy, when it comes to joint support, painkilling and natural remedies for the musculo-skeletal system, we really are spoilt for choice. Better still, many of these are the remedies that science has now been investigating for twenty or even thirty years. This means we can report that research, explain in detail how and why these remedies work and give well-documented specific advice on therapeutic dosages.

Bone – How It Is Made

The most fascinating thing about bone is that it is a constantly changing tissue that has several key jobs to do. As well as providing strength and stability, and a framework for the muscles to move against, bone is also used to protect the body's most sensitive tissues, including the brain and the spinal cord.

Many people assume that if you get enough calcium in the diet you will build and keep a strong skeleton, but this is not the case. To understand why not, you need to know how new bone is made.

First, you need a mesh of microfibres for the calcium and magnesium minerals to cling on to. This mesh, called the osteoid, is made up of proteins, collagen, elastin and various glucosamine polymers (which is why lots of joint support supplements include glucosamine, which has been shown, in independent trials, to perform just as well as conventional arthritis and joint medications). To build these proteins, the body also needs vitamin C, vitamin B6, copper and zinc. To make glucosamine polymers the body needs glucosamine and manganese, and to activate the whole matrix, you need vitamin K.

Once this matrix is built and active, it is then impregnated with the calcium and magnesium salts the body uses to form solid bone. But one of the most important substances the body needs to make and keep strong bones is one few people have even heard of: **ipriflavone.**

This flavonoid, in supplement form, is a semi-synthetic isolate of soya, which has been shown, in adult clinical trials, to reduce bone loss and promote bone building. However, following a decision by the UK Medicines Control Agency (MCA) that this was not a natural substance but a medicine (a dictate that followed concern that long-term usage may increase the risk of asymptomatic lymphocytopenia, or abnormally low lymphocyte counts, which has been reported in about 10 per cent of patients taking it for more than six months), you can no longer buy ipriflavone in supplement form here. What you can still do is eat more of those foods that are rich in a phytochemical called daidzen, which is used to make ipriflavone, including soy products and the herb red clover. (See I is for, page 220, and Meno-Herb, page 405.)

Back To Basics . . . Calcium

The most important mineral for strong healthy bones is, of course, still calcium, which is so important that the body will maintain homeostasis of calcium in the plasma at the cost of bone integrity. What this means is that if calcium levels drop, the body will leach calcium from the bones.

There is more of this than any other mineral in the body – about 3lb/1.3kg in an adult – and most of it is stored in the bones and teeth. Some 20 per cent of the calcium in our bones is re-absorbed and replaced every year, as old bone cells break down and new ones form to keep the skeleton strong. This is an ongoing process, and what it means is that the whole skeleton is replaced once every seven years (in children this process takes just two years).

If you plan to take individual calcium supplements, you must take magnesium too, since levels of one will affect levels of the other. The correct ratio is 2:1 in favour of the calcium.

The typical diet provides only a third of the amount of calcium the body needs not just for strong bones and teeth but for proper nerve functioning, muscle contraction and blood clotting too. Calcium supplements are also especially important for women who have a history of yo-yo dieting and who will be deficient, but, again, you need to know what you are doing. Do not be tempted to buy cheaper forms of calcium supplements – we know from clinical trials that you get what you pay for. In one study, for example, women aged twenty-five who were taking calcium in the form of calcium dolomite supplements were shown to absorb just 20 per cent of the calcium. When they switched to calcium in the form of the more expensive **calcium glycerate**, absorbency more than doubled to 50 per cent. (The reason the absorption rate is so low is that it is totally dependent on the existing calcium-binding proteins already circulating in your bloodstream.)

The recommended daily dosage for calcium supplementation is 1200mg but since we now know that with cheaper supplements the body can only absorb up to 25 per cent (and usually only absorbs about 10 per cent) of the calcium available, what is clear is that you may not be getting the protection you think.

The One to Watch – BioCalth

The solution lies with a new, patented US supplement called **BioCalth,** in which the calcium is *already bonded* with a metabolite of vitamin C called threonic acid (or L-threonate), to boost absorption rates to an impressive 95 per cent. Thanks to this bonding, the mineral is then delivered through the intestinal mucosa, thus improving bioavailability.

This supplement, which has no side effects, is relatively new to the UK and is going to be huge. All women from the age of thirty should think about taking calcium supplements in this form for prevention (take one tablet a day), and if you are post-menopausal or already have osteoporosis, you need to take a higher dosage of three tablets a day.

BioCalth is currently only available in the UK from Victoria Health (0800 389 8195; www.victoriahealth.com).

Fixing Broken and Fractured Bones

The common name for the bone-healing herb **comfrey** is knit-bone, which tells you just what it does in the body. Herbalists here, however, no longer recommend taking it internally following recently reported fears that ingesting preparations made from the root of the plant could cause cancer. Other parts – the flowers and leaves – are still deemed safe but if you still want to use the root, as is traditional, you will now have to take it home-opathically. And of course, if a fracture is covered with a plaster cast, you cannot massage a cream where it is needed either.

The homeopathic version of comfrey is called **Symphytum** (taken from the Latin name of the herb, Symphytum officinale), and if you have a fracture that is taking time to heal, you need to take this together with **Calcium phosphate**. Take a 6c potency of both remedies but take the Symphytum in the morning and the Calcium phos. at night.

The herb **horsetail** (or shavegrass) is rich in the trace mineral **silica**, which works in the body to strengthen bones and cartilage, making it critical for bone healing too. European studies have found that fractured and broken bones heal better when both calcium and silica are present than when the patient is given calcium alone, suggesting the mineral works in some way to facilitate the absorption of calcium.

Oats are another excellent source of silica so starting your day with my breakfast cereal (see page 68) or a herbal porridge (see page 15) can help keep bones, teeth and cartilage strong and healthy. This grain is also rich in magnesium and phosphorus, two other important bone-supporting nutrients.

Reversing Bone Loss . . .

. . . can you get back the skeleton you had at twenty-five?

Clinical trials on post-menopausal women in China have shown how regular acupuncture sessions (three times a week for six months), along with calcium and vitamin D supplementation, really can help increase bone density.

The study, reported in the *Journal of Chinese Medicine*, highlighted three important acupuncture points to stimulate, two of which relate to supporting the kidneys. This is because TCM links osteoporosis to kidney functioning.

This report is timely because lots of women who have been taking HRT to help prevent osteoporosis after menopause are now seeking alternatives (see Meno-Herb, page 405), following an admission by mainstream science that the benefits of hormone replacement do not outweigh the increased risks of heart disease and breast cancer. And neither does HRT protect against osteoporosis.

If you are too squeamish for needles, you can still not only stop but reverse the loss of bone density by taking a supplement of **genistein**, a compound found only in soya. This is one of a group of compounds known as isoflavones and is a phytoestrogen, which means it acts like a weaker oestrogen molecule in the body, where it can help reduce oestrogen-withdrawal symptoms during menopause, including loss of bone density, hot flushes, night sweats and insomnia.

Soy milks are obviously an excellent source but (1) a lot of soy has been genetically modified, and (2) the genistein content will vary between different brands. Lentils are another wonderful source, as are kidney and haricot beans, but in clinical trials researchers used a therapeutic daily dose of 54mg in supplement form (far more than you could get from eating lentils) over twelve months.

In placebo-controlled, double-blind trials comparing the effects of genistein supplementation and HRT on the bones of ninety healthy post-menopausal women, researchers found that genistein significantly increased serum levels of both phosphatase and osteocalcin, substances that are known indicators of new bone formation.

The results of the year-long trial led the researchers to conclude that the isoflavone (genistein) reduced bone reabsorption and increased bone formation and bone density in the hips and lumbar spine. These results were consistent with similar findings in animal studies. Furthermore, both HRT and genistein reduced bone loss but only the latter promoted new bone generation.

The sugar substitute xylitol (see page 197) has also been shown to reverse bone loss in animal trials. In a study where the skeletons of twenty-four rats who had been given xylitol in their diets for two years were compared with age-matched animals who had had no xylitol, researchers found the supplemented group had better bone density and concluded: 'A continuous moderate dietary xylitol supplementation leads to increased bone volume and to increased bone mineral content in the long bones of aged rats. This indicates xylitol-induced protection against aging-related osteoporotic changes.'

Try It Lying Down . . .

. . . or is that too good to be true?

If you hate skipping – which really can help build increased bone density; just fifty jumps a day can confer a 4 per cent increase – but like the idea of building bone density in your sleep, then a mat that is said to create a natural energy field to prevent the loss of bone density while you sleep could be the solution for you.

Health Mat – which is now a trademark – was first developed by the Nyvatex Oil Corporation, a company that specializes in the detection of new deposits of oil and gas. It is made up of interspersed layers of aluminium and polyester and is as thin as a light blanket.

The idea is to place it under your bottom sheet and sleep on it. The theory is that as the sleeping body moves around, it causes these layers in the mat to move against each other and thus create a natural energy field to enhance the body's own intracellular repair mechanisms and help prevent osteoporosis.

Scientists at the University of Connecticut Health Center are currently investigating this claim. In the meantime, to find out more, suspend your disbelief and visit www.health-mat.com.

The Wrong Kind of Six Packs

If your fridge is full of diet Coke six packs or any of the other popular soft drinks then do your bones a favour and pour the whole lot down the sink right now. I know they taste good and the kids love them, but by the time I have worked my way through the list of their ingredients and the effects they have in the body, you won't want to drink them.

We know that many soft drinks are loaded with sugar but let's look at another equally damaging but less well-known ingredient that is also present – **phosphoric acid**, a chemical which, in another context, is so strong it can dissolve teeth.

What is it doing in soft drinks? It provides an acid medium that enhances the absorption of carbon dioxide (which is also acidic), thus reducing the pressure required to keep the fizz contained and allowing the mix to be bottled with a metal cap. It also helps keep the drink fizzy for longer. The downside is that it has a nasty, sour taste, but this is simple enough to hide if you load the mix with lots of sugar.

The real downside is what this ingredient does in the body, which, naturally, has to maintain a concentration of phosphorus and calcium in the bloodstream at the correct ratio for building new bones. The shock of a sudden influx of phosphorus with no accompanying calcium triggers a slump in blood-calcium levels and an increase in the excretion of this mineral.

This slump, in turn, causes another system to leach extra calcium from the bone, first from the spine and the pelvis, to redress the balance. Even worse, the body leaches more calcium from the bones than it really needs to in anticipation of your next soft drink (another assault of phosphoric acid). If this process continues over time, then younger people drinking lots of these types of drinks can expect the same weakened bone density that would be more typical of an elderly person suffering from osteoporosis.

If you're still not worried about your bones, then what about your weight? Phosphoric acid is so strong, it reduces the body's own secretion of hydrochloric acid (see betaine hydrochloride, Chapter 2, page 55), the chemical we produce in the stomach to break down proteins and fats. This will disrupt normal digestion and can cause both bloating and flatulence.

The high sugar content of soft drinks will do you no favours either. It too increases urinary excretion of calcium by impairing its reabsorption in the kidneys. This then triggers the parathyroid gland to secrete hormones, which, again, tell the body to release more calcium from the bones.

The carbon dioxide (which our body treats as a waste product of metabolism) is probably the least noxious thing in a soft drink,

yet a US health official knew enough eighty years ago to pro-
nounce in *Good Housekeeping* magazine that 'any child who
drank three or four Cokes a day would probably ruin their health
for life'. And the stuff we drink today is even worse.

Soft drinks should be dished out the way they were in my childhood – as an occasional treat.

Joint Stiffness . . . Wear and Tear and Uric Acid

Cartilage is the connective tissue that normally protects your
joints, but with age and overuse or misuse it can start to wear
away, leaving bones exposed, prone to inflammation and, of
course, very painful. Another cause of pain and stiffness is a
build-up of uric acid in the body (see Gout, page 231). Stiffness
in a joint is a clear sign that cartilage is degrading there, and uric
acid is the by-product of that deterioration. Lots of herbal remedies can help counter both the degradation and the pain. The
better known ones include devil's claw, white willow, yucca,
celery and feverfew, and several of these are combined in the new
Bastyr Formula A joint-support supplement from Eclectic
Institute (www.eclecticherb.com).

Bastyr University is America's leading naturopathic college and
so its endorsement or involvement in any formulation is worth
noting, but the clever little remedy that can help prevent stiffness
is the new **Cherry Fruit Extract** from Enzymatic Therapy, which
can not only reduce uric acid levels, but also provides a therapeutic dose of antioxidant flavonoids in each capsule to help
prevent further degeneration of the joints.

If you want a good painkilling cream, check out the **Drs A–Z
Glucosamine and Boswellia** (see pages 211 and 208 for more on
how these agents work). You can also now get glucosamine in a
skin patch (see page 216) and, talking of patches and pain, the

new **Pain Ease Patch** from Lifes2Good (www.lifes2good.com) is an excellent drug-free solution not only to painful joints but to all types of discomfort, including period pains (see Chapter 8, page 411).

If you cannot find these specific remedies in your local health store, mail order from Victoria Health on 0800 389 8195; www.victoriahealth.com.

What About Magnets?

Lots of people swear by magnet therapy, claiming that wearing magnets or magnetic jewellery, or even lying on 'magnetic' mattresses overnight, can help relieve joint pains. The theory is that magnetic polarities have opposing effects on biological systems. Negative magnetic fields, for instance, are reported to normalize the body's pH balance, oxygenate tissues, prevent accumulation of too much fluid in cells, slow down the rate of infection, reduce pain and inflammation, and increase relaxation by slowing down the brain's electrical activity. Positive magnetic fields, by contrast, are said to promote disease and increase pain.

Researchers have commented that, in healing itself, polarity plays a role. When you first injure or hurt yourself, the energy surrounding that body part is positive. The body then draws healing negative magnetic energy to that site to accelerate the healing process, which is where magnet therapy comes in. Magnets are used to provide an additional and stronger negative magnetic field and are believed to be useful when a person cannot generate and maintain enough negative magnetic energy around an injury site to trigger and complete the healing process.

What this tells me is that magnet therapy is a lot more complex than most consumers may realize. If, for example, you are using magnets that provide both polarities, you may be doing more harm than good. What you need is a magnet that will provide a negative field only.

Patients with cancer or any type of infection should avoid using magnets with both polarities since generating a more positive magnetic field is believed to accelerate tumour growth and encourage microbe replication. Pregnant women should not use magnets near their abdomen and people with pacemakers should avoid them too.

Inflammation and Pain Relief . . .

. . . or how chicken stock will keep you on your feet.

If you have ever suffered from inflammation of the musculo-skeletal system in any form you will have had the misfortune to experience crippling pain. In my researches for cutting-edge, new-generation natural products designed to alleviate this type of pain and its root cause, I stumbled across an intriguing new supplement called FYI (For Your Inflammation)*, formulated by US naturopathic physician and researcher Dr Jordan Rubin.

To work out precisely what best to include in the supplement, he thought long and hard about the possible causes of inflammation and came up with the following less-than-magnificent (since you don't want to be suffering from them) list of seven key triggers.

Dr Rubin's Seven Key Causes of Inflammation

Cartilage/Collagen Degeneration

This will come as no surprise to any of us but what is appealing is Dr Rubin's beautifully simple solution: **chicken stock**. Stock, he explains, supplies hydrophilic (water-loving) colloids to the diet,

---

* FYI is made by Garden of Life; www.gardenoflifeusa.com.

i.e. substances that attract liquids. Real homemade soup stocks also supply high quality collagen and gelatin, which are, in turn, rich sources of glycosaminoglycans including chondroitin sulphate. Collagen works to draw water or synovial fluid to the joints, which further helps to cushion them.

So, FYI contains chicken collagen sourced from French chickens raised naturally.

Overacidity

Russian researchers have made a positive correlation between increasing body acidity and the severity of damage and inflammation to joints. They studied the acidity of joint fluid in some sixty-five patients suffering from rheumatoid arthritis and concluded that **potassium** levels are frequently too low in older arthritics. (Potassium plays a key role in maintaining the naturally, slightly alkaline pH of the healthy body; see page 136.)

So, FYI includes **alfalfa grass juice**, which is a naturally alkalizing agent.

Chronic Low-grade Infections

You may not be wilting under the duvet, but you might still have an undetected low-grade infection. Telltale signs include persistent tiredness and skin eruptions. If you suspect you may be a sufferer, Live Blood Analysis (Chapter 3, page 113) can confirm your hunch. Since the link between infection and inflammation is indisputable, it may be worth getting checked, especially if you are beginning to suffer arthritic-type problems.

So, FYI includes **wild oregano** and **bayberry bark**, herbs that have potent antimicrobial properties to tackle the bacteria, viruses and fungi that may be causing your infection.

Immune Dysfunction

As we have seen in previous chapters and as we will see again and again, you cannot divorce the immune system from anything that is happening in the body. There is plenty of evidence to suggest that persistent inflammatory conditions can be caused by both an overactive and an underactive immune system, and lots of conditions, including arthritis and ankylosing spondylitis (see page 227), are now believed to be what are termed autoimmune complaints.

Cat's claw is an excellent immune-supporting herb. It has been shown in trials to block several inflammatory pathways and will work in an adaptogenic way (see page 203) to harmonize the immune system by either boosting an underactive immune response or by toning down one that is stuck in overdrive. This is one of the active agents in the FYI formulation.

Overproduction of Inflammatory Enzymes

Conventional painkilling drugs for arthritic and inflammatory-type conditions fall into two categories: non-steroid anti-inflammatories (NSAIDs), which come with a pretty nasty list of side effects (see the alternative, Nexrutine, page 212), and the so-called Cox-2-inhibiting drugs, which, although originally promoted as being less harsh than the NSAIDs, are not without their side effects too. The good news is that there are lots of natural Cox-2-inhibitors which work just as well as ibuprofen and aspirin, and one of these is one your granny could have told you would work: **cod liver oil**.

Nothing 'second generation' about this natural remedy, I know, but what is new is that scientists in Cardiff have finally been able to tell us how it works – by switching off those enzymes that cause inflammation and switching on those enzymes that protect joints from the destruction of cushioning cartilage.

This action is thanks to the presence of **essential fatty acids** (essential always means the body cannot make it but must glean it from the diet). The two key fatty acids are omega-6 and omega-3 and while lots of foods (including nuts, seeds and avocados) contain omega-6 fats, very few provide omega-3.

Oily fish and flax (or linseeds) are the best sources – some will argue the body can better use those fatty acids sourced from fish, but if you are vegetarian, you will definitely want to take the flaxseed route – and whichever you do choose, it is still hard to make sure you eat these fats in the correct ratio. Our ancestors, for example, ate a healthier ratio of 5:1 in favour of the omega-3 fats. In the modern diet, that ratio is now closer to 24:1 in favour of omega-6. This is unfortunate, too, because it is the omega-3 fats (not the omega-6) that are doing most of the work in helping protect against arthritis (by switching off the enzymes which would otherwise help make those chemicals that destroy cartilage and cause pain and swelling of the joints).

Other natural anti-inflammatories include **turmeric** and **ginger** (see Top Ten Natural Remedies to Help with Musculo-skeletal Problems, pages 207–214), and both these are included in the FYI supplement.

Enzyme Deficiencies

Again, if you take a truly holistic approach, you cannot focus on one or two systems and ignore the fact they are all interlinked and related. Cleverly, FYI includes **bromelain,** which works as an anti-inflammatory at living tissue sites (see page 208), and **papain,** an enzyme found in unripened papaya that can help reduce inflammation at sites where dead or diseased tissue is present.

Oxidative Stress

There is an argument which goes that all sickness and disease is the result of oxidative tissue damage over time, and so any self-respecting formulation for inflammation should include good antioxidants. FYI includes a botanical extract of **rhododendron caucasicum,** which, Dr Rubin believes, is several times more potent than both Pycnogenol and grapeseed extract, thanks to better bioavailability.

So, FYI . . . Does It Work?

In trials by the maker (therefore, not independent, but then neither are drug trials), FYI was shown to boost immune function by increasing levels of both macrophage and natural killer cells. And in placebo-controlled trials, where seventy rheumatoid arthritis patients were given FYI for three months, 30 per cent of participants had achieved clinical remission by the end of the study.

Patients who were given FYI also reported a host of other benefits including better sleep patterns, improved skin, no more migraine headaches, fewer digestive problems, no more constipation, and even, for three male patients suffering some degree of impaired hearing, significant auditory improvement.

It's a Dog's Life

Here's a tale that could stop short the wag in the tail of your older dog. In 1996 – the year before an anti-arthritic drug for dogs called Rimadyl was launched – the FDA recorded a total of some 3000 animal drug-adverse reactions. In the first twelve months since coming to market, Rimadyl, which was originally intended for humans, produced that number of adverse reactions alone.

While initial testing had thrown up some unusual liver function results, nobody seemed too concerned until the owners of older arthritic dogs started reporting a range of horrible side effects including vomiting, diarrhoea, lethargy, liver problems and even death. Pfizer, manufacturer of the drug, has now been asked to add 'death' as a possible side effect to its marketing literature and TV ads, but since some pet owners have reported very positive results, the drug has not actually been withdrawn.

If your vet is offering Rimadyl as a solution to your pet's painful joint problems, visit the website of the US Senior Dogs

Project (www.srdogs.com) to learn more. Better still, make the trek with your pooch to the UK's best alternative veterinary centre, run by Christopher Day (www.alternativevet.org). My Jack Russell terrier Ellie absolutely loves him – probably because, as he checks your dog out, he throws in an osteopathic realignment for free. He is the only vet who has ever asked me to bring a urine sample from my animal and, in my dog-loving opinion, this man should be cloned . . . around the world.

The Spine – Are You Sitting Comfortably?

A healthy spine, in standing position, is a very gentle S-shape, with an inward curve at the lower end. This curve is known as the lordorsis.

Sitting, unlike standing, squatting or lying down, is simply not a natural thing for the human body to do, and bad posture, especially when sitting, can exaggerate this curve, leading, at worse, to a prolapsed disc and even osteoarthritis of the spine.

Those most at risk are people who are obese and those with weak abdominal muscles but office workers spending most of their waking day at computer terminals are clearly sitting on more than badly designed chairs, they are sitting on a health time-bomb too.

What happens when you sit on a flat-seated chair without the proper back support is that the spine slumps into a C-shape that then places too much pressure on the lower back. An ergonomically designed chair has a sloping seat to prevent this. Instead, it tilts the pelvis forward so that the spine is lengthened, even in the sitting position. The back of a good chair will mould to the spine to provide full support and there should be armrests to take the full weight of those limbs off the shoulders. This is especially important for those who suffer neck and shoulder tension.

If you are worried about your back and are concerned your office chair may be exacerbating the problem, you are going to have to look at spending upwards of £500 for an ergonomically designed chair. As well as tilting the pelvis forward – and at first, this feels very odd, almost as if you are going to slide to the floor – a good chair should recline. Make sure, though, that the whole chair, not just the back, reclines since this means, when you are on the telephone, you can lean back and give your spine a good stretch.

If you look around an office, you will see some people sitting perched on the very edges of their chairs. They may not even be aware they are sitting this way but this is actually the body's natural and usually subconscious response to an uncomfortable chair, and provides the same relief as a good chair by tilting the pelvis forward in the same way. It does not, though, support the lordosis and so is not a cheap and cheerful long-term solution to back pain.

At the top end of the market, you can spend almost twice that £500 figure on a chair that has a specially designed 'bladder' incorporated into the height-adjustable back support. This comes with an attached pump that you use to inflate the region to fit snugly into the curve of your own lordosis.

This may sound like a gadget too far but I have seen grown men and women, including a family doctor and the head of an NHS trust, on their knees and crying with the pain of a bad back so, personally, I would pay whatever it takes to avoid being similarly incapacitated.

When you do decide to invest in a decent office chair, you should undergo a simple postural assessment that will include a brief medical history and take into account your body proportions, height and weight. The chair you choose should then be adjusted for your shape so that once you are sitting at your desk, your palms will lie level with the keyboard you are working at so there is no bend or lift in the wrist.

Sorting your chair out is only one step in the right direction, and poor workplace design, especially the idea of a standard desk height, has to take a major share of the blame for the nation's back troubles. It is just silly to think that an 8st, 5ft 3in woman will be as comfortable at a standard 72cm high desk as a 16st, 6ft 2in man.

In Scandinavia, stand/sit desks are all the rage. Again, to take pressure off the back, you simply adjust the height of the desk and work from the standing position for a while. Here in the UK, although there is an EC directive recommending that we too work from height-adjustable workstations to avoid repetitive strain injuries (RSI – see page 230), nobody is paying too much attention.

Where to go for more help? BackCare is the new name for the UK's National Back Pain Association. Contact the charity on 020 8977 5474 or visit www.backpain.org. Although there are other shops specializing in selling back-support chairs and gadgets, in the UK, there is still *only one* **The Back Shop** (020 7935 9120), which has been in London's New Cavendish Street for twenty years. For a decent chair, expect to pay upwards of £500. Frequent travellers or long-distance drivers – ask about the inflatable Archi Air cushion which will support the lordosis when you are on the move.

Tried and Applied

Your partner's reaction to your back problems can affect how much pain you experience, according to research by psychologists at the University of Heidelberg, which compared two groups with chronic back pain. One group had 'solicitous' spouses who reacted to signs of pain by fetching medicine and waiting on them, and the other had 'non-solicitous' partners who, at the same signs of pain, either tried to provide a distraction or simply left the room. They found the more solicitous the partner, the worse the experience of pain!

Teeth and Gums – the Fluoride Debate

If, like me, you grew up in the 1970s, you will remember endless TV ads of clean-cut young men and women whose dazzlingly bright white smiles and perfect happy lives were testament (apparently) to the power of . . . fluoride in their toothpaste.

Of course, back then nobody thought to ask precisely how it is that we know this is such a good thing. Who has done the long-term research? Or even, as we sipped our fluoridated water from the tap, what gives a government the right to 'mass medicate' the population? The fact was, we all believed fluoride was good for our teeth because everyone, including the dentist, told us so.

What nobody told you back then is that fluoride is a poison. It is used to kill rats and mice. It is highly corrosive, and animal studies now suggest that, far from promoting health, this chemical is a possible carcinogen, especially in tissues such as bone and liver. Water fluoridation shows a positive correlation with an increased risk of hip fracture in the over-65s – scientists at Yale University have reported that doses as low as 1 ppm (parts per million) of fluoride decrease bone strength and density, making fracture more likely – and the truth is, most studies show little or no difference in the incidence of dental cavities in children living in areas where the water is fluoridated and where it is not.

Ironic, then, that one of the more widely accepted treatments for osteoporosis was once fluoride therapy.

To learn more about the health hazards of fluoridation, check out www.fluoridealert.org and www.fluoridedebate.com. In the meantime, here are some of the ways in which you can minimize your exposure from now on, according to Barry Groves, the author of a new book called *Fluoride: Drinking Ourselves To Death?*

- Avoid toothpastes that contain fluoride.

- Avoid drinking apple and grape juices; these are the fruits most commonly sprayed with high-fluoride pesticides, so peel raw apples and grapes before eating them.
- Avoid nonstick cookware with Teflon and Tefal coatings since these are made from fluoride too.
- Avoid using aluminium saucepans if you live in an area where the water is fluoridated, since they usually have the same fluoride coatings, which then doubles your exposure/risk.
- Fit a fluoride filter on your tap (these usually need to be installed in tandem with the more common carbon-blocking filters). Check out the National Pure Water Association at www.npwa.freeserve.co.uk.

Tried and Applied

Drink your tea with milk. Tea contains about 4.4ppm fluoride, but if you drink it with milk, the calcium content of milk will mitigate the effects.

OK, we now know fluoride is not the answer, so what does work for teeth and gums?

What you are looking for are remedies that will (1) help stop the formation of plaque in the mouth and (2) prevent gum disease which can, if left unchecked, progress to affect the bone and, in the latter stages, cause teeth to fall out. Here are my 1, 2, 3 . . . best remedies to protect the teeth and gums.

Top Three Remedies to Protect Teeth and Gums

Xylitol

Tooth enamel is the single strongest substance in the human body, but it will wear away if constantly exposed to sugar. Eating sugar before bedtime has been linked to higher numbers of dental cavities, and so introducing a sugar-free zone last thing at night and especially for children will help prevent decay, as will eliminating soft drinks or 'liquid candy' as they are sometimes scathingly but deservedly known (see page 184).

A better substitute for sugar is xylitol, which the body produces naturally when metabolizing glucose, and which is also found in berries, plums, mushrooms, lettuce, hardwoods and corn-on-the-cobs. Made from birch tree bark, it can have an adverse effect on the digestive tract but only if ingested in very high doses. Unlike pure sugar, it protects teeth by creating an alkaline environment in the mouth that is inhospitable to the bacteria that cause tooth decay; hence its widespread use now in chewing gums and candy bars. Studies have shown xylitol can inhibit plaque formation and decrease dental decay by 80 per cent. Even better, it may work to promote the remineralization of tooth enamel. Visit www.xylitol.org.

Gingigel

After tooth decay, the second most common disorder in the mouth is inflammation of the gums (gingival), a condition known as gingivitis. Dental experts believe that although some 95 per cent of the adult population suffer from some form of gum (periodontal) disease, only 10 per cent develop serious problems. Early warning signs include bleeding gums, unpleasant tastes or odours in the mouth and sensitivity of the teeth to hot and cold foods.

Gingigel is a biological mouth and gum-care gel based on hyaluronic acid, a natural substance found in the connective tissues of the body, which can help stimulate the production of new, healthy tissue when applied to the gums. In university trials in Germany, researchers found this agent could double the rate of tissue healing, increase blood supply to the gums and reduce inflammation. You can buy a tube of gel to apply direct to the gums, or a mouth rinse to use morning and night. (If not on sale in your local UK health store, mail order from Victoria Health on 0800 389 8195; www.victoriahealth.com.)

Co-enzyme Q10 (CoQ10)

Japanese research suggests that co-enzyme Q10 can help maintain healthy gums. You need to take a therapeutic daily dose of 60mg a day.

Tried and Applied

Use myrrh for mouth ulcers. The active agent in myrrh is the resin, which contains both a volatile oil and mucilage substance to provide anti-inflammatory, deodorizing and antimicrobial protection. It has a long tradition of use for oral problems including mouth ulcers, gingivitis, chapped lips and even loose teeth. You need a bottle of myrrh tincture, which you use topically, and undiluted (1–2 drops), on the affected areas, or which you can dilute (5–10 drops in a glass of water) to make a rinse or mouthwash gargle. You can buy myrrh tincture in all good health stores.

Exercise – the Girlie Stuff

According to the American Heart Association, only 10 per cent of the US population exercise regularly, despite the fact that 54 per cent are deemed clinically overweight. If you know you should exercise more but cannot find the will or the motivation to get started, check out the 10,000 Steps-A-Day Program (www.newlifestyles.com/challenge.html), which is a great kick-start to getting the body moving. Ten thousand steps equates to about 5 miles and the idea is that where you can, you walk.

For example, instead of getting a taxi to take you two miles from the train station to an office, if the weather is fine, then walk. This programme involves wearing a small pedometer that counts those steps for you and participants report that using this device helps them set and then realize achievable goals that keep the body moving.

My trainer starts every session with the maxim 'Use It or Lose It'. I start with a grimace, but I know she is right. I am over forty and still spend long hours sitting writing, and I am now counting the cost of that lifestyle in stiffness and musculo-skeletal imbalances, so it's hard to argue with her.

Macho men may shudder at the thought but those girlie core-strength-building exercise regimens, such as yoga and Pilates, really will help you build longer-lasting strength and help to correct musculo-skeletal imbalances that will otherwise cause problems as you age. Research has also shown how light weight-bearing exercise coupled with deep yoga breathing can help keep arthritic bodies moving and alleviate serious stiffness in damaged joints. If you have serious stiffness or arthritis, rub your muscles to warm them before you do any form of exercise.

Tried and Applied

When you exercise, your body generates more tissue-damaging free radical molecules and toxins. Counter these by taking a good quality antioxidant such as Pycnogenol (see Chapter 3, page 148), plus a good quality probiotic to help accelerate the detoxification of these substances. Farmers know that feeding animals probiotics in high dosages works to decrease body fat and increase lean muscle; common sense and natural healers suggest the same could work for humans too.

Endurance, Performance and the Body-building Stuff

The single most popular sports supplement is still the energy-boosting nutrient **creatine**, which has been around for several decades and gets sold under names like Muscle Power, which tells you pretty much what it will do for you. It is now so popular that surveys show over 40 per cent of US high-school athletes use it, but what you may not know is how much you can safely take, what are the risks of side effects (which are real enough to have made the over-the-counter sale of this supplement illegal in France) and, if you still want to use it, which form is the best to take.

Creatine is a non-protein amino acid that is made in the kidneys, liver and pancreas from two other amino acids: L-arginine and L-methionine, so you may find these two cropping up in combination formulas too. Once the body has made its supplies, these are shipped to the skeletal muscles, the heart, the brain and other tissues, where it is then converted to another chemical called phosphocreatine.

The reason this conversion is important is that storing phosphocreatine is one of the main ways the body stores energy. And if you have more energy, you can work out for longer, build bigger muscles and wipe the floor with the competition.

During exercise, the working muscles must break down a compound called adenosine triphosphate (ATP) to release energy. This process converts the ATP to adenosine diphosphate (ADP), inorganic phosphate and energy. What phosphocreatine (PCr) is able to do is to combine with the inactive ADP to turn it back into high-energy ATP and it is this that translates into more strength and stamina for the muscles during high-intensity brief bursts of activity such as weight training.

The creatine you swallow will be absorbed in the small intestine and then taken to the liver from where, along with the creatine the body has made itself, it is despatched to the body tissues, including nerves and muscles. In normal health, up to 67 per cent of the creatine entering these cells is converted to energy-boosting PCr but in animal studies, chronic (long-term) creatine supplementation has been shown to *reduce* the amount of creatine entering the cells. The solution is to take it for a month and then give it a rest for a couple of weeks before starting again.

To get started, most users take what is called a 'loading dose' of 15–30g, four times a day for one week. This will overburden the liver so it would be better to start and stick with a lower (5g a day) maintenance dose, but if you insist on the higher loading doses, then after this first week definitely cut back to a less burdensome maintenance dose of 2–5g a day. If you do go ahead with a high loading dose, you should also take steps to protect the liver by taking an additional supplement of amino acids.

Although there is little good quality clinical research to prove the many health claims that are made for it, creatine is said to improve muscle size, overall strength and performance, especially when taken in conjunction with exercise. There are, though, risks, and reported side effects include not only diarrhoea, which is common, but mood disorders including depression, anxiety, edginess and even temper flare-ups. Creatine might give you the muscle but, as most top sportsmen and women will tell you, performance demands something else: it demands that when it really counts, you be the very best you can possibly be.

How Humble Herbs Can Give You the Competitive Edge

The herbs that are going to give you the psychological and physical advantage over your competitors in the gym, at work, at college and even on the nightclub dance floor are known as **adaptogens**. What they do is make every single biological system in your body – your immune system, your hormonal system, your cardiovascular system – and thus you, the very best it and you can be.

Even better, according to newly released Russian research, some of these incredible herbs can be combined to make them work together for even more effect. This is known as synergy and if you're wondering why on earth Russian scientists would even stoop to look at herbs, they turned to plants and plant chemicals to make sure their elite athletes and their cosmonauts would achieve the very best performances – again, physically and mentally – despite being subjected to the kind of stress in training that most of us will never have to face.

Here then are some of the better-known adaptogens you will find in the health store and throughout this book (check the index). These are the often bitter-tasting herbs your grandmother and her mother before her would have called tonics, so you may need to hide them in juices to get the full health benefits, while disguising the unpleasant taste.

- Astragalus
- Cat's claw
- Ginseng
- Liquorice (not the sweet strings that kids used to chew but the dried and powdered root)
- Pycnogenol or pine bark (which is actually a group of bioflavonoid compounds)
- Green tea (which also has weight-loss promoting properties)
- Ginger (which is great for joints too)
- Suma (also known as Brazilian or Amazonian ginseng)
- Agnus castus (*the* key hormone-balancing herb)
- Rhodiola rosea
- Tribulus terrestris

All these herbs will make the body more resistant to stress, infection and energy slumps. Usually you would only use adaptogens when you know you are coming under pressure and when, for example, you have to perform. (For more on this subject, see Chapter 5.)

Leg cramps, when exercising, can be a sign of deficiency in either or both magnesium and calcium, or even potassium or zinc. Check the A–Z of Foods (page 217) to find out how to increase your dietary intake of all these nutrients, and think about taking a good quality joint support supplement.

Tried and Applied

One of the most important adaptogenic herbs for males is the east European herb tribulus terrestris, which is now on sale in the west. In clinical trials, healthy males who took 750mg a day for five days were found to have a 40 per cent increase in testosterone, the key anti-stress and performance-boosting hormone in men.

Sports Injuries

Lots of people use **arnica** (leopard's bane) to help reduce the swellings and bruises caused by accidents, including sporting injuries, but the evidence for its effectiveness remains mixed. If you already know it works for you, then great. If not, make sure, if you plan to put it to the test, you are using a homeopathic remedy (that you take internally) as well as any topical gel you may be applying; and take three x 30c potency homeopathic pellets every four hours until you see an improvement.

The other remedy you should be using is one you may not have even heard of: **bromelain** is an anti-inflammatory mix of enzymes sourced from the stems of fresh pineapple, and is one of my top ten musculo-skeletal remedies (see page 208). In trials, seventy-four boxers who emerged from a boxing match with serious bruises to their faces, lips, ears, chests and arms were given bromelain, while another seventy-two boxers were given a placebo pill. In almost 80 per cent of those boxers given bromelain, all signs of bruising were gone in just four days. Among those given a placebo, just 14 per cent reported the same healing rates.

Musculo-skeletal Testing

The fact is, until you get an assessment, you will not know how much damage you may have already done to your musculoskeletal system. You may be the fittest person in the gym and utterly obsessed with exercise but if you are not maintaining proper alignment, you will be doing more harm than good.

Lots of private health insurance companies now offer full musculo-skeletal screening, or visit one of the new integrated health centres such as the Diagnostic Clinic in London (020 7009 4650), where qualified holistic physicians and a range of practitioners, from reflexologists to osteopaths, can help you start to remedy some of the problems identified.

Or drop the macho image and get down on the yoga or Pilates mat to build core strength and stability that will serve you much better in later life than beefy biceps or tight buns. In other words, forget what's on the outside and start thinking about training from the inside out.

Tried and Applied

The 'placebo effect' is always talked about in derogatory terms when you could, in fact, argue it is an indisputable sign of the power of mind over matter. In one bizarre* trial, where patients with knee injuries were given either real or sham surgery, researchers concluded outcomes were no different whether you had the real operation or a pretend one.

* Bizarre because it is hard to believe that this trial, where both groups of patients underwent skin incisions, was passed by any ethics committee.

Seven of the Best . . . Hands-on Therapies for Joint Problems and Pain

As in all fields, there are good, bad and indifferent practitioners. There are also beginners who, unfortunately, are not required to wear learner L-plates, and while there is nothing wrong with being a guinea pig if you know in advance that's what you are, you do not want someone 'practising' on you without your prior consent.

In my experience, many of the best practitioners simply work 'through' their chosen techniques; in other words, they may have trained and become very experienced in, say, acupuncture or the Bowen Technique, but they are also working from intuition and a good holistic understanding of how the body works.

All of the following techniques can help relieve joint problems, but only if you get a good practitioner: Acupuncture/Acupressure, the Bowen Technique, Chiropractic, Kinesiology, Kosmed/Scenar, Mora Therapy, Osteopathy.

The best way to choose a practitioner is always word-of-mouth from another satisfied client. Failing that, contact the accreditation and referral organizations for each discipline (see Useful Contacts, page 447). When you telephone to make an appointment, make sure you get to speak in person to the practitioner who will be treating you, and quiz them about their qualifications and relevant experience in this field.

Your health is not in their hands. It's in your hands.

If you are not sure what a treatment will involve, check out my website, www.whatreallyworks.co.uk, where I have free fact sheets explaining each of these therapies and how they work. Simply key the name of the technique into the search and print off the information that comes up.

Top Ten Natural Remedies to Help with Musculo-skeletal Problems

In the UK, the NHS bill for treating gastric bleeding caused by anti-inflammatory drugs is currently running at £367 million a year. I'd say that was pretty good reason to investigate what the natural world has to offer.

Borage

This herb is an excellent source of the joint-protecting anti-inflammatory essential fatty acids (see Cod Liver Oil, page 190), making this a good alternative for anyone who wants a vegetarian and not a fish-oil source of these nutrients. Borage seed oil is, of course, extracted from the seeds, but you can also get supplements and creams made from the above-the-ground parts of the plant, including the flowers.

The primary agent is a fatty acid called gamma linoleic acid (GLA), which is also the primary agent in evening primrose oil supplements. In humans, GLA is quickly metabolized to dihomogammalinoleic acid, which is a precursor to a potent anti-inflammatory agent called prostaglandin E1.

Therapeutic dose

The dosage used in clinical trials to tackle rheumatoid arthritis is 1–1.5g of borage seed oil, daily.

Do not mix this remedy with prescription medications for liver disorders, blood thinning or schizophrenia.

Boswellia

One of the less well-known anti-inflammatory agents now incorporated into joint supplements is Boswellia serrata or Indian frankincense, which can inhibit the enzymes that would otherwise trigger the inflammation causing arthritic conditions. The active agents in this herb are boswellic acid and alpha-boswellic acid, which both have a painkilling as well as anti-inflammatory action, but if you look for a supplement, make sure you do not confuse it with Boswellia carterii or Bible frankincense, which has different properties. Boswellia works to increase blood supply to the wound/injury and so can accelerate healing.

In trials where Boswellia serrata was compared with the prescription drug, sulfasalazine, patients taking the herb reported similar improvement to those taking the more conventional medication. Sulfasalazine is prescribed both for patients with rheumatoid arthritis who have not responded to any other treatment and for patients with ulcerative colitis (see Chapter 2, page 103), suggesting boswellia may be useful for both conditions.

Therapeutic dose
400mg, 3 times a day.

Contraindications
None reported.

Bromelain

Known as the **tissue healer**, this increasingly popular anti-inflammatory agent is derived from the stems of fresh pineapples.

It is not a single chemical but rather a family of sulfhydryl prote-olytic enzymes that work to reduce swelling and bruising by triggering the release of a chemical called kinin, which then stim-ulates the production of anti-inflammatory prostaglandin compounds in the body.

If you are scheduled for surgery, do not leave home without this remedy, which has fantastic post-operative and post-traumatic anti-swelling properties and which has also been used, in cream form, for keeping wounds clear of infection and dead tissue in burns cases. It has been shown to reduce swelling, pain at rest and during movement, and tenderness following both surgery and injury. If you are having an operation, start taking it before you check into hospital and carry on for ten days. For spinal injuries, slipped discs, dislocations etc, take it with Nexrutine (see below).

Therapeutic dose
500mg, 3 times a day, half an hour before eating.

Contraindications
Do not combine with zinc, which can inhibit the activity of bromelain, and avoid potatoes and soy products, which can do the same thing. Avoid altogether if you know you are allergic to bee venom.

Cetyl Myristoleate CMO
This is, in effect, another fatty acid found in small quantities in foods such as nuts, vegetables and butter, and in animals as diverse as whales and mice. There is very little scientific evidence proving efficacy but the reason for all the excitement (and not a little hype) is that what has been clearly shown is that Swiss albino mice, which are born with unusually high levels of CMO, never get arthritis and seem to be protected from it

when exposed to factors that would cause the condition in other breeds.

Sales of this supplement are on the rise, thanks to good anecdotal evidence, and if you do plan to use it, the recommended dosage is 10–15g a month for three months. The problem is that it's expensive, especially if you have fallen into the trap of thinking more is better, which, in the case of this supplement, research suggests is not the case. Most of the supplements (which are made from bovine marrow, by the way) vary in strength from 12 per cent CMO to 40 per cent, but in this instance, the higher strength is not necessarily better. The lower strength is better because it allows for more of the important essential fatty acids the supplements also supply.

Therapeutic dose

Most 500mg capsules provide 12 per cent CMO which is the equivalent to 60mg, so you would have to take 6–7 capsules daily, making this an expensive option.

Contraindications

None reported.

Ginger

This herb has lots of different actions in the body, but in this chapter we are specifically interested in its potent anti-inflammatory properties. In double-blind, placebo-controlled, multi-centre trials (and they don't come much more scientific than that), involving some 250 patients suffering from osteoarthritis of the knee, those taking ginger extract for just six weeks reported much less pain when standing and were also able to cut back significantly on the use of prescription painkilling drugs.

In a smaller trial – just fifty-six patients of whom twenty-eight had rheumatoid arthritis, eighteen had osteoarthritis and ten had general muscular pains – scientists again concluded ginger was effective for the relief of joint pain and swelling. You can dilute ginger oil in a carrier oil and massage directly over stiff joints, which is especially helpful if you want to do any stretching exercises such as yoga or Pilates.

Therapeutic dose
250mg, 3 times a day.

Contraindications
None reported.

Glucosamine

Glucosamine is produced naturally in the body, where it is then used to make cartilage. The reason it is so effective in supplement form is that it does not simply treat the symptoms, but can actually slow the progress of joint diseases caused by wear and tear, especially osteoarthritis. Glucosamine supplements are usually made from chitin, a substance found in the shells of shrimps, lobsters and crabs, and you will often find combination formulations that include **chondroitin**, another naturally occurring substance which can protect the joints from wear and tear.

There is now a large body of evidence comparing glucosamine with both placebo and conventional medications that proves it really does work to relieve the pain and inflammation of arthritic conditions, including rheumatoid arthritis. For best results, look for a supplement that combines glucosamine with chondroitin and collagen (see Collagen Plus, page 215).

Therapeutic dose
500mg, 3 times a day.

Almost all the clinical trials have been conducted on glucosamine sulphate but if you are on a sodium-restricted diet then take it in the form of glucosamine hydrochloride (HCl).

Methylsulphonylmethane (MSM)

This is a naturally occurring form of organic sulphur which is present in all living organisms, and which plays such a key role in tissue healing it is often prescribed by surgeons. You can get MSM from lots of foods, including fresh fruit, cow's milk and fresh vegetables, as well as meats and seafoods, but it is easily destroyed by both cooking and food processing techniques, making it impossible to get a therapeutic dose from your diet.

Instead, you need to take a supplement of 1g a day (with food) to promote internal healing and alleviate inflammation. Arthritis sufferers who take this supplement report the welcome side effects of thicker, glossier hair and stronger nails too.

Therapeutic dose

No typical dose has been specified so take as directed on the bottle or use the cream or powder forms as suggested on the packet. Aim for 1500mg a day for staying flexible and 3g a day if you already have joint problems.

Contraindications

None reported.

Nexrutine

Developed to prevent the stomach bleeding and gastric irritation that is a common side effect of anti-arthritis drugs, Nexrutine is a brand new anti-inflammatory agent now available as a supplement. The active ingredient comes from the rue – a plant most gardeners would treat as a weed but whose name comes from the

Greek word 'reuo', which means to set free, as in free from disease. In clinical trials, nine out of ten volunteers who took 250mg of Nexrutine three times a day for two weeks reported no gastric side effects. In fact, Nexrutine is so gentle, you even take it between meals and not with food.

Therapeutic dose
Each Lifetime capsule provides 250mg (see page 215); take one, 3 times a day.

Contraindications
None reported.

Papain
Used industrially as a meat tenderizer and as an ingredient in cosmetics, papain is, like bromelain, a mix of enzymes, but this time sourced from papaya (pawpaw) fruit. It is used in Chinese medicine to help alleviate the pain of rheumatism but is also a good digestive aid that can help break down plaque deposits on the teeth (see page 197). This fruit is also a good source of bone-building nutrients, including calcium, magnesium, manganese, phosphorus and vitamin C (see Bone – How It Is Made, page 178), and can help flush out excess uric acid that can otherwise cause joint problems.

Therapeutic dose
1500mg a day is the dosage used in clinical trials to treat swelling and injuries following trauma and surgery.

Contraindications
If you are allergic to kiwi fruits or figs, you will probably be allergic to papain too. Do not use this remedy alongside anticoagulant herbs or drugs, including garlic, ginkgo biloba, red clover or turmeric.

Turmeric

A member of the ginger family, turmeric has many medicinal actions including anti-inflammatory properties that can help alleviate the pain of arthritis. The key active ingredient in the spice is curcumin, which gives it its distinctive yellow colour and which has been shown to be an even more potent antioxidant than vitamin E.

Turmeric, which is also an antimicrobial agent, contains between 0.3 and 5.4 per cent of this active ingredient, which is said to work as well as the steroid cortisone in relieving acute cases of inflammation. It works only half as well as the conventional treatments when the condition is chronic, but you need to weigh this up against the fact that, unlike many of the orthodox treatments, at the recommended safe dosages (400–600mg, three times a day) it has no toxicity.

Curcumin works in the same way as capsaicin, the active ingredient in chillies, to deplete nerve endings of substance P, a neurotransmitter that carries pain signals in the body. Curcumin also works to stabilize cell membranes and thereby prevent the release of inflammatory agents, and, according to Ayurvedic practitioners, works specifically to help relieve shoulder injuries.

Therapeutic dose
400–600mg a day.

Contraindications
In some arthritic patients, turmeric in the diet can exacerbate arthritic-type conditions. Unfortunately, there are no predictors for who may be adversely affected in this way; you will have to monitor your reactions and stop using this remedy if your symptoms worsen.

Top Three Over-the-Counter Combination Remedies for Joint Problems

Advanced Joint Support Formula

This supplement, which is part of the Lifetime range, is the only joint remedy that has been researched by scientists at Harvard and endorsed by Boston Medical School. It contains bromelain, MSM, glucosamine and chondroitin, plus type II collagen, a form that contains hyaluronic acid (see Gingigel, page 198). Type II collagen forms well over 80 per cent of the body's collagen network and the tissue-regenerating properties of hyaluronic acid have been well documented. Take this alongside Cherry Fruit Extract by Enzymatic Therapy (see page 186), which will help flush excess uric acid from the body. If you cannot source either locally, mail order from Victoria Health on 0800 389 8195; www.victoriahealth.com.

Collagen Plus

Collagen is needed to build bone. Glucosamine then strengthens that bone, but the clever active ingredient that completes this hat trick is chondroitin, which works to attract more fluid to the space around joints to help keep them lubricated.

Even better news for those who hate popping tablets that look like horse pills, all three of these active ingredients come in a powder form with vitamin C (which is also crucial for healthy bones and cartilage), plus calcium and magnesium. To take it, you simply dilute the powder to make an orange-flavoured drink, which you take once a day after breakfast.

Collagen Plus is made by the Preston-based company Arthrovite (mail order on 0800 018 1282). Take it for at least three months to give it a chance to kick in.

Solgar's Bone Support

This supplement is part of the impressive Gold Specifics range. It includes every nutrient you might have on your wish list for helping to maintain bone density, and in all the right ratios, which takes the guesswork out of supplementation. Unfortunately, because it contains ipriflavone, it is not for sale in the UK, so you will have to source elsewhere in Europe or America. Take alongside the Joint Modulators supplement from the same range. Call 01442 890355 (www.solgar.com) for local stockists. Solgar is a huge champion of independent and specialist health stores and the range is widely on sale in these kinds of outlets. The range is expensive but you get what you pay for and the price reflects a commitment to quality, stability testing, quality control testing, investment in research to find natural preservatives and other hidden costs which translate to better quality products.

Tried and Applied

Glucosamine Skin Patch: This clever idea from joint specialist Health Perception was developed in Japan, in conjunction with the School of Pharmacy at the University of Brighton in the UK. It is the brainchild of the founder of the company, former Olympic swimming champion

David Wilkie, who first introduced the benefits of glucosamine and chondroitin into the UK in the 1980s, and completes a range that includes a non-sticky topical glucosamine and horse chestnut extract gel for additional pain relief. For best results, use the skin patch in conjunction with glucosamine and chondroitin supplements. Check it out at www.health-perception.co.uk.

A–Z of Bone and Joint Nourishing Foods

As we have seen, what you put on your plate can have a lot more impact on your body than making you feel full at the end of a delicious meal. Just as some foods can help protect against joint inflammation and problems (e.g. soybeans; see genistein, page 182) others will exacerbate those conditions. Candida (see Digestion, page 94) is often linked with these types of complaints so you may need to avoid fermented foods, including alcohol, which can trigger an outbreak, but a less obvious food which we now know can, when ingested, worsen arthritic-type pain in some sufferers is hot chilli peppers.

This is thought to be because of the presence of capsaicinoids, those stinging hot flavours it is now suggested may be responsible for activating certain nerve centres, which then trigger a more painful response and burning sensation to inflammation. This is ironic, because capsaicin has also been used successfully topically with some patients to help stop pain (see page 229).

What this proves is that what works for one person may not work for another, and with conditions as multi-factored as arthritis, you may need to try two or three remedies in consultation with a qualified health practitioner, such as a homeopath, nutritionist or naturopath specializing in joint complaints, before finding the one that's right for you.

Cayenne pepper, made from the seeds and pods of chilli

peppers, contains the same capsaicinoid chemicals and so could exacerbate your pain too. For a full list of foods likely to cause this adverse reaction if you have joint problems, visit www.arthritistrust.org and search for the guidebook, *Food Pain*. For a more positive list of foods that will help support the musculo-skeletal system, read on.

A is for alfalfa and vitamin A. Alfalfa is rich in vitamin D, which can boost the absorption of calcium in the diet, plus vitamin K which can help protect against osteoporosis. It is also traditionally used, in tincture form, to help treat muscle spasms and cramps. Vitamin A plays a key role in the repair of healthy tissues and in maintaining healthy bones, skin, gums and teeth. Good food sources include yellow fruits, tomatoes, dark green vegetables and eggs.

B is for broccoli, another good vegetable source of vitamin K and vitamin B6, which the body needs to make strong bones. Bananas, legumes, meats, poultry, potatoes and leafy greens are all good sources, but for an extra boost take brewer's yeast, which you can buy from your local health store.

C is for copper, which is also needed for bone regeneration but which is more tricky to source from the diet. It is doable, though, and the foods you need to eat more of include seafood – especially oysters – legumes, wholegrains, potatoes, meats, almonds and, unexpectedly, raisins. Also cucumbers, which provide silicon (silica) in the diet, and celery, which can help flush out excess uric acid that would otherwise cause stiffness in joints.

D is for vitamin D, without which the body cannot use the calcium you ingest. Butter is a good dietary source and so is cod liver oil. Also eat more eggs, fatty fish and organ meats if you need to increase your intake. Alternatively, stick with salads but get out in the sun more since sunlight (at the right wavelength; which in the UK is only between April and October, which is your best excuse ever for flying off to the winter sun) helps the body make the vitamin D it needs.

E is for eggs, which are an excellent source of vitamin K, vitamin A and magnesium, so you get a triple-whammy bone-building boost. Also a good source of muscle-building protein, of course, and sulphur, which the body needs to maintain healthy connective tissue structures.

F is for fats, which support the musculo-skeletal system, and which are the essential fats – omega-3 and omega-6 – that the body cannot make but must get from the diet. Good sources of omega-6 include sesame oil, nuts and seeds, and meats. Sources of the even more important omega-3 fats (see Cod Liver Oil, page 190) include dark leafy greens, fish oils, pumpkin seeds, soybeans, walnuts, tuna, salmon and anchovies.

G is for grains, which have been shown to be the No. 1 bone-healing foods. Buckwheat, for instance, is rich in magnesium and manganese, while brown rice is a good source of that all-important silica (see Fixing Broken and Fractured Bones, page 181), and millet provides both calcium and magnesium in a form the body can easily assimilate. Gooseberries are high in vitamin A to help repair healthy tissues, and ginger has impressive anti-inflammatory properties.

H is for hemp and herring: both provide the omega-3 fatty acids the body needs to maintain a healthy musculo-skeletal system, and which also have an important anti-inflammatory role to play in helping alleviate joint stiffness that is the result of cartilage degradation. Also sulphur-rich horseradish (eat more sushi with wasabi horseradish sauce), which will support the connective tissue that forms joint tendons and ligaments.

I is for ipriflavones (see page 179) which you can no longer get in supplement form and so have to get from food. Since this is a semi-synthetic bone-supporting substance made from a phyto-chemical called daidzen, which is present in soy products, start stocking up on tofu and other soy-based foods, but check they are organic and have not been genetically modified. Surprisingly, and good news for growing kids, baked beans are a good staple food source.

J is for juicing: mix vitamin-A-rich carrots with celery to flush out excess uric acid and help prevent joint stiffness, add silica-rich red beetroot and a teaspoon of warming grated ginger. Sweeten to taste with antibacterial manuka honey to make a potent joint-protecting tonic to drink every day.

K is for kelp, the health-promoting seaweed that provides vitamin K (as do cauliflower, soybeans, broccoli, Brussels sprouts, oats, rye, eggs, yoghurts and wholewheat; all good dietary sources of this important nutrient). To make a snack from kelp, simply toast it for two minutes in the oven (at 180°C/350°F), or serve as a complement to vegetables, grains, legumes and seafood. Kale is a good source of calcium; lightly steam the younger leaves, which should be bright green and tightly curled.

L is for lentils, a good source of the bone-protecting phytochem-ical genistein (see page 182), especially useful after menopause, and also bone-protecting copper. Also lassi (see page 81 for the basic recipe, and to protect joints use anti-inflammatory papaya instead of bananas and make with organic soya milk instead of dairy); to warm in winter and make a slurp rather than a smoothie, make the lassi and then blend with gently warmed (or steamed) porridge oats. Sweeten to taste with honey.

M is for meat, which will provide vitamin B6, and molasses, a by-product of the refining of sugar cane which is a good vegetarian source of B6 and other important vitamins and minerals, including vitamin K and calcium. Molasses is often used as a sweetener in baked produce, especially rye bread and ginger cake, which is a good excuse for a teatime treat or two.

N is for nectarines, whose rich colour is a dead giveaway for a high vitamin-A content. When buying fresh nectarines, look for richly coloured, plump fruits that feel soft along the seams and avoid any that feel hard, look slightly shrivelled or are cracking along the seams. Also nutmeg, which in India and in Ayurvedic medicine is a topical antirheumatic remedy prepared by frying in oil, then cooling and straining the oil before massaging into the affected body part.

O is for silica-rich oats (see Fixing Broken and Fractured Bones, page 181). You can gently simmer oats to make a porridge to thicken smoothies (see 'L' above; I call these 'slurps'), but you can also buy oats in tincture form to add to juices, herbal drinks or take neat. Remember, studies have shown the body can better absorb calcium in the presence of silica than when it is given on its own.

P is for pears, which provide boron, one of the bone-building trace minerals which can help improve calcium absorption by up to 40 per cent, and, just as importantly, aid its retention. It plays a key role in maintaining healthy bones and muscle growth because it helps the body make its own natural steroid compounds. It also boosts the absorption of other bone-building nutrients, including phosphorus and magnesium. Raw nuts, carrots, grapes, apples and wholegrains are other good sources.

Q is for quinoa, the vitamin-K-rich grain that is one of the best natural foods for supporting musculo-skeletal functioning, and the only grain that is a complete source of protein, making it an important staple for vegetarians; other good dietary sources of this nutrient include yoghurt, alfalfa, egg yolks, kelp, leafy green vegetables and fish oils.

R is for rye and red beetroot, both of which will help increase your intake of bone-building silica; plus rose hips, one of the vitamin-C-rich bioflavonoids that is often included in herbal tea bags, and raisins, which are a surprisingly good source of calcium.

S is for sprouted wheat (see Sprouting, page 69), which is traditionally used to keep joints flexible by attracting more synovial fluid to the spaces around bone, and organic soy products (see below), which are an excellent food source of the phytochemicals we now know can help prevent bone loss after menopause, without the risk of adverse side effects.

T is for tofu and tempeh; both are made from soybeans. Tofu is rich in bone-protecting vitamin A, phosphorus and calcium, while tempeh (a fermented food that has been pre-digested by bacteria, yeast and moulds to change its composition) provides no vitamin A, half the calcium but almost a third again of the phosphorus, if you match portions. Tempeh also has a meatier taste, making it a good substitute for meat, including hamburgers.

U is for uric acid, an excess of which can cause joint problems and stiffness, including gout. Parsley works to flush it out of the body and tomatoes can help neutralize uric acid ingested from animal products. Papaya fruit can help break down unwanted toxic compounds, including uric acid, and the humble turnip will also flush uric acid out of your system. Juice with cabbage or carrots for a joint-protecting breakfast drink.

V is for vegetables – the brighter and richer the colour, the better the supply of tissue-protecting antioxidants. Dark-green leafy vegetables are a good source of both calcium and magnesium. Kale is known as the 'king of calcium' and mustard greens can help flush out excess uric acid (see above). Yellow vegetables are a good source of vitamin A and the bioflavonoids that are sometimes collectively known as vitamin P.

W is for antioxidant- and sulphur-rich watercress, which has the highest nutritional value of all greens. For musculo-skeletal support, juice with carrots, green pepper, dandelion and cucumber to make a superjuice that will support hair, skin, nails, bones, collagen formation and muscle tone. Also winter squash, which contains four times more betacarotene than carrots and which is delicious lightly steamed.

X is for xylitol (see page 197), a natural alternative to sugar, which can help protect teeth by preventing the formation of plaque. If you suffer from diabetes or any milder form of insulin resistance (see Syndrome X, page 122) you may have side effects, primarily diarrhoea, which is also a risk at very high doses.

Y is for yams, which can help heal inflammation; if you're not sure what to do with yams and squash, the basic guideline is if you can think it, you can do it: bake, steam, sauté, scallop, mash; use in sweet and savoury foods, including omelettes, sauces, soups, pancakes, cakes, muffins, puddings, pickles and relishes.

Z is for zimmer frame, which is what you will need if you don't take care of your musculo-skeletal system by eating the right foods and, just as importantly, avoiding the wrong ones (see pages 184 and 217). What's the point of a long life if you can barely put one foot in front of the other because your body, through neglect and lack of care, has effectively seized up? Eat to keep your joints flexible and make sure you stretch and exercise those joints, including the spine, each and every day.

Ancient Wisdom, 21st-century Healing

Traditional Chinese Medicine (TCM)

TCM treats rheumatoid arthritis as an allergic reaction that is passed through the blood to the joints, following a streptococcal infection. Traditional Chinese doctors call this 'pi cheng', which means numbness disease, and it is exacerbated by cold climates and cold foods.

Chinese **wolfberry** (gou ji dze) is used to help alleviate all forms of arthritis and, in particular, back pain, including lumbago. You can buy this herb in Asian supermarkets and add it to winter casseroles, stews and soups, or make your own herbal tea, which, in China, is given to the elderly to help strengthen weak legs and knees. You can chew on the raw berries, too, since they are quite tasty, but they are also quite strong so don't eat more than three or four at one time.

The Planetary Formulas range includes a Lower Back Support supplement that features a number of traditional joint-supporting Chinese herbs, including angelica, which works as a painkilling tonic.

For maximum therapeutic benefits with TCM, find an accredited practitioner in your area. To do this, contact the Register of Chinese Herbalists (see Useful Contacts, page 448).

Ayurvedic (Indian) Remedies

If you want to practise yoga but are worried that stiff joints are going to leave you flailing around at the back of the class, make your own Ayurvedic flexibility paste, which is recommended by the US herbalist Michael Tierra, founder and formulator of the excellent Planetary Formulas range which draws on both TCM and Ayurvedic traditions.

First, boil a quarter of a cup of **turmeric** powder in half a cup of water until a thick paste forms. You can put this in the fridge to keep. Now boil a cup of milk and add a quarter of a teaspoon of your turmeric paste, 1 teaspoon of sesame oil and honey to taste. Drink one cup of this every day. (Don't get hung up about quantities, the ratio is more important than the liquid volume of the cup you are using. Since you are keeping the paste in the fridge and drinking the turmeric drink, you do not have to worry about wastage.)

If you don't have time for DIY remedies, the Pukka Herbs range includes an organic Turmeric Joint Formula (which I successfully used for a crippling shoulder pain which stopped me writing for two weeks). To mail order, call 08456 585858 (www.pukkaherbs.com). Health Perception's Back-O-Samine supplement cleverly combines glucosamine with turmeric to do what it suggests on the box (www.health-perception.co.uk).

Native African Remedies

Devil's claw has been used for centuries in Africa to help relieve joint pain and alleviate the symptoms of a range of musculo-skeletal conditions, including arthritis, gout and rheumatism. It is a rich source of both calcium and magnesium to help build muscle tone and skeletal strength, but also contains those extra magic ingredients: silicon, vitamin A, phosphorus, manganese and zinc.

It is one of the agents in the Bastyr Formula A joint support supplement (see page 186) and, in clinical trials, was shown to perform as well as one of the slow-acting conventional drugs prescribed to treat osteoarthritis. Patients who use it are also able to cut back on the use of painkillers, including the non-steroid anti-inflammatories (NSAIDs), which can cause gastric bleeding.

The part of the plant used is the tuber, and the primary active agent is an anti-inflammatory glycoside called harpagoside, so if you are opting for a supplement offering a standardized extract, this is the ingredient you need to look out for.

The typical dosage is 100mg, twice a day. Although the Bastyr formula contains more (137.5mg), you are not at risk of overdosing if you take a higher dosage. There have been no toxicity reports, although this herb could interfere with the action of blood pressure and antacid medication, so avoid it if you are taking either of those types of prescription drugs.

Native New Zealand Remedies

One of the prized remedies in my bathroom cupboard is a **comfrey** ointment made from both the leaves and the root of the plant (Symphytum officinale). Commonly known as knitbone, the reason I prize it so highly is that in the UK we can no longer buy creams made from the root (see Fixing Broken and Fractured Bones, page 181). I brought this back from one of my trips to New Zealand and am very mean about dishing it out to (literally) bruised family and friends. It is part of the exciting new Kiwiherb range so you can easily buy it if you are either resident or travelling in that part of the world. You can also try to get it direct from the company's website, www.kiwiherb.com.

Also in the same range, the ginger and **kawakawa** tincture can help maintain flexible joints. This is an especially warming winter formula, which will work wonders if you take it diluted in warm water.

What Really Works for Musculo-skeletal Problems

Ankylosing Spondylitis

This is a connective tissue disorder, characterized by painful inflammation of the spine and larger joints, resulting in both stiffness and pain. It is three times more common in men than women and is most likely to first strike between the ages of twenty and forty. It is also up to 20 times more common in people whose parents or siblings have it, suggesting a strong genetic risk.

1, 2, 3 . . . Easy Steps to Help Cope With Ankylosing Spondylitis

Use Nexrutine (see page 212), which has been shown to be more effective than standard non-steroid anti-inflammatory prescription drugs. Mail order from Victoria Health (0800 389 8195; www.victoriahealth.com).

Boost the immune system with cat's claw (100mg daily).

Practise shakti bhandi (see page 237) and simple yoga asanas, such as the crocodile (see page 235), to help keep the spine flexible.

Arthritis

Arthritis – which is really an umbrella term for more than two hundred different joint conditions – is anything but new; archaeologists have found evidence of this disease in the skeletons of Neanderthal man, Maori tribesmen and even dinosaurs.

There are two main forms – osteoarthritis and rheumatoid arthritis – which together will affect an estimated 50 per cent of the population over the age of sixty-five. Osteoarthritis is caused by the physical wear and tear of the connective tissue, especially cartilage, around the joints. This tissue normally retains water to act as a shock absorber, and when damaged can no longer do this. Instead it degrades to leave the bones exposed, resulting in pain, stiffness and swellings.

There is no single cure for arthritis, whatever its form – and what works for one person will not work for another – but avoiding chemicals in your food by switching to an organic diet, and managing the symptoms with a programme of moderate exercise, anti-inflammatory herbs and foods and collagen-building supplements, may help. Lots of people already take a fish oil supplement, which provides omega-3 fatty acids to alleviate stiffness. If you do find relief with these, make sure you are taking a product that comes from an unpolluted source.

1, 2, 3 . . . Easy Steps to Help Relieve Osteoarthritis

Take any of the top three over-the-counter remedies for joint problems, highlighted on page 215.

Boost the immune system with cat's claw (100mg daily) and take cod liver oil or, if you prefer a vegetarian source, flaxseed or borage oil to provide anti-inflammatory essential fatty acids.

Use it or lose it – gentle exercise, combined with deep breathing, has been shown to help stop the wear and tear but you need to be doing the right kind of exercise and maintaining correct alignment. For advice on remedial fitness training, visit www.annthompson.org.

Back and Sciatic Pain

Spiritually, chronic back pain is interpreted as a lack of support in your life. If the lower back is affected, then perhaps the problem lies in a lack of financial support. Whatever the trigger, back pain is now so common, it is the biggest single cause of long-term sick leave from work, and will affect some 40 per cent of all adults at some time in their lives.

1, 2, 3 . . . Easy Steps for Dealing With Chronic Back Pain

Chronic pain in the joints is a sign of degradation and excess uric acid, so take the Lifetime Advanced Joint Formula with the Cherry Fruit Extract as recommended on page 186.

To tackle the pain, take nexrutine (see page 212) alongside the Advanced Joint Formula and use the Drs A–Z Boswellia, Capsicum and Glucosamine cream from Victoria Health (0800 389 8195; www.victoriahealth.com).

For pain caused by trapped nerves, including sciatica, take 500mg of magnesium, which is a muscle relaxant; Nature's Plus (www.naturesplus.com) makes a food state supplement which is better absorbed by the body.

Bruising

Some people bruise more easily than others, thanks to fragile capillaries in the skin. Each time these small blood vessels break, a little blood leaks out, leaving tiny red dots in the skin and bluish-purple bruises. Women are more prone to bruising from minor injuries than men, especially on the thighs, buttocks and upper arms. Older people are especially susceptible to easy bruising after bumps and falls because they have more fragile blood vessels and a thinner layer of fat under the skin, which would normally serve as a cushion to protect against injury.

1, 2, 3 . . . Easy Steps for Treating Bruising

Bashed-up boxers who were given bromelain supplements (see pages 204 and 208) reported faster bruise fading and healing than those with similar lesions who took a placebo pill.

Homeopathic arnica does work, but only if you take it internally and at the right potency (see page 204). Remember, if you are using homeopathic pills, avoid touching them since this can affect their potency. Simply tip the required number of pills into the lid of the bottle and then drop them under your tongue. Do not eat or drink for thirty minutes before taking them, or thirty minutes after.

If you bruise easily, you need to use a topical cream rich in the antioxidant oligomeric proanthocyanidin (OPC) compounds, which work to stabilize the walls of blood vessels and reduce bruising. Clear Vein Cream from the American Derma E range includes grapeskin extract, which is one of the more powerful OPCs. Mail order from Victoria Health on 0800 389 8195; www.victoriahealth.com.

Carpal Tunnel Syndrome/RSI

The carpal tunnel is the passageway through the wrist that protects the nerves and tendons that extend into the hand. The meridian nerve that passes through it is close to nine tendons and if any of these become injured or if the tissues of the tunnel become swollen and inflamed, this nerve will get compressed, causing numbness, tingling and, often, an incredible pain that shoots up and down the arm and is always worse at night.

This is the single most common occupational illness now reported and is always the result of repetitive movements causing repetitive strain injuries (RSI), such as typing on computer key-boards.

1, 2, 3 . . . Easy Steps for Coping With Carpal Tunnel Syndrome

Some sufferers have been shown to be deficient in vitamin B6 and in trials, a number of patients taking 100mg, twice a day, for 12 weeks were able to reduce their intake of painkillers and avoid surgery.

Since this condition is caused by inflammation, you need to take one of those anti-inflammatories highlighted in the Top Ten Natural Remedies to Help with Musculo-skeletal Problems (see page 207).

Take cod liver or flaxseed or borage oil to switch off those enzymes causing continuing inflammation.

Gout

Gout is another form of arthritis, and while we tend to think of it as only affecting older men who have grown too used to the good life, it can strike both sexes as young as thirty.

It is caused by an accumulation of **uric acid** in the blood, urine and tissues. This excess solidifies in the joints to form sharp, needle-shaped crystals, which then jab at the surrounding tissue when the body moves. Inflammation and severe pain may be the first signs of a problem, especially in the big toe where gout is most common. It can, though, also occur in the joints in the middle of the foot, in the ankle or the knee, the thumb, wrist, finger or elbow joints, and even, in chronic cases, in the cartilage tissue of the ear.

It is true that gout is linked to a high consumption of rich and fatty foods, heavy meats and alcohol. The trouble with heavy meats, for example, is that they are rich in substances called purines, which promote the production of uric acid in the body. As well as red meats, sweetbreads and all organ meats, purine-rich foods also include consommé, asparagus, shellfish, mussels, herring and sardines, but vegetarians may be at risk too since yeast products, white flour, sugar, mushrooms, oatmeal, spinach, cauliflower and even lentils can all increase uric acid in the body.

Slimmers are another group at risk because crash and yo-yo dieting, like extended fasting (more than three days), also works to increase the production of uric acid. Gout sufferers have also been found to be lacking in the digestive enzyme uricase, which oxidizes the relatively insoluble uric acid into a highly soluble form to prevent it from crystallizing.

1, 2, 3 . . . Easy Steps to Help Prevent Gout

Celery seed supplements have been shown to have an antiarthritis action in the body. The theory is that this herb can help stop the formation of and accumulation of uric acid in the joints. Celery juice can work the same way but this herb is not an anti-inflammatory, so you will need to take one of those agents (see below) as well.

The bioflavonoid quercetin is an anti-inflammatory agent that has been shown to inhibit the enzyme xanthine oxidase, which triggers the production of uric acid. The therapeutic dosage is 250mg, three times a day. Since vitamin C has been shown to increase urinary excretion of uric acid, too, take Source Naturel's Activated Quercetin, which also contains vitamin C (to mail order, call Revital on 0800 252875; www.revital.com).

Cut out those foods that we know can exacerbate this condition and also switch from dairy to soy milk (dairy contains xanthine oxidase, which we know triggers the production of uric acid).

Osteoporosis

Known as the 'silent' epidemic or killer because bone loss occurs with no symptoms, osteoporosis is the term used to describe a generalized loss of bone in both sexes. Over the age of fifty, one in two women and one in eight men will suffer a fracture linked to loss of bone density.

There are now reckoned to be two types of osteoporosis. Type 1 is linked with a midlife loss of hormones (oestrogen in women; androgen in men) and type II is the inevitable age-related loss of bone density that starts from the age of thirty.

Bone weakness, loss of height and back pain are some of the symptoms that may manifest but, generally, you only know you have this problem when a simple fall results in an osteoporotic fracture or if you have a bone density scan (see Testing, page 205).

1, 2, 3 . . . Important Steps to Help Prevent Osteoporosis

If you are female, take Meno-Herb (Victoria Health: 0800 389 8195; www.victoriahealth.com), which is rich in red clover, which can help slow down bone loss after menopause.

If you are male, take Lifetime's Advanced Joint Formula. Whatever your sex, do some form of weight-bearing exercise to build bone density. Even skipping can help. Just fifty jumps a day can increase bone density by up to 4 per cent.

Supplement your diet with silica in the form of horsetail tincture or tablets. Also vitamin K (45mg a day). Studies of osteoporotic female patients showed they had 75 per cent lower levels of this crucial bone-building nutrient than other women.

Rheumatism

Rheumatoid arthritis is an autoimmune disease in which the synovial membranes in the joints become inflamed, resulting in swelling and pain. This condition affects about 1 per cent of the population; women are affected two or three times more than men. It usually starts first between the ages of twenty-five and fifty, and while most sufferers can rely on treatments to manage their symptoms, in one in ten cases it will become so bad it is deemed disabling.

1, 2, 3 . . . Easy Steps to Help Manage Rheumatoid Arthritis

Take Lifetime's Advanced Joint Formula (page 215), which provides type II collagen to help stop the further deterioration of joints.

Take 50mg of zinc, and boost the immune system with cat's claw (100mg daily).

Take anti-inflammatory fatty acids in the form of cod liver or flaxseed or borage oil; and for pain relief, one of the new generation of natural analgesics, such as nexrutine, bromelain or boswellia (see pages 212 and 208).

Shoulder Injuries – Including Frozen Shoulder

Six out of ten people who start working out drop out in the first six weeks because of an injury. Since the shoulder joint will always sacrifice its stability for motility, it is one of the more common sites of such accidental injury, caused by damage and subsequent swelling of the muscles and tendons that hold the upper arm in the shoulder joint.

1, 2, 3 . . . Easy Steps to Help Deal With Shoulder Pain

Turmeric is the anti-inflammatory agent that is specific to shoulder problems; Pukka Herbs (08456 585858; www.pukkaherbs.com) now do an excellent organic Ayurvedic turmeric joint formulation.

Find a Bowen Technique practitioner who has experience of shoulder injuries (to learn more about this technique, visit my website, www.whatreallyworks.co.uk, and to find a practitioner, contact Bowtech: www.bowen-technique.co.uk).

To relieve the pain, take anti-inflammatory essential fatty acids in the form of cod liver, flaxseed or borage oils and use Lifetime's StopPain, a topical analgesic spray that includes glucosamine, boswellia and MSM. Not for the fainthearted, the shock of the cold you will feel when you spray it on the affected body part will take your mind off your underlying pain. (Mail order from Victoria Health: 0800 389 8195; www.victoriahealth.com.)

Roll Out Your Yoga Mat

You don't need to be a rocket scientist to understand that any system of postural patterning that has the effect of strengthening and keeping joints active is going to pay dividends in terms of keeping flexible and mobile in later life. But just in case you need convincing, here are just a handful of reported results from clinical trials that put yoga to the test for the relief of a number of musculo-skeletal conditions, including osteoarthritis and carpal tunnel syndrome.

For instance, when researchers monitored improvements brought about by yoga exercises in patients suffering from osteoarthritis in the hands, they found those practising supervised yoga for eight weeks showed a better range of finger movement and less pain and tenderness than those who suffered the same condition but had no therapy at all.

Similarly, when patients with carpal tunnel syndrome who practised yoga postures and relaxation, again for two months, were compared with sufferers who simply relied on the use of a splint, those in the yoga group showed significant improvement in grip strength and pain reduction when compared with the splint control group.

Astonishingly, even simple yoga postures such as the prayer greeting, Namaste (which you can do at both the front and back of the body), can help rebuild musculo-skeletal strength and flexibility in those parts of the body that are engaged in moving into and holding the posture.

Here are my **1, 2, 3 best yoga postures** for the spine and joints.

In its true sense, yoga was only ever employed to help strengthen the spine and maintain its flexibility so that the yogic practitioner could sit comfortably for long hours in meditation. And it is perhaps ludicrous to imagine you can highlight just three asanas (from more than 840,000 poses; of which eighty-four are the most important) as being better than any of the others. What I want to do here is show how relatively simple asanas will work to build that strength and flexibility which is as important for everyday life as it is for meditation.

Makarasana (Crocodile Pose)

Nothing could be simpler or more relaxing for the spine than this easy posture, which is designed to relieve tension from the spine, especially the lower back. Of course, as with all forms of exercise, you will get out of this asana what you put into it. You could adopt the pose and then lie there watching television, but you will derive more health benefits if, once you are in position, you close your eyes and move your awareness slowly up the spine, starting from the base. Imagine you are relaxing every single vertebra and imagine that your breath is moving slowly up the spine as you relax it.

To get into the posture, lie on your stomach on your yoga mat, allowing your legs to stretch out behind you. Raise the head and shoulders and rest the chin in the palms of your hands, propping yourself up on your elbows.

If you feel tension in the neck, your elbows are too close together, so widen the space between them. If you feel tension in the lower back, you have your elbows too close to the chest, so move them away.

Once you are comfortable, close your eyes and practise relaxing the spine.

Hold this posture for as long as you feel comfortable, and when you finish, counter by folding the body forward into the pose of the child, then rest.

Namaste (Prayer Posture)

Bring both hands to the front of the chest. Bend the elbows. Push the palms together in the prayer position and bring the hands, in this posture, into the sternum. This looks just like praying, except you have your elbows out to the sides and are pressing the palms together to create resistance and make it an active posture.

This is namaste, an everyday greeting in India, which means 'I honour the higher self in you'.

Again, you will only get out of this practice what you put

in. You need to keep the palms pushing against each other to help strengthen the wrists and shoulder joints.

Now try to do the same thing behind your back. This is much more of a strain on both the wrists and shoulders. You will need to keep the spine straight and the chest open to achieve it.

Again, hold this position only for as long as the body feels comfortable and do not use any force or strain.

Shakti Bhandi Pawanmuktasana (anti-arthritic exercises)

These joint exercises may not have the wow factor in a busy yoga class but they are critical for helping to keep joints moving (in the right way) and flexible. You can use them to warm up for other postures, but just because they don't look as impressive, don't think that doesn't make them as valuable as those more advanced and convoluted postures – if not more.

You will run through all these exercises sitting on your mat. Try to keep the spine erect and try not to race through each exercise just to get on to something that looks more like yoga. Try not to move any muscles other than those involved in each exercise. If you do these practices with awareness, you will find they also generate rejuvenating feelings of deep inner tranquillity and stillness.

Toe bending

You are going to start this series of anti-arthritic exercises with simple toe bending. As you sit, become aware of your musculo-skeletal system: your bones, your skeleton, your muscles, your ligaments, and how these body parts move in relation to each other. Take your awareness to your toes and, one foot at a time, simply bend your toes backwards and forwards. Do this slowly, 10 times on each foot.

Foot bending

Now do the same thing with the whole foot. Again, bend each foot backwards and then forwards again. Count 10 forward and backward bends for each foot. Concentrate on your breathing, on the muscles you are using and on keeping the rest of the body still.

Ankle rotation

Now part the legs a little to give you the space to rotate both ankles in first one direction (10 rotations) and then the other. Drop back to 5 rotations if your ankles are very stiff and this is too demanding for you. Again, do this exercise slowly and deliberately, with awareness. Now, slowly rotate both ankles, again at the same time but this time in opposite directions. Aim for 5 or 10 rotations, depending on how stiff these joints feel.

Ankle cranking

To rotate the ankle this time, you are going to bring your foot up towards the top of the thigh of the opposite leg and cradle it with your hands. It sounds brutal but is actually very comforting. Take hold of the ankle with one hand and the toes of that foot with the other and gently rotate the ankle, first one way (10 times), then the other. This is the same rotation as above but this time your hands are doing the rotating. After 10 rotations in each direction, swap ankles.

Knee swings

Ever since a yogi told me this exercise worked to draw more synovial fluid into the space around the knee joints, I have practised it every day. Staying in the sitting position, with your spine erect, bend the knee of your right leg and bring it into the body. Release it out straight again, hold it straight for a second or two and bring it back into the body. Repeat 10 times, then do the same with the other leg. I think of this as being similar to the knee swings you did as a kid when you sat on chairs that left your feet dangling above the floor.

Knee cranking

This time, you are going to rotate the lower leg from the knee. If it helps, imagine how the joint is working to do this. Again, rotate one leg 10 times in one direction and 10 in the opposite direction before switching to the other leg. Keep the rest of the body still and your bottom firmly on the yoga mat. The knee joint supports the whole weight of the upper body but has no strong muscles to help it do this. This rotation helps build strength into the muscles and ligaments around these important joints.

Half butterfly

Here you need to bring the foot as high up the opposite leg as you can. If you know what a half-lotus position looks like, aim for that, but do not strain. Once you are comfortable with the foot up on the opposite leg, gently push the knee of that raised leg down towards the floor. It is important that you do not force the knee down. Instead, think about allowing it to release down from the hip, which is the joint you are now working with. Once you feel comfortable with the motion, allow the leg to 'rock' up and down. Repeat on the other side.

Hip rotation

Keeping the leg in the same position as above, now take your awareness to your hip, and using the muscles in your arm, rotate the right knee in as large a circle as you can. Again, you are moving the knee to rotate the ball and socket joint of the hip. You must do this slowly, with awareness and, again, avoid using force or straining to complete the rotation. Keep in mind what you are trying to achieve: a release and rotation of each hip.

Full butterfly

To complete your session of working your ankle, knee and hip joints, you are going to bring the soles of your feet together and allow the hips to open out and the knees to fall out to the sides. If you are a beginner or have stiff joints, gently allow the knees to release down to the ground and back up again. If you are more experienced, gently bounce the knees to the floor and back again.

Hand clenching

We are now moving on to the wrist, elbow, shoulder and neck joints. Remain sitting on your mat with your spine straight and your legs stretched out in front of you. Stretch both arms out too, keeping them strong and straight. Now work the joints in the hands by clenching your fingers into a fist and releasing them. Allow the fingers to make a fist round the thumb and really stretch each one as you release. Breathe in as you open the hands and breathe out as you close them again.

Wrist bending

Remember how we bent the toes and the ankles? Now we're going to do the same with the wrists. Again, work slowly and do not race through the practice. Keep your movements strong and deliberate. Bend the hands upwards and imagine you are pressing a wall with the palms; now drop the hands down and point the fingers to the floor. Repeat 10 times with both hands together and keep the fingers straight throughout the practice.

Wrist rotation

This time we are working one wrist at a time. Keep the arms and elbows still and simply rotate the hand from the wrist, 10 times in a clockwise direction and then 10 times anticlockwise, before switching to the other hand. Keep your arms strong and stretched out at shoulder height and keep your movements slow and deliberate.

Elbow bending

This is as simple as it sounds and is a good counter practice for having held your arms outstretched through the preceding exercises. Keeping both arms stretched out, tip the palm up towards the ceiling and bring both arms in towards the body. Touch each shoulder with your fingertips and stretch the arms out again. Repeat 10 times. Breathe in as you straighten the arms out and breathe out as you bend them back in again. Remember, you are working the elbow joints.

Shoulder socket rotation

We do this exercise one arm at a time. Keep your fingertips resting on each shoulder joint and make a rotation of your right arm, using the elbow to make as big a circle as you can. Rotate 10 times in one direction and then 10 in the other before switching to the other arm. As you rotate, close your eyes and become aware of how big and how strong the shoulder joint really is. This asana can relieve muscle tension and strains incurred from spending the day in front of the computer screen and will also build strength back into the shoulder joints following inflammation or injury.

Neck movements

If you make time for no other yoga practice in this book (or any other), make time for these movements, which relieve both physical and mental tension faster than anything I can think of.

Keeping the rest of your body still and your spine straight, slowly release your chin down onto your chest. Really think about the muscles and bones in the neck that are moving to allow you to do this. Now, slowly take the weight of the head backwards and feel the stretch along your throat. Only take the head back as far as you feel comfortable and do not strain. Repeat this action 5 times forward and 5 times back.

Now you will be feeling more connected to your neck. Keeping your chin parallel to the floor (in other words, don't drop it for this exercise), slowly turn your head to the right, back to the centre, to the left and back to the centre again. This counts as one round. Do 5. Close your eyes and keep your awareness on maintaining a straight neck.

Neck rotation

This last exercise will take you as close to heaven as anything I can think of that you can do in a quiet room on your own. If you know your neck is strong, simply release the chin to the chest as before but this time, allow the neck to sweep across the top of the body to the right and up to the top of the right shoulder. Release back to the centre and do the same thing to the left side of the body.

If you have a stiff neck or have not practised this before, you must raise the shoulders into a hunch position before you do it. This then acts as a cushion to keep your neck safe as you start to build strength back into all those tiny joints.

Once you feel comfortable with this side-to-side sweeping

action, rotate the neck 360 degrees, all the way round on its axis, moving first in a clockwise direction and then reversing it.

When I feel I cannot take any more of the outside world and its demands, this is the yoga posture I use to recentre myself, shut all that nonsense out and relieve all the tension that has crept into my back and shoulders, but especially my neck, during the day.

Try it. It really is bliss.

PART TWO

CHAPTER FIVE

Stress and Immunity

In this second part of the book, we start to look at those conditions that are more difficult to define and which, previously, might have been dismissed as being 'all in the mind'. The single most damaging of all these is the one you may not even realize you are suffering from until something else, something tangibly physical, goes wrong. I am talking, of course, about **stress**.

What Is Stress?

Like you need me to tell you!

If you think about it, stress is not a condition at all, but an experience, i.e. your experience of tension. In other words, if you feel it (stress), then you have it, and what is important is not the stressful event itself but how you and your body respond to and handle it.

This explains why factors that may stress one person will not stress another, and why circumstances that did not stress you yesterday may become serious stressors tomorrow. In other words, stress is not only accumulative, it is also, for most of us, a movable feast.

As long ago as 1974, Canadian researcher Dr Hans Seyle, then professor and director of the Institute of Experimental Medicine and Surgery at the University of Montreal, and author of a book called *Stress Without Distress*, explained: 'The word stress, like success, failure or happiness, means different things to different people.'

There are lots of telltale signs of stress creeping up but the two that should convince you that you need to do something to reduce the amount of stress in your life are (a) excessive sweating and (b) waking up in the wee small hours at night and being unable to get back to sleep.

Excess sweating is always a sign of **adrenal glands** under pressure – when the body experiences chronic stress, these glands pump out excess cortisol, the stress hormone that also plays a role in the metabolism of carbohydrates and the regulation of blood sugar levels. The other three major stress hormones are adrenaline, dehydroepiandrosterone (DHEA)* and norepinephrine, and in good health, levels of all four are naturally higher in the morning and lower in the evening.

When stress becomes prolonged and chronic, levels may remain too high all day. Cortisol also has an immunosuppressive effect in the body so this is not a hormone you want circulating in the bloodstream when you do not need it. Also, when stress goes on and on, the adrenal glands will become so overworked they can

---

* DHEA supplements are sold over-the-counter in America but banned in Europe. Use with caution since reported adverse reactions include causing acne, hair loss, voice deepening and insulin resistance (see Syndrome X, page 122).

no longer pump out normal levels of any of the stress hormones, including cortisol (see page 253).

What this all means is that supporting these triangular-shaped glands, which sit on top of the kidneys, must be the place to start with any holistic approach to reducing stress levels (see page 268). This may also necessitate important lifestyle changes, since smoking, poor nutritional choices, alcohol and drug abuse can all contribute to adrenal failure.*

How Stress Creeps Up On Us

We often talk about stress as something insidious which has us in its grip before we quite realize it, and the reason for that is that when we first start to experience stress, the body has no problem adapting to it. Lots of people thrive on and respond well to more pressure and, in fact, we can seemingly cope with stress for quite long periods of time without appearing to suffer. That is because the damage that is taking place when the stress goes on and on is, mostly, hidden.

There are three very distinct phases of stress, and if you recognize yourself as being in any one of these, now is the time to act. Do not think that because you are still in the first phase, you are safe. You will not stay in this 'alarmed . . . but still coping' phase for ever. Unless you reduce the impact of the stressors in your life, it is inevitable you will move into the more harmful adaptive (resistant) and, finally, exhaustive phases described (with their consequences) below.

* Addison's Disease is a serious autoimmune condition, characterized by adrenal failure; with the proper medical supervision, sufferers can enjoy a normal life expectancy, but clearly this is not a condition to try to self-treat.

Alarm Phase . . . the First Few Hours

Regardless of what is causing your stress, your initial reaction will always be the same. This response, which occurs within the first six to eight hours of a stressor, is known as the alarm phase, and here is what happens in your body: the activity of your sympathetic fight-or-flight nervous system becomes heightened, the adrenal glands enlarge, levels of the stress hormone cortisol increase, but the weight of the thymus, spleen and lymph nodes actually decrease.

Resistance (Adaptive) Phase . . . the Next Few Days

If the stressor and your experience of stress continues over the next two or three days, your body will move into the second resistance phase. You will recognize this – it feels as if the mind is willing but the body is dragging itself. That does not mean you will not get to the end of your long 'to-do' list; you will, but only by gritting your teeth and calling on sheer bloody-mindedness and willpower. What happens internally is that all those changes that occurred so rapidly in the alarm phase become 'the norm'. Your body adapts and remains in this state of optimal adaptation so your adrenals remain enlarged and levels of stress hormones stay high. Your body starts to think this is normal.

Exhaustive Phase . . . Weeks or Months of On-going Stress

This is the one we often call burn-out, and if you have ever got this far, you will know that stress is not for wimps but can bring grown men and women to their knees. This happens when the stressor continues and, having survived the resistance phase, the body can no longer maintain its adaptive survival mechanism. Those organs that change during the alarm phase will become damaged and willpower alone will not be enough to keep you on your feet. It is critical, if you have already reached this phase, that you now get help and support and find some way to cut down on the stress in your life.

Even if you would like to insist that stress is solely emotional in its origin, you have to accept, because science can prove it, that the body reacts to physical, electromagnetic, chemical, nutritional and microbial stress in the exact same manner – with the excessive release of the stress hormones, overactivity of the nervous system and depletion of energy reserves described above; all of which cause a great deal of wear and tear on the body, leaving it, unless the stress and the body's reaction is managed, less well able to adapt and cope with the next (inevitable) stressful event.

This is where natural remedies, especially **adaptogens**, really do come into their own; for less than the cost of a good meal out, you can buy and use one of the adaptogenic herbal supplements that really will work to protect the body from the worst ravages of stress.

Adaptogens . . . What Are They?

The term 'adaptogen' was first used by Russian scientists in the 1940s, who defined them as: 'Substances designed to put the organism into a state of non-specific, heightened response in order to better resist stresses and adapt to extraordinary challenges.'

Understanding what happens as the body moves into a

permanent state of stress is important because it helps explain how **adaptogens** really work – they cannot stop the stress that is causing you problems, of course, but they change how the body copes by reducing its reactions during the initial alarm phase and delaying the transition from the second, resistant or adaptive phase through to total exhaustion and burnout.

The most widely studied of all the adaptogens to date are the **ginsengs** (see page 280), which have been shown in both animals and humans to help prevent the internal changes that occur during the first few hours of the alarm phase of stress. None of these herbs are ones to use every day but only when you know times are about to get more stressful and when your system needs extra support. **Astragalus** (page 276), for instance, will bolster the immune system, while **schisandra** (page 283) has been shown to help support adrenal functioning in patients undergoing both chemo- and radiotherapy treatments. **Tribulus terrestris** is the adaptogen-of-choice for men who want to improve performance (in and out of bed, as it happens) but if you plan to take a supplement, make sure it is made from the leaves of herbs that have been harvested in Bulgaria, and not cheaper, less potent imitations.

The One to Watch – Rhodiola

According (again) to Russian research on stressed-out students chewing their fingernails and tearing their hair out at exam time, the best stress-busting herb, especially when you need to crank up for the performance of a lifetime, is **rhodiola,** an adaptogenic herb that enhances the body's physical and mental work capacity and productivity. In placebo-controlled, double-blind, randomized trials (and they don't come much more scientific than that) students who took the herb for twenty days outperformed those taking a placebo, were less fatigued and reported higher levels of well-being.

In Siberia, it is said that if you drink rhodiola tea every day of your life you will live to 100. In Mongolia, it is used as a cancer treatment. Brewing a tea is a chore for most of us and thankfully the herb is now available here in supplement form on sale in good independent health stores. Take the equivalent of 50mg, twice a day, but do not use this herb if you are pregnant or breastfeeding your child. This herb is also an excellent mood booster since it works to disable the enzyme that would otherwise be breaking down serotonin, the body's own feel-good brain chemical.

Tried and Applied

Social isolation has now been clearly linked with poor survival rates in patients with coronary artery disease (CAD). In a survey of over 400 cardiac patients, researchers found those with three or fewer people in their social support network had a mortality rate that was twice as high as those with more friends.

What Happens When Stress Goes On . . .

. . . and on . . . and on?

We have looked at the psychological definition of stress, now for the physiological one: it is that state where the body is expending energy faster than it can be regenerated.

In Chapter 7 (Energy and Fatigue) we explore further how natural remedies can help rebuild energy levels. Here, I want to introduce a novel idea about what happens in animals when the stress goes on and on and on, and suggest the same could be true for humans too.

When we experience chronic stress, the body responds by producing excessive levels of the hormone cortisol from the adrenal glands. This can then result in a catch-22 situation, because although cortisol is one of the anti-inflammatory stress hormones that can help the body to better cope with stress, when we produce too much, it can actually work to suppress the immune system and thus reduce our natural defences to sickness, disease and – ironically – stress. Also, the continued, increased production of cortisol triggered by chronic stress will result in exhausted adrenals, which can no longer pump out this hormone, causing an eventual deficiency.

American veterinary surgeon Dr Alfred Plechner has written several thought-provoking articles about a condition he calls Common Variable Immunodeficiency (CVID) in dogs, which, he suggests, could be relevant to their owners too since they can also suffer from this syndrome. His theory is that the reason chronic stress underlies most diseases is because it leads to an eventual decrease in the production of the stress hormone cortisol by the adrenal glands; a deficiency which then has the knock-on effect of causing a hormonal imbalance where oestrogen levels rise and where the chain reaction to this includes a disruption to thyroid functioning, a slowdown of the metabolic rate and, again, suppression of the immune system. In other words, too little cortisol will adversely affect the immune system in the same way as too much cortisol; hence the catch-22.

Dr Plechner reports: 'In thousands of cases – now well over 50,000 – I have repeatedly observed the same endocrine-immune dysfunction operating in dogs. It undermines homeostasis and sets the stage for malabsorption and digestive disorders, allergies, lung and urinary tract problems, sluggish liver function, strange or aggressive behaviour, epilepsy, obesity, deadly viral and bacterial infections, periodontitis, vaccine reactions, autoimmune problems and cancer.'

This theory may not yet be proven (and will not be, until someone decides to test it) in humans, but it does nicely fit the holistic model, which refuses to separate body parts and systems, and recognizes that they are all inextricably linked. It also reflects the theory that the adrenal gland is the endocrine organ (for more on which, including the thyroid, see Chapter 8) that is most vulnerable to damage by stress and toxins, and that disturbances to this important part of the body can fundamentally and adversely affect the whole body's physiology and bio-chemistry.

Stress and Your Sex

Women cope better with stress for the simple reason they know how to ask for help . . . and how to give it.

According to American researchers reporting their findings in the journal *Psychological Review*, the females of many species, including humans, react differently to stress than males. While the latter will adopt an aggressive fight-or-flight response, or simply withdraw altogether from a stressful encounter, females facing stressful conditions will first seek to protect their young (the so-called 'tend response') and then seek social contact and support from others (the so-called 'befriend response').

Both men and women secrete a hormone called oxytocin in response to stress. This is the same hormone that helps women cope with childbirth, and we now know that both animals and people with higher levels of oxytocin are calmer, more relaxed, more social and less anxious than those with lower levels.

What leaves men at a disadvantage relative to women in terms of coping with stress is that while the calming effects of this hormone are enhanced in the presence of the female hormone oestrogen, they are reduced in the presence of the male hormone testosterone.

According to researchers, this fact, coupled with the female tend-and-befriend response, could account for why women generally live longer than men, and why good social connections increase longevity too. In other words, they help one sex cope better than the other with stress, which has an accumulatively adverse effect in the body.

The Immune System

You cannot talk about stress, or any other condition, including cancer, without thinking about the immune system. In fact, in addition to those problems defined as autoimmune diseases (see Chronic Fatigue Syndrome, page 362, Chapter 7), you can blame virtually every other severe and chronic health condition you can think of on some degree of immune dysfunction.

Your immune system accounts for approximately 1 per cent of your body's 100 trillion cells but what marks immune cells out as being so extraordinary is the fact they are not confined to a single space or organ, but are mobile units able to travel and act at sites far from their origin in the bone marrow.

Immune system cells mature in the thymus (see Cell-mediated Immunity, page 263) spleen and lymph glands, and while there are different types of immune cells, they all share the common goal of seeking out and destroying those substances, dead or alive, that should not be present in the body.

In essence, the immune system has a three-fold brief:

- To recognize substances which are foreign to the body;
- To respond quickly enough with a counterattack to neutralize any invader;
- To remember previous invasions so that, if the same thing happens again, the response time is even faster.

To achieve this, the immune system and its component parts must function as a highly complex information super-highway, comprised of the cells and organs detailed above, but also biochemical messenger substances known as cytokines and neuropeptides. Together, all these parts must maintain a healthy state of dynamic equilibrium to enable the immune system to respond rapidly and adjust to an ever-changing environment.

The premise of any natural healing is that you cannot embark on a treatment regimen for any chronic health condition which ignores the critical role of an immune system that may need rebuilding; and that to keep the body's natural defences strong and healthy, you need to be aware of what lifestyle factors, avoidable and unavoidable, will cause it the most damage.

There are, in no particular order, five things that will do most harm to your body's defences and weaken its ability to protect you. The most important of these (since it is probably the hardest to address) is stress, which we have already looked at, but here is the full list.

Stress We have already seen how prolonged stress will compromise your immune system. The B vitamins are known as nature's own stress-busters, and while the most important of these is vitamin B5 (panthothenic acid), which is crucial for adrenal function (see page 248), all the B vitamins are synergistic and work best when taken together, so take a good B-complex supplement and turn to page 277 (Top Ten Natural Remedies) for advice on other natural remedies that will help the body maintain its natural defences and better counter stress.

Infection Ever wondered why some people are prone to repeated fungal or thrush infections while others, whose bodies carry the exact same micro-organisms responsible for these infections, never suffer any kind of nasty rash? The reason for repeated infections of any kind is a weakened immune system; see my 1, 2, 3 . . . Easy Steps (page 298) for advice on boosting the immune system to eliminate, and prevent, these types of recurring health problems.

Trauma (including medical treatments) When researchers questioned almost 300 volunteers about the stresses in their lives and then inoculated them with the common cold virus, they found those who had been severely stressed for over a month by major events, such as unemployment or, conversely, too much work responsibility, were the most at risk of disease. Family problems and trouble with friends also increased the risk, as did smoking cigarettes, having trouble sleeping and a low vitamin C intake (see page 277). The fact is, anything you perceive as being traumatic will have a negative effect on your immune system, and the longer the stressor goes on, the worse its impact.

Toxins (environmental and dietary) One of the most overworked organs in your body is your liver, which has to detoxify every toxic chemical you take in. Your mind may consider a food-colouring ingredient a perfectly acceptable molecule to ingest with your lunch, but to your liver this is a toxin that will have to be cleared out. The reason the liver has an impact on the immune system is that, if it has become overburdened dealing with a daily onslaught of dietary and environmental toxins, it will be less efficient at processing the stress hormones the body pumps out, which means stress hormones will stay in the bloodstream longer than needed, providing enough time for their negative effects to kick in. Cortisol, for instance, which is pumped out by the adrenal glands, has an immunosuppressing effect when it hangs around for too long in the bloodstream.

Nutritional deficiencies The immune system is highly prone to free-radical damage. Free radicals are those unstable and highly reactive lone molecules that are the normal by-product of metabolic processes. Foods that produce the greatest numbers of damaging free radicals include fried and junk foods, and while antioxidant nutrients can help counter this, if you are deficient in any of these, including vitamins A, C, E and the trace mineral selenium, you will not be getting the protection you need.

We may now know a lot more about the immune system than previous generations did – knowledge about how your body's natural defences work is reckoned to double every five years – but the truth is that there is a lot we still do not know. The science of immunology is relatively young, and, compared to the knowledge that is still to come, what we know today could be written, metaphorically, on a postage stamp.

To future generations, whose understanding of the body's natural defences will be as refined as the system itself, the assertions that we make today will seem crude and basic. We are only at the beginning of our understanding, which is just one reason why it is right that we should, for example, continue the UK debate on the triple vaccination of our children, whose immune systems are not even mature until the age of fourteen. (For more on this controversy and advice on what to do, whether you have vaccinated or not, or remain undecided, see my previous book, *What Really Works for Kids – The Insider's Guide to Natural Health for Mums & Dads*.)

The Lymphatic System

A crucial component of the immune system, this has to be one of the most overlooked and ignored of all the body's secret workings – that is until, of course, something goes wrong with some part of it. The lymphatic system includes the lymph vessels and nodes, the tonsils, adenoids, appendix, spleen and thymus gland: all organs and tissues that provide much of the body's natural defences to sickness and disease.

Lymph vessels carry lymph fluid, which contains all types of toxins and waste, from the body's tissues and organs to the veins under the collarbones, where this fluid then enters the bloodstream. This waste is eventually filtered out of the body by the liver and kidneys. Unlike the circulatory system, the lymphatic system has no pump to move its fluid around, which means it is entirely dependent on movement and exercise.

According to American exercise specialists, the single best form of exercise for encouraging healthy lymph flow is any movement that combines muscle movement with deep breathing. (Again, think yoga.) Muscle movement effectively squeezes the lymph vessels to shift lymph fluid towards the subclavian veins close to the heart, and deep breathing squeezes the lymphatic thoracic duct, which dumps most of the body's lymph into the bloodstream.

The single most effective movement for encouraging lymph flow is rebounding – jumping or jogging on a mini-trampoline. All the rage in the early 1990s, this fitness fad may have had its day in trendy gyms, but the sheer fact of being propelled into a state of weightlessness at the top of the bounce and then landing with twice the force of gravity creates hydraulic pressure that moves these lymphatic fluids more effectively around the body. Plus, it's great fun. Do not, though, be tempted by cheap rebounders that can do more harm than good by jarring joints. Instead, save up for one from Wholistic Research (01707 262686), a UK company that specializes in these and other health-promoting devices.

Natural Killer Cells

The immune system is both complex and sophisticated but one critical aspect that we know we can easily bolster using natural remedies are those cells known as the natural killer (NK) cells. These protect us from both virally infected cells and cancer cells, and represent the body's last line of defence.

These are, in effect, large white blood cells or lymphocytes that circulate in the blood, where they account for up to 22 per cent of all the circulating white blood cells, and their name – natural killer – reflects their ability to selectively seek out and destroy a wide range of abnormal cells. I think of them as the immune system's equivalent to the army's special SAS or paratrooper forces: an elite defence mechanism, designed to outwit even the most cunning enemy invader.

In organs where there is a continual onslaught from toxins, especially the liver, levels of NK cells are twice as high (some

45 per cent of all those immune cells present in liver tissue, for example, will be NK cells). What is extraordinary about these cells is that not only are they capable of rapid responses to the signals of attack, they appear to be able to coordinate their own counterattacks even when the rest of the immune system is, effectively, switched off or looking the other way.

The Other One to Watch – BioBran

BioBran, a Japanese product which is sold as MGN3 in the United States, is a patented formula of rice bran, broken down using enzymes from immune-boosting shiitake mushroom extract. In trials, this food supplement, now supported by the Bristol Cancer Help Centre, has been shown to bolster every single critical component of the immune system but especially the production of the cancer-killing NK cells, whose activity increased by 300 per cent.

Nobody knows precisely how this works but the theory is that BioBran triggers an increased production of cytokines, the body's messenger proteins that stimulate the immune system and inhibit virus replication and cancer proliferation. In new test-tube studies by immunologists at the Drew University of Medicine and Science in Los Angeles, researchers also demonstrated that BioBran increases the effectiveness of chemotherapy too.

When multi-drug-resistant tumour cells were exposed to the chemotherapy drug Adriamycin, the killing dose could be reduced from 25mg to just 7mg if the researchers added BioBran. Nobody is claiming this is a cure for cancer but the consensus is that this could mean doctors could give lower doses of chemotherapy to induce the same level of cancer cell death. Also, unlike other immune boosters, BioBran does not cause 'hypo-responsiveness' where there is an immediate significant improvement that then tails off over time.

It is non-toxic, remains effective over long-term use and in further trials has been shown to increase the lifespan of terminally ill patients by almost 60 per cent. In the study, over two hundred patients with a variety of terminal cancers were monitored over eighteen months; those given BioBran (MGN3) recorded a 59.9 per cent survival rate, while those on conventional therapies alone recorded 33.9 per cent. Again, please remember this does not make this supplement a cancer cure. What it may do is help a cancer patient survive a little longer than expected.

In the UK, BioBran is available from the Really Healthy Company on 020 8480 1000 (www.healthy.co.uk). If you are well but want to give your immune system a boost, the maintenance dose is 250mg a day; for support during cancer therapies, patients need a start-up dose of 3g a day for two months before cutting back to 1g a day. Unfortunately, this is a costly exercise. At the time of going to print, the price of just 30 x 1g sachets in the UK was £105. You can also get this supplement direct from the US maker, LaneLabs-USA Inc; for more information visit www.lanelabs.com.

The Thymus Gland and Cell-mediated Immunity

The thymus gland is one of the major players in the immune system and, in effect, determines the health of this whole system. Located at the front of the chest, under the breastbone, it lies just below the thyroid gland and just above the heart. It is strongly linked with the adrenal glands (see page 248) and makes at least seven different thymic hormones of its own, low levels of which are associated with suppressed immunity and an increased risk of infection.

Critically, the thymus produces the immune system's T-lymphocytes, those white blood cells that are responsible for **cell-mediated immunity** – in other words, all those aspects of immunity not controlled or mediated by antibodies. This is the crucial built-in part of the immune system that is important in fighting off all manner of conditions, from repeated fungal and viral infections, such as herpes, to autoimmune problems including allergies and rheumatoid arthritis. Cell-mediated immunity also plays a role in protecting us from cancer, which tells you just how important it is. Repeated infections (see page 298) are a sign that this aspect of your immune system is working under par and needs supporting; so too are everyday health problems such as hay fever and migraines.

Although its activity declines naturally with age, the thymus can be easily rejuvenated with the use of thymus extracts, which you can buy over the counter in health stores. Thymus (and other gland) extracts used in supplements are usually taken from lambs and calves, or sheep and cow embryos, and while I personally always prefer, where possible, to use a plant substitute,* this type of cell therapy is anything but new and is simply the modern version of a long-established technique, where animal tissues from organs as diverse as monkey testicles and tiger sex glands have all been used in traditional rejuvenating medicines for humans.

Cell therapy was first popularized by the world-famous Clinique La Prairie in Montreux, Switzerland, where suspensions of cells from the various organs of sheep foetuses were given, via

---

* New Chapter's Host Defence medicinal mushroom supplement, which combines the maitake, reishi and cordyceps Asian mushrooms, can help support the thymus. For details, visit www.newchapter.info. The body also needs zinc, vitamin B6 and vitamin C to make the thymic hormones; see A–Z of Stress-Busting and Immune-Supporting Foods (page 285) for ideas on how to get more of these nutrients in your daily diet.

intra-muscular injection, to humans for the sole purpose of repairing and rejuvenating corresponding cells.

Today, the use of fresh cells, which is expensive, has been replaced in the mainstream by supplements, for which enthusiastic devotees make many anecdotal claims of improvement in symptoms caused by conditions as varied as osteoarthritis (see page 227) and chronic fatigue (page 362), and there are now companies, which have their roots in agriculture, making tissue extract products to meet this renewed demand for cell therapy.

The Spleen

The fist-sized, spongy spleen is the largest lymphatic organ in the body. For centuries, physicians believed the spleen had no real role to play.

Today, we know it plays an important role in the reticuloendothelial system (RES), which is that portion of the immune system responsible for filtering blood and signalling other parts of the defence mechanism.

I always think of the spleen as the body's housekeeper because, as well as acting as a blood reservoir for the storage of red blood cells, it has a major 'mopping up' role in the body, where, as well as producing white blood cells, it has to engulf and destroy invading bacteria and cellular debris and get rid of worn-out red blood cells and platelets.

Practitioners of traditional Chinese medicine (TCM) pay far more close regard to the spleen and its workings than western doctors, and will use both acupuncture and herbal medicine to bolster the physical and energetic workings of this lymph organ.

It's All In the Imagination . . . Right?

Wrong. Psychoneuroimmunology is the science of the impact of the mind on the immune system. True, if immunology is still in its infancy, then psychoneuroimmunology is a premature baby, but that does not mean we should ignore this fascinating field, which I believe will become ever more relevant, especially to natural healers.

Researchers have shown, for example, how the stress of hospitalization effectively down-regulates the immune response of chemotherapy patients even before treatment has begun; in other words, the very act of being taken to a place of sickness increases your risk of sickness before the doctors lay a finger on you. (Natural remedies that can help support the patient and the immune system through the stress of medical treatments include BioBran, page 262, and the Chinese herb schisandra, page 283.)

Stressful events can even take their toll on the elite troops of the immune system: the natural killer cells (page 261). In a study of 116 breast cancer patients who had recently been treated with invasive surgery, clinicians found that the sheer stress of being a cancer patient lowered NK and T-cell activities against specific antibodies, thus decreasing the body's defences against the cancer itself and increasing the risk of the cancer spreading to other sites. And in another study, investigating the link between life stress and colorectal cancer, the researchers found that among over 500 colo-rectal cancer patients, matched with over 500 healthy controls, those that said they had experienced serious and on-going job aggravation in the previous ten years were more than five times as likely to have developed this cancer, compared with those who had no such stress in their history.

What this tells me is that even if stress starts in the mind, it does not stay there, and if you are currently in a stressful job, or any other stressful situation, you have to ask whether the rewards are worth such a serious risk to your health.

The Immune System's Role in Cancer Protection

We now know that a strong immune system is critical in protecting the body against cancer because of the case of two kidney patients who developed melanoma after being given kidneys donated by a woman who had been 'cured' of the disease many years before.

The case, reported in the *New England Journal of Medicine*, told how the donor had had a melanoma lesion removed sixteen years earlier and was believed to have been completely cancer-free. And while she died, at the age of forty-seven, of a brain haemorrhage, the suggestion now is that melanoma cells had lain dormant in her kidneys and had been allowed to flourish after transplant because of the drugs used to suppress the recipient's immune systems in order to prevent rejection of the kidneys. Without a fully functioning immune system to stop it, the dormant cancer was able to reassert itself.

While one of the organ recipients died eighteen months later, the other recovered but the incident was enough to prompt medical researchers to suggest that nobody who had ever suffered from melanoma should be accepted as an organ donor, and that while donor-related cancers remain rare, doctors should check a donor patient's full medical history before accepting organs for transplant.

There are lots of excellent books devoted specifically to natural health and cancer, written by both survivors and clinicians, but if you or your family are looking for more support and advice in the UK, contact the doctor-run Dove Clinic of Integrated Medicine

(01962 718000) or the Bristol Cancer Help Centre Helpline (0117 908 9505).

Tried and Applied

Researchers reporting their findings in the journal *Clinical Infectious Diseases* claim that taking a simple multivitamin supplement each day can boost the immune systems of seniors – men and women over the age of sixty-five – to better protect them from infections and further enhance the action of vaccines in the body. Aim for an intake of selenium (100mcg), zinc (20mg) and vitamin E (200mg) to get the same protective benefits.

Relaxation Techniques . . . Take Your Pick

It doesn't really matter what form of relaxation you introduce into your daily life – from getting a pet to chanting along with a Tibetan singing bowl – as long as you do something.

We saw in the yoga studies I reported in Chapter 3 how active postures *alternated with relaxation practices* had greater health benefits than those same active postures practised alone, but what you need to remember, and what most people forget, is that we all need to learn how to relax.

It can take weeks and sometimes months to learn and fully grasp some of these relaxation techniques, and even when there is a therapist in the room, which means all you have to do is relax, it can be hard to resist the urge to fill the silence with chatter and difficult to really let go; but while this learning-to-relax process will require both effort and commitment from you, the health benefits will be more than worth it.

Unmanaged stress can cause a wide range of physical and emotional disorders ranging from anxiety and depression to headaches, asthma and insomnia. And while you may be able to control environmental stressors (e.g. change a demanding job, end a broken relationship), what is harder to control is your own reaction to prolonged stress, which is where the following relaxation techniques come into their own.

Aromatherapy

If an aromatherapy person approaches with promises to cure you of every ailment you have ever suffered, run fast in the other direction. If, however, you meet one who can explain the value of using essential oils to soothe and calm an overstressed body and mind, book a series of weekly visits and make those trips a priority each week because, in the right hands and with the right – realistic and achievable – goals, aromatherapy is hard to beat on results. To find a qualified therapist who can take the strain of a session while you bliss out, contact the International Federation of Aromatherapists at 4 Eastmearn Road, West Dulwich, London SE21 8HA, and ask for a local referral.

There are lots of excellent books on aromatherapy explaining how you can choose various oils to burn and create different relaxing moods at home, but my basic rule is to follow your own nose and use those oils you find the most soothing. Rose is a real winner, especially if you are feeling depressed, overemotional or are coping with grief, and one of the most uplifting oils I currently use is grapefruit, which I buy in both room-spray and bath-oil form from Ancient Roots (www.ancientroots.com), a UK company specializing in well-being and remedies drawn from ancient healing systems.

Autogenic Training

Too much stress produces too much adrenaline in the body, high levels of which overpower the serotonin that would normally help you get a good night's sleep, so bringing your stress levels under control is important. The technique that has proved the most effective in bringing the disturbed sleep patterns of pilots under control is a technique called Autogenic Training. Said to work at the deepest levels, it alters the body's stress chemistry to encourage deeper relaxation and to reduce anxiety and lower stress levels. Autogenic means 'self-generated' and the technique teaches a series of simple mental exercises that help you to switch off at will.

For more information and to find a practitioner in the UK, contact the British Autogenic Society (020 7383 5108; www.autogenic-therapy.org.uk).

Breathing

I know it sounds daft, because if you weren't breathing you wouldn't be reading this, but by breathing I mean proper breathing and not the shallow, top-of-the-lung inhalations and expirations that most people get by on. Stress triggers shallow, panicky breathing, which will not get a rich supply of oxygen to the body's tissues, and the best way to learn to breathe properly is – again – to find a yoga practitioner who teaches pranayama (the science of breathing) in his or her class.

Chanting

This is not as bonkers as it sounds because words (as you will know if you were ever teased or bullied as a kid) have the power to both wound . . . and heal. Chanting plays an important part in both Sivananda and Vini yoga (see page 51), and the real power of a chant will lie in the words you choose. You can buy chanting tapes with accompanying books to learn to chant yourself or simply play Indian chants as you relax in savasana – the corpse pose (see page 300).

Hypnotherapy

A powerful tool in the right hands and a complete waste of your time and money in the wrong ones, so find a practitioner who has had more than a weekend course by way of training and who specializes in stress management. Some of the new integrated health clinics offer hypnotherapy alongside doctors specializing in complementary medicine. The Integrated Health Partnership in London (020 8332 9265) has pioneered this combined approach, and co-founder Charles Montagu is one of the best hypnotherapy practitioners in town. He specializes in anxiety disorders, including panic attacks and stress.

Incense

The neighbours may think you've gone 21st-century pagan but there is nothing more soothing and meditative than burning your own incense (just be careful not to set off your smoke alarm). You can choose your incense according to smell – let your nose guide you to the one you respond most strongly to – or learn more about how to use different incenses to create different moods. You can even develop the art of blending your own resins to create the effect you want.

Creative Nature is a small UK company that specializes in exotic incense blends from around the world to burn at home and help change your mood. For more information, call 020 8941 7485.

Meditation

When researchers decided to investigate whether a gentle audio-tape meditation session, concentrating on stress reduction, could enhance the effectiveness of ultraviolet phototherapy among psoriasis patients, they found the answer was a resounding yes. Those subjects who listened to the tapes during treatment found their psoriasis cleared more quickly than those who had the light treatment alone.

If you are a psoriasis sufferer, you can ask your holistic health practitioner to make a tape that is specific to you and use this to visualize your skin improving; in fact, you can have a tape made and tailored to any chronic health condition you are currently coping with. What the study reported here tells us is that meditation may start in the mind, but the health benefits do not stay there.

Music

Listening to music will reduce stress levels and any music will do – just as long as it sounds good to you. In Japanese trials, where levels of stress hormones were measured before surgical patients were given anaesthesia, researchers found those who listened to classical music immediately before their operation showed a drop in stress hormones of more than 50 per cent from the baseline. Conversely, patients who did not listen to classical music showed a rise in levels of the same stress hormones of more than 50 per cent.

Doctors have also used music to promote healing and recovery rates after major surgery and studies have again shown that patients in coronary care units, for example, suffer fewer complications, less rapid heartbeats or arrhythmias and fewer problems with blood pressure if they listen to soothing classical music within the first twenty-four hours after surgery. In another trial, premature babies who were sung to every day gained weight faster and left intensive care sooner than those who were not lullabied back to health.

Pets (or, if you're allergic to animals, find a Qi Gong practitioner)

Did you know that a cat's purr can help heal human bones? Many domestic cats purr at a frequency of between 27 and 44 hertz, which, according to scientists at the Fauna Communications Research Institute in North Carolina, exactly matches the frequency that helps human bones strengthen and grow. Cats also purr when they are injured themselves, suggesting there is more to the idea of healing with sound than even the Ancients realized.

Qi Gong healers, measured by scientists at the Beijing Acoustics Institute, have been found to work in much the same way since they emit up to 100 times the level of ultrasonic waves as the average well person, and 1000 times more than people who are sick. The Chinese researchers went on to build a device that replicated the patterns and frequencies of Qi Gong healers for use on people and animals, including horses. For more on their fascinating findings, visit www.chinahealthways.com.

Qi Gong

Talking of Qi Gong, another study showed how HIV-positive patients not only increased their T4 cell counts but also suffered less depression when they agreed to practise Qi Gong meditation for at least three months. This reverses the normal trend for T4 cell counts to drop over time, and Qi Gong, a combination of controlled martial arts and meditation practised by millions of Chinese people to help maintain good health, is clearly a promising enough tool for enhancing the immune system to merit more investigation in the west.

Spiritual Healing and Prayer

You may feel resistant to the idea of any form of relaxation and be tempted to dismiss it all as a load of hippy hype put about by people with nothing better to do than listen to whale music, but scientists have identified what they call a relaxation response, which is a physical and tangible thing. This includes a decreased metabolism, heart and respiratory rate, decreased responsivity to plasma levels of the stress hormone norepinephrine, a lowering of systolic and diastolic blood pressure and a slowing down of the alpha, theta and delta brainwaves. Spiritual healing is reported to achieve this same relaxation response, especially through the power of prayer. One of the UK's leading specialists is Yvonne Ferrell (07071 780229; or, if calling outside the UK, 00 44 1753 889528), who also works on a regular basis in India and France.

Walk In The Countryside . . .

. . . or sit on top of a mountain. And if you cannot get out in nature for real, invest in a coffee-table book of fantastic images because just looking at pictures of nature can help counter both stress and pain. American scientists, reporting their findings in the *Journal of Environmental Psychology*, induced a stress response in volunteers by showing them images of gory work-related accidents and then compared the physical recovery rates between groups who were subsequently shown (a) scenes from nature, (b) scenes of urban traffic, and (c) scenes from a shopping mall. They found, of course, that those watching the nature video recovered significantly faster from the trauma of the grisly video than those in the other groups. We also know that hospital patients staying in beds which have an outside view of trees spend less time in hospital and need less pain medication than those whose rooms overlook brick walls.

Top Ten* Natural Remedies to Beat Stress and Support the Immune System

The cost of bringing a new pharmaceutical drug to market is now an estimated $802 million – and even a small clinical trial can cost as much as $160,000, which would be way beyond the budget of most small herbal companies. There are companies who invest in researching natural products but they are few and far between, not least because nobody can patent a natural product (see

*Plus Two Too Good To Be Left Out.

Hoodia and Weight Loss, page 86), which means you cannot recover those costs or keep ahead of the competition by preventing them from using your findings.

This explains why there is still relatively little hard science – double-blind, placebo-controlled trials – proving that all those supplements on sale work, but that does not mean they are not effective. There is plenty of empirical (anecdotal) evidence for all the remedies recommended here and, increasingly, the science to back this evidence up and tell us how these agents are working.

The important thing, if you want to use natural agents, is to do your homework first: find out which form works best, what dosage you should be taking and, since it may be impossible to know just what you are getting for your money, which are the reputable suppliers (see Echinacea, below).

Avoid the rest like the proverbial plague.

Vitamin A

This immune-boosting nutrient is so important it plays not one but multiple roles in supporting the body's natural defence systems. The anti-infection properties of vitamin A have been known for more than seventy years and the reason it plays such an important role is because, once in the body, it can be converted into a wide range of different metabolites.

A deficiency in vitamin A can lead, for instance, to a loss of ciliated cells in the lungs, which are an important first-line defence against invading pathogens. Vitamin A also promotes the secretion of mucin and the formation of the micro villae in the gut, which, again, work to regulate nutrient absorption and keep the body's system clear of toxins that would otherwise place an extra burden on the immune system. Retinoids, which are important derivatives of vitamin A, have been shown to play a role in the programmed death of the immune system's disease-fighting

T-cells, and this derivative also increases the activity of natural killer cells (see page 261) and macrophages.

Therapeutic dose
Up to 25,000 IUs.

Contraindications
Pregnancy and breastfeeding: use products that have been specifically formulated for pre- and post-natal development. Check out the Pregnancy Planning range by UK acupuncturist and midwife Zita West (www.zitawest.com).

Astragalus
This Chinese herb is, in my opinion, a better single winter immune-booster than echinacea because you can take it for months on end (i.e., in the UK, from October to the end of March) without any risk it might lose its potency.

This is one of several of the remedies in this list that trigger the production of interferon, the antiviral protein produced by white blood cells that has been made synthetically in the lab and touted as a miracle drug for cancer. (The other remedies that do this are vitamin C, Siberian ginseng and schisandra.) Interferon will act against viruses and cancer cells and also help regulate other immune cells by increasing the production of T-cells.

A fever is a sign of the body producing more interferon and should not be suppressed unless it becomes dangerously high.

In traditional Chinese medicine, Astragalus is often combined with immune-boosting ginseng (see page 280). For the same kind of double- or even triple-whammy immune booster, use a supplement that combines astragalus with echinacea, or, even better, with echinacea and goldenseal.

Therapeutic dose
500mg–1.5g a day.

Contraindications
Do not use any of these immune-boosting stimulants if you have an autoimmune disease or are already taking prescription medicines.

B-complex Vitamins

Known as nature's own stress-busters, all the B vitamins work best when taken together. That said, the key antistress member of this nutritional dynasty is vitamin B5 (pantothenic acid), which can help improve wound healing (see page 299), is used to make infection-fighting antibodies, can help treat post-operative and post-trauma shock, and can reduce the toxic effects of prescription drugs, including antibiotics.

All the B vitamins are water-soluble and so cannot be stored and must be replenished every day. If you smoke or drink heavily, you will have a greater need for some of the B vitamins, especially B1, which the body also uses more of during times of great stress, including sickness and surgery.

Therapeutic dose
Take as directed on the bottle.

Contraindications
None, since any excess will be flushed out.

Vitamin C

One of the three big-hitting ACE antioxidants (the others are vitamins A and E), vitamin C has been shown in clinical trials to help the body recover better from the stress of life-threatening trauma followed by life-saving surgery. Of 595 patients admitted to the intensive care unit, 91 per cent were victims of trauma. Doctors randomly assigned antioxidant supplementation to these patients for either twenty-eight days or their stay in intensive care, depending on which was shorter.

Supplementation was started twenty-four hours after either trauma or surgery and consisted of 1000 IUs of vitamin E, administered every eight hours by a tube through either the nose or straight into the stomach, and 1000mg of vitamin C in 100ml of 5 per cent dextrose, also administered every eight hours and intravenously.

After twenty-eight days, the incidence of multiple-organ failure was 57 per cent lower among patients given antioxidant therapy; these patients spent less time in the intensive care unit and the mortality rate among them was 44 per cent lower than among those not given supplementation.

If you do nothing else to support your immune system and help ward off stress, take vitamin C.

Therapeutic dose

1g a day, split into three or four equal doses, to take throughout the day. Look for a supplement that combines vitamin C with a bioflavonoid such as rosehip or quercetin, which will work synergistically to enhance its immune-boosting action in the body.

Contraindications

Do not take vitamin C if you suffer from kidney stones; do not exceed 2g a day since higher doses can cause stomach upsets, including diarrhoea.

Echinacea

The name of this best-selling immune-boosting herb trips nicely off the lips now we have all heard of it but be warned: in a US survey of fifty-nine echinacea-only products, researchers found that 10 per cent contained no measurable echinacea chemicals at all, and that the species specified on the label was present in only half those brands investigated. In addition, of the twenty-one products labelled as containing 'standardized extracts', only 43 per cent provided the standard dosage promised on the label. If self-dosing and taking pot-luck sounds appealing, carry on. If not, make sure you buy from a reputable maker who will guarantee the capsules provide what it says on the label.

Gaia Herbs based in the Appalachian mountains of North Carolina, for instance, have a 250-acre herb farm that the company is using to analyse different species of echinacea and work out which allow for better standardization processes. For example, the company has discovered that drying the root of the Echinacea augustifolia species at temperatures higher than 70°C causes a significant loss of the bioactive compounds. In phase one of a two-phase study, Gaia Herbs also developed a reliable method of encouraging echinacea seed germination during dry storage, which will allow growers higher and more consistent yields.

With this level of commitment to research on a single herb, I would be happy to be getting my supplies from this company: www.gaiaherbs.com.

Therapeutic dose
600mg a day of standardized extract or use a good quality organic tincture.

Contraindications
Do not use this herb with immunosuppressant prescription drugs; if in doubt about what you are already taking, check with your doctor.

Elderberry

An extract of black elderberries and raspberries, which is sold in health stores as a tincture called Sambucol, has been shown in test-tube studies to inhibit the replication of seven different strains of the flu virus. In subsequent tests on humans, researchers found this antiflu, antiviral agent performed just as impressively. After just two days, the symptoms of 93 per cent of the twenty-seven individuals taking part in the trial had dramatically improved, compared with just 25 per cent of the control group.

The mean duration of sickness among those taking Sambucol was 2.7 days. The mean duration of sickness among the control group was 4 days; results which, because the figures are small, could statistically be due to chance, but which do reflect early trials of this remedy in Israel, where researchers at the Department of Virology at the Hebrew University Hadassah Medical School in Jerusalem reported that flu patients taking Sambucol recovered twice as quickly as those given a placebo. The scientists concluded that the active ingredient of the black elderberry could shorten the duration of a flu attack to just two days.

Therapeutic dose

Children should be given 2 tablespoons of Sambucol a day; adults need to take 4 tablespoons a day. You can also buy elderberry in supplement form; take these tablets as directed on the bottle.

Contraindications

None.

The Ginsengs

There are three types of ginseng on sale in health stores, which can give rise to confusion. They are Siberian ginseng (Eleutherococcus senticosus), which technically is not ginseng at all but works in a similar way, panax ginseng (Panax pseudoginseng) and the somewhat milder American ginseng (Panax quinquefolius). In Mandarin, the word 'ginseng' means 'root of man'; in Greek, the word 'panax' means 'panacea', and all three varieties work in the body as adaptogens (see page 251). The differences between the three, all of which are used to enhance stamina and performance, are subtle, making them interchangeable.

Therapeutic dose
400mg a day.

Contraindications
Ginseng has an oestrogenic effect in the body and should not be used by anyone with hormone-related disorders including fibroids.

Goldenseal

Break the stem of this native American plant and the scar that forms is said to resemble a golden wax letter seal, hence its common name. The parts used in natural supplements and tinctures are the dried roots and rhizomes, which contain an active antifungal, antimicrobial, antiviral and immune-enhancing alkaloid called berbine.

What is interesting about this alkaloid is that its immune effect has been found to be specific to epithelial mucous membrane tissue, such as that found lining the mouth, vagina and stomach, which, together with its antimicrobial activity, makes it an excellent remedy to tackle vaginal thrush, as well as bacteria such as Escherichia coli (which causes bladder infections, including cystitis) and Staphylococcus aureus (which has been implicated in skin conditions including eczema and acne). In other words, this is an excellent, broad-spectrum antibacterial and antifungal immune-booster, which you can now buy in tincture, tablet and even therapeutic tea-bag form from independent health stores.

Therapeutic dose

No more than 3g a day. If taking a tincture, use as directed on the bottle. To make an antibacterial mouthwash or eyewash, steep 6g of the dried herb in boiling water for 10 minutes, cool and strain before using the yellow liquid wash.

Contraindications

Do not use this herb if pregnant or breastfeeding. Doses providing more than 500mg of berbine (which would be the equivalent of 8–10g of dried root, depending on the concentration of berbine in the plant), can cause toxicity and adverse reactions including spasms, cardiac damage and even death. In any event, take care when handling goldenseal tincture, which is bright yellow and will stain anything it comes into contact with.

Magnolia

With calming kava kava now off the market in Europe (following unsubstantiated reports of liver toxicity), the best of the new generation of antistress calming alternatives is a supplement called **relora**. Made from an extract from the magnolia plant, in clinical trials supplements reduced levels of cortisol in stressed-out volunteers by 37 per cent in just two weeks. Taking up physical exercise to give stress hormones an outlet can help you stay calm too, and, according to sports researchers at Loughborough University, ten-minute bouts of exercise are just as effective – if not more so – than prolonged sessions.

Therapeutic dose

750mg a day; take 3 x 250mg; mail order from Victoria Health

(0800 389 8195; www.victoriahealth.com) if you have problems sourcing it elsewhere.

Contraindications

Do not give to anyone under the age of 18 and avoid if pregnant or breastfeeding. If already taking prescription medication, consult your doctor.

Maitake

Also known as the 'dancing mushroom', this is one of the powerful immune-boosting Asian mushrooms; the others are reishi, shiitake and cordyceps, all of which are now sold either on their own or in combination in supplement form. Maitake has been shown to activate the natural killer cells (see page 261) and kick-start the immune system's cytotoxic T-cells, and – a welcome side effect for some – it can help maintain weight loss too.

Therapeutic dose

Take 500mg to 1g with water, 2 or 3 times daily between meals, unless it causes stomach upset, in which case take it with food.

Contraindications

If you are diabetic, do not use maitake or any of the immune-boosting Asian mushrooms, which can all affect blood-sugar levels, without medical supervision.

Schisandra

This is the adaptogenic herb to take if you are facing any form of traumatic medical treatment, from surgery to chemotherapy. Look for supplements made from the seeds of the fruits, which are the most potent – so potent, in fact, that as an antioxidant this herb is now considered superior to any of the vitamin or nutrient antioxidants, including the big ACE three (vitamins A, C and E).

Schisandra (which is sometimes spelt schizandra) works to support the adrenal glands and help improve the liver's detoxifying powers. It will help increase concentration, coordination and stamina, even if you are not sick, and researchers are now investigating how nigranoic acid, one of the agents extracted from the stem of the plant, has proven itself useful in HIV therapy.

Therapeutic dose
500mg to 2g a day.

Contraindications
Do not mix with prescription drugs without medical supervision and avoid if you suffer from epilepsy or gastroesophageal reflux disease (GERD).

Zinc
This mineral is critical to healthy immune functioning and even a mild deficiency can decrease the action of disease-fighting T-cells and the production of cytokines by lymphocyte cells. Zinc deficiency is fairly common and may affect up to 70 per cent of the adult population; white flecks across the nailbed are a telltale sign. One reason we no longer get enough in our diets is our increasing reliance on processed foods. Processing means we get less and less of these important minerals on our dinner plates.

Since even a mild zinc deficiency can reduce immune function, it makes sense to supplement the diet, especially if you are prone to repeated infections and slow wound-healing. Zinc is involved in around two hundred different biochemical processes – it acts, if you like, as the body's traffic policeman, directing and overseeing the actions of dozens of enzymes – and its impact on the immune system is now widely accepted.

Therapeutic dose

30mg a day, sold as zinc sulphate and zinc gluconate: both will work but the latter appears to be better tolerated.

Contraindications

Taking antibiotics will affect absorption of zinc; so can drinking coffee. Its absorption is also lower in people suffering from rheumatoid arthritis.

A–Z of Stress-Busting and Immune-Supporting Foods

Just as certain foods will provide nutrients that can help ward off stress and further support the immune system, others can have an adverse effect on the body's ability to defend itself. If you know your fats, then you will know that the ones to avoid are the saturated fats in meats, and the ones to increase in your diet are the unsaturated ones – right? Unfortunately, it is not always that simple. Unsaturated fats can support the immune system since they provide the essential fatty acids you have to get from the diet, but if you eat too much, they can have the opposite effect and suppress immunity.

In some studies, where, in a bid to increase their calorie intake, cancer patients were given unsaturated fats intravenously, doctors were shocked to learn the condition of these patients worsened as these fats suppressed the immune system and increased the risk of the cancer spreading. The reason for this, we now know, is that cancer cells preferentially use unsaturated fats for fuel because (and this is clever) these fats also inhibit those enzymes that would otherwise break down the cancer cell's protective connective tissue capsule that helps hide it from the immune system.

Both coconut and butter – fats we have been advised to avoid in the past – prevent this by stimulating the differentiation of cancer cells, thus helping the immune system to recognize and destroy them.

If you are old enough, you will know the reason we have been on the receiving end of a 'Welcome Back to Butter' marketing drive is that for several years health experts told us to avoid butter and eat margarine instead. Again, they could not have got it more wrong, because the fats you really need to avoid are the trans fats (processed fats). These do damage the immune system and, even in moderation, are the only *really* bad, bad fats.

So bad that, according to new guidelines published by America's Institute of Medicine, there is no known safe-intake amount of artery-clogging trans fatty acids in the diet; findings which, hopefully, will prompt food experts to demand the listing of previously hidden trans fatty acids on food labels. Until that happens, **avoid excessive intake of any product that lists hydrogenated fat** among its ingredients, since it is likely to include trans fats; these include, commonly, biscuits, cookies, cakes, crisps, crackers, margarines and some vegetable oils.

Palm oil, which is a naturally trans-free fat, is a better alternative and a good source of vitamin E. With all the other fats, the key word is moderation.

A is for vitamin A (see page 275), which plays several roles in protecting tissues from stress and boosting immune function. The liver converts betacarotenes from food into vitamin A; good sources of the former include red and yellow vegetables, liver, prunes and dairy products.

B is for the B vitamins, nature's own stress-busters. These nutrients are synergistic, which means they work best when taken together, but the one that is most important for protecting the body against stress is vitamin B5 (pantothenic acid), which has been shown to support the adrenal glands (see page 248). Food sources include fish, fruits, legumes, meats, nuts, eggs, vegetables, salmon and, from your local health store, royal jelly.

C is for cabbage, one of the most potent of all immune-boosting agents. In animal studies, cabbage juice was shown to stimulate the immune system and boost production of a substance called tumour necrosis factor. Researchers believe the key agent is glutamine (see page 61), which is present in beetroot too, although there must be other agents working as well.

D is for dairy products, which are a good source of tryptophan, one of the chemicals the body uses to make the antistress, mood-boosting brain chemical serotonin, which also stimulates the immune system. (If you have a dairy intolerance, switch to soy, which also contains tryptophan.) Other good food sources of this amino acid include alfalfa, fennel, celery, chicken, turkey, spinach and sweet potato.

E is for eggs, which also provide tryptophan (see above), and vitamin-C-rich elderberries (see page 280), which can help ward off coughs, colds and even flu. Even the lacy white flowers of this humble hedgerow plant can help bolster the body's natural defences thanks to high levels of vitamin A, plus vitamin C and bioflavonoids, all of which work together to protect against germs and viruses.

F is for fennel, a good source of immune-boosting magnesium, and another plant that provides the B vitamins, along with vitamins A and C. Roast and serve with fish, brew into a therapeutic tea or chew on the seeds after a meal to get the health benefits. Fennel can also help support the immune system by detoxifying the body and cleansing the liver.

G is for wholesome grains and greens; those complex carbohydrates and nutrient-rich vegetables (which should form the basis of any vegetarian diet) can help counter the daily onslaught of toxins, both environmental and dietary, that can, if it goes on unchallenged, reduce resistance to sickness and disease. Plus vitamin-C-rich gooseberries.

H is for herring, which provides selenium, a trace mineral that has been shown to help boost resistance to infection too. Other foods that provide selenium include brazil nuts, sesame seeds, tuna, wholegrains, oysters, clams and organ meats.

I is for Indian gooseberry (see Ayurvedic Remedies, page 293), which you can now take as a hot or cold drink made from an immune-boosting paste.

J is for jujube dates, a Chinese fruit used in TCM to support the spleen and lymphatic system. According to this system of healing, low energy is usually a sign of low spleen energy, the symptoms of which include loose stools and a dragging downward feeling in the abdomen. Remedy this with a combination of uplifting astragalus, combined with ginseng (see Top Ten Natural Remedies, page 274).

K is for kale and kohlrabi, two of the most powerful immune-boosting cruciferous vegetables (the term cruciferous is used to describe plants whose flowers have four petals, which historical botanists described as resembling the cross or crucifix). Kale is rich in both vitamins C and A and chlorophyll; kohlrabi, which tastes like mild turnip, helps support the lymphatic system.

L is for L-carnitine, the over-the-counter supplement form of the antistress, energy-boosting nutrient carnitine, which is found in red meats and dairy foods. It is taken in supplement form to enhance physical performance, although a review of clinical studies investigating this claim concluded there was no real scientific evidence that it could boost athletic performance in this way.

M is for medicinal mushrooms – maitake, reishi, shiitake and cordyceps – which all support the immune system. To use them in everyday cooking, chop and add to recipes requiring mushrooms, but avoid using too much salt or soy, which can spoil the flavour. For a therapeutic cough mixture, boil the fresh mushrooms with water to make a tea, add a teaspoon of manuka honey and drink.

N is for nori, the dusky jade-coloured sea vegetable that is rich in immune-boosting vitamin A. Add to soups and stews, sprinkle dried flakes over grains, crumble into casseroles or use the dried strips to make your Californian sushi rolls.

O is for omega-3, one of the immune-enhancing essential fatty acids that you have to get from the diet. Supplement your diet with spirulina (see page 70) and other chlorophyll-rich foods to increase your intake, and eat more cold-water oily fish such as mackerel and salmon, and walnuts, purslane, soybean products and pumpkin seeds.

P is for zinc-rich pumpkin seeds, which are also a good source of the antistress B vitamins. Add them to homemade breakfast cereals (see my recipe, page 68) or roast and toss into salads and grains. Also papaya and peas, both good sources of vitamin C, and poultry, which provides more soothing B vitamins.

Q is for quercetin, the anti-cancer bioflavonoid found in apples, onions and shallots, which also enhances the action of immune-boosting vitamin C in the body. Studies from Beijing University show that eating an apple a day can help keep cancer (as well as the doctor) at bay; just one onion a day is said to protect from malignant cell growth and, thankfully for those who do not relish eating raw onion, cooking does not destroy the quercetin content.

R is for raspberries, a good dietary source of immune-supporting folic acid, and which also have an antiviral action in their own right, helping to protect against winter colds and flu. Plus radish, which can help the body fight off bacteria thanks, again, to the plant's in-built antimicrobial properties. Also reishi, the immune-boosting medicinal mushroom (see M is for . . .).

S is for spelt, the best tolerated of all the wholegrains and the one that is highest in stress-busting B vitamins to help keep your immune system strong. Also high in complex carbohydrates, it contains all eight essential amino acids that cells need to stay healthy. The subtle, nutty flavour makes this grain an excellent alternative for those sensitive to wheat.

T is for tuna, a good source of selenium, which has been shown to better help support immune function and improve resistance to disease, especially among the over-65s (see Tried & Applied: a multivitamin-a-day, page 268). Also tyrosine, the antistress non-essential amino acid found in nuts, oats, beans, eggs, fish, dairy foods and meats.

U is for unsaturated fats, which provide the essential fatty acids the immune system needs to stay healthy. Best food sources are nuts and seeds; to avoid the rancidity of oxidized fatty acids, shell and eat them fresh. Pecan and almond nuts are the very best sources but the high concentration of these fats can make them difficult to digest, so eat only in small quantities.

V is for vitamin B6, one of the nutrients the thymus needs to make its hormones; good dietary sources include bananas, fish, grains, legumes, meats, poultry, potatoes, leafy green vegetables and brewer's yeast.

W is for watermelon and winter squash, two antioxidant foods that will help keep the immune system strong and protect tissues from oxidative damage by marauding free radical molecules. Also walnuts, which are a good source of the omega-3 fats the body needs to support the liver and the immune system.

X is for X-rays and other radiation exposures, which can take their toll on immunity. Foods that can specifically help to counter these health risks include buckwheat, which contains a glucoside called rutin that protects against the effects of radiation; apples and sunflower seeds, which contain pectin, a substance that binds with radioactive residues to flush them from the body; mung beans which remove lead; miso soup, and all chlorophyll-rich foods including spirulina, wheatgrass and barley grass.

Y is for yellow fruits and vegetables, providing the bioflavonoids that enhance the action of antioxidant nutrients such as vitamin C, and which also provide a healthy dose of vitamin A.

Z is for immune-boosting zinc, found in foods as diverse as mushrooms and shellfish, tuna and veal, crab and eggs, and oatmeal and oysters. The liver needs adequate supplies of zinc to release stored vitamin A, which is another immune-supporting nutrient (see page 275). Excessive sweating can cause the loss of as much as 3mg a day, and pregnant women carrying a male foetus will lose five times more zinc to the baby than those carrying a female foetus.

Top Three Over-the-Counter Combination Stress-busting Immune-boosting Remedies

Calm & Calmer

Formulated to replace the now withdrawn antistress herb kava kava and to combine three of the most powerful stress-busters in the natural arsenal, Lifetime's aptly named Calm & Calmer provides rhodiola (see page 252) with calming relora (see page 335) and theanine (glutamic acid gamma-ethylamide). The latter is one of the more soothing and calming active ingredients; also found in a nice cup of antioxidant green tea. Clinical trials have shown how taking a theanine supplement increases alpha brainwave activity, which is precisely what happens during meditation and relaxation. (Mail order from Victoria Health, which specializes in US supplements, on 0800 389 8195; www.victoriahealth.com.)

Supercritical Cold 'n' Flu

New Chapter's new immune-boosting winter supplement combines echinacea, goldenseal, astragalus and melissa (see page 309) with the less-well-known Ayurvedic immune-enhancing herb andrographis paniculata, which is known in Bengal as the 'king of bitters', and which in animal studies has been shown to boost the immune system. This formulation also includes purple willow, a natural analgesic, which can help soothe the aches and pains of a nasty flu attack. This is one of my all-time favourite American ranges not least because there are no hidden 'nasty' preservatives or other agents in the formulations. For details visit www.newchapter.info and to order in the UK call Victoria Health (0800 389 8195; www.victoriahealth.com).

Sambucol/Elderberry

I always have one bottle (and a spare) of this amazing immune-boosting tincture in my medicine chest and I use it to dose my young daughter up at the first signs of trouble, including coughs, colds, snuffles, sickness and cold sores. In other words, any sign of a struggling immune system. See page 280 for more on the preliminary university trials showing how this mix of antiviral black elderberries and raspberries can halve the duration of a flu attack, and to try it yourself, mail order from Revital (0800 252875; www.revital.com).

Ancient Wisdom, 21st-century Healing

Traditional Chinese Medicine (TCM)

Since we spend at least a third of our lives sleeping, **herbal**

pillows are an ingenious and simple way of using this time to benefit from the therapeutic properties of herbal remedies. The way it works is that the heat from your head as you sleep on the pillow warms the herbs you are lying on to release their aromatic vapours and essential energies, which you then breathe in as you sleep. You can now buy these pillows from specialist suppliers or even make your own, which should last for a good six months. You will know the pillow is 'spent' when it no longer smells aromatic in the morning.

The Chinese herb that is used to help counter adrenal deficiency caused by ongoing and prolonged stress is a plant called anemarrhena asphodeloids or jih mu, which has a bitter taste but a pleasant odour. Remember, illegal suitcase imports mean you may not always get the herb you think you are buying (mix-ups are common), so get your supplies from a reputable qualified practitioner or an organization such as the UK's Register of Chinese Herbal Medicine (01603 623994).

Ayurvedic (Indian) Remedies

Ashwaganda, which is known as Indian ginseng, is one of my favourite Ayurvedic herbs. Said to make a man 'potent as a horse', it is another stress-busting adaptogen (see page 251), which is also said to have anti-ageing properties for both sexes. It has also been shown in trials to increase bone marrow cells and white blood cell count in animals that have been treated by radiation. Because it can help stimulate immune function, it should not be taken with immunosuppressant drugs, and because it has sedative properties too, do not take it with antidepressant medication. Mail order from Pukka Herbs (www.pukkaherbs.com; 08456 585858).

Chy-wan-prash is a wonderful immune-boosting tonic

made from another potent plant, the Indian gooseberry, along with another forty or so Ayurvedic herbs. Formulated by an Ayurvedic doctor in India and high in vitamin C, it works to cleanse the body of toxins and regenerate all systems at the cellular level, and comes in the form of a thick paste, which you simply dilute with water to make a hot or cold drink. For more details and to order it, contact Jiva-Living (www.jiva-living.co.uk).

Native American Remedies

The **Essiac** formula is a combination of herbs said to have been passed to a Canadian cancer nurse called Renee Caisse (Essiac is her name spelt backwards) by a Native American Indian healer in the 1930s. She never published her exact formula, and even today there are bitter disputes about what should be in it and who owns the rights to the true formula to what has become the most popular herbal mixture used to treat cancer in North America.

Essiac contains just four herbs: sheep sorrel, a cytotoxic herb which is believed to help reduce radiation damage and strengthen cell walls; plus burdock root, an excellent immune-strengthener shown to have anti-tumour properties; turkey rhubarb, which cleanses the liver and has an anti-tumour action too, and slippery elm, which disperses swelling and supports the liver, spleen and pancreas. All these herbs work to purify the blood, an action some practitioners enhance by the addition of red clover too (see Chapter 1, page 7), which works to purify the blood.

You can either buy a dried herbal mix (mail order on 01225 833150) and brew your own tea, which you take twice a day on an empty stomach, or buy a ready-made liquid formula from your local health store, which is more expensive but which takes the fag out of making your own remedy.

Native New Zealand Remedies

Colostrum is the fluid that new mothers produce during the first few days after birth to provide infants with a rich mix of antibodies and growth factors.

The colostrum on sale in supplement form in health stores is collected from cows, and whether cow antibodies can do the same for the human immune system remains unproven. What has been shown is that patients deliberately infected with bacteria who took colostrums as well were more protected than a control group, which suffered more diarrhoea and more fever symptoms, making this an excellent immune-boosting protective remedy for travellers.

With its impressive agricultural background, what better country for researching and producing immune-boosting colostrums from its farm animals than New Zealand? Check out the NZ colostrum range from BioActive Technologies: www.bionz.com.

What Really Works in Helping Manage Immune-related Problems

For advice on specific autoimmune conditions and other health problems that are linked with compromised immunity, go to the index at the back of the book and look up the health complaint you are interested in. Chronic fatigue and fibromyalgia, for example, are both covered in depth in Chapter 7. Here, and unlike in previous or subsequent chapters, I am giving advice for more general immune-related symptoms. This reflects the statement on page 256, that with almost any chronic condition you can think of, some degree of usually hidden immune dysfunction will be to blame.

Allergies

An allergy is simply the immune system's extreme reaction to a substance it perceives as an allergen – pollen or dog hair or cigarette smoke – so you can use natural remedies to both counter this reaction and restore normal immune function.

1, 2, 3 . . . Easy Steps to Restoring Normal Immune Function in Allergies

Take 1g of vitamin C but split your dose into three or four to take throughout the day.

Air Power can help reduce a build-up of mucus in the bronchial airways, which is a common allergic response. It contains Guaifenesen, an expectorant herb, which will stop the accumulation of mucus.

Allergy Relief is a homeopathic preparation, which is safe to give to children too. It combines the Indian herbs Cardiospermum, Galphimia glauca and Luffe operculata to reduce the body's allergic response.

You can get both Air Power, made by Enzymatic Therapy, and Allergy Relief, made by Boericke & Tafel, from UK supplier Victoria Health on 0800 389 8195; www.victoriahealth.com.

Coughs, Colds and Flu (including SARS)

A healthy adult should succumb to no more than two colds a year (a child should get no more than six), and so repeated coughs and colds are always a sign that the immune system needs extra support. The problem with flu is that, although you may have developed resistance to an earlier strain, the virus can mutate to produce a pathogen – often more virulent, as was the case with the SARS virus – the body does not recognize, which means your immune system must start again.

When SARS first grabbed the headlines in November 2002, US supplement-maker Quality of Life shipped hundreds of bottles of its ImmunoKinoko AHCC to the Hong Kong Ministry of Health to dispense. Clever PR? Of course, but the fact is, a healthy immune system should be able to fight off new as well as more established pathogens.

ImmunoKinoko contains a substance called Active Hexose Correlated Compound (AHCC): a Japanese medicinal mushroom extract derived from a manufacturing process that relies on the hybridization of several species of immune-boosting mushrooms.

It is cultivated in Japan where, currently, over 700 hospitals and medical clinics recommend it to patients who need to bolster their immune system. You can learn more about AHCC by visiting www.ahccresearch.com.

1, 2, 3 . . . *Easy Steps to Help Prevent Coughs, Colds and Flu*

If you travel frequently and are concerned about SARS, use ImmunoKinoko, which you can mail order from the NutriCentre on 0800 587 2290; www.NutriCentre.com.

If you are looking for general protection and immunity-boosting, take vitamin C and zinc supplements, alongside elderberry, which is included in the Nutrition Now range and sold as Sambucol in some health stores.

If you do succumb, a light chicken broth can help reduce mucus production and is often used in Chinese medicine to treat colds. To make it, boil leftover chicken plus the bones in a large pan of water with an onion, carrot, bay leaves and peppercorns for flavour. Turn the heat down and simmer for an hour. Sieve to remove the bones (but keep the chicken meat), and add chopped spring onions before cooking on a low heat for another hour.

Emotional Trauma

An emotional shock can depress the immune system as dramatically as a physical trauma; use the Australian Bush Essence Calm & Clear tincture to help you recover your emotional equilibrium, and see Chapter 6 for mood-boosters and additional support during times of extreme psychological stress.

Medical Treatments

Supercharge the immune system before any type of treatment and recharge your body afterwards.

1, 2, 3 . . . Easy Steps to Support Your Immune System Through Medical Treatments

Take 30mg a day of zinc.

Use schisandra (see page 283).

Use the Australian Bush Emergency Essence from Ancient Roots (www.ancientroots.com). Take seven drops under the tongue in the morning when you wake and seven again at night.

Nutritional Deficiencies, including Dieting and Eating Disorders

Getting all the nutrients you need to support immune function is hard enough without extreme diets that eliminate fats or carbohydrates or other food groups. If you are concerned that your immune system may be lowered because it is not getting the nutritional support it needs, either because of the quality of your diet or weight watching, then take the Natural Nutrition Center's Perfectly Balanced formulation, which combines all the vitamins and minerals you need with immune-supporting bioflavonoids and essential fats, plus concentrated superfoods, including spirulina (see page 70) and wheatgrass juice. If you are a fan of the Atkins Diet, which bans all carbohydrate foods, or any other programme that does not recommend eating a balanced diet from all food groups, you should definitely take this supplement, available from US supplement specialists Victoria Health on 0800 389 8195; www.victoriahealth.com.

Repeated Infections

Cold sores, styes, mouth ulcers, earaches, athlete's foot and candida infections are all signs of lowered cell-mediated immunity (see page 264).

1, 2, 3 . . . Easy Steps to Stop Repeated Infections

Take Host Defence, a formulation from New Chapter that combines the medicinal Asian mushrooms maitake and shiitake (see page 283), to support the thymus gland.

Take zinc (30mg a day) plus a good quality B-complex supplement.

Use horopito or colloidal silver topically on fungal infections (see page 41).

Slow Wound Healing

This is another sign of impaired immunity, which is, again, easily remedied with natural agents.

1, 2, 3 . . . Easy Steps to Accelerate Tissue Healing

Take tissue-repairing sulphur in the form of methylsulphonyl-methane (MSM), which is often used by surgeons to help the body repair itself; from Higher Nature, 01435 882880.

Zinc is critical to healing; take 30mg a day.

Manuka honey is now used in hospital wards in Australia to keep wounds free from infection. You can now buy it in a superstrength wound-care cream from New Zealand specialists Comvita, (www.comvita.com) but watch out for its stickiness, which means you need to cover the area you apply it to.

Toxic Overload

Dietary and environmental toxins can overburden the body's major systems, including the immune system.

1, 2, 3 . . . Easy Steps for Clearing Toxic Overload

Use Ultimate Liver Cleanse from Victoria Health (0800 389 8195; www.victoriahealth.com).

Take a good quality probiotic every day (see page 65).

Supercharge cells and energy levels with spirulina, which you can take in powder or supplement form. For details, contact the UK specialists Xynergy (08456 585858; www.xynergy.co.uk).

Roll Out Your Yoga Mat

We have seen how a combination of deep breathing with the movement of major muscle groups works to encourage better lymphatic flow (see page 260), and for the technique that best achieves this, look no further than yoga.

Here are my **1, 2, 3 best yoga asanas** for boosting the immune system and relieving stress. Your aim, with all three, is to relax the muscles, slow the breath and calm the mind.

Savasana (Corpse Pose)

Probably the most important asana you will ever practise since it works to trigger the parasympathetic nervous system, which is all about rest and repair.

You should make sure you practise the corpse pose in between more active postures to give the body a chance to assimilate the resulting physical and energetic changes, and then again at the end of your practice.

This posture is not as easy as it looks, and it is not just a case of lying on the floor with your eyes closed. You need to maintain the body in the correct position, relaxing every single muscle while keeping your correct alignment.

To do this, lie flat on your back on your yoga mat with your arms about 15cm away from your sides, palms facing upwards. Move your feet to hip-width apart and allow the feet to fall out to the sides. Close your eyes but keep your body still. Think about keeping the head and spine in a long straight line, and bring your shoulders up to the ears before allowing them to fall back on the mat and relax. Think about becoming completely still and bring your awareness to your breath. Concentrating the mind on the breath is the quickest way to allow the rest of the body to relax.

Lie in savasana for at least 10 minutes at the end of every yoga practice, longer if you can. You can use candles, incense and soothing music to create the right atmosphere for this relaxation. Do not attempt it with the family bursting in and out of the room asking for things or the telephone ringing incessantly. This is a time for peace, quiet and relaxation for you.

Bhujangasana (Cobra Pose)

This posture, which helps keep the spine supple and strong, also tones the adrenal glands (see page 248) and can help relieve tension and stress, not least because you cannot achieve the full posture without using the breath to release muscle tension. You need to inhale deeply before you lift the chest as you exhale and this simple act of concentrating on the breath will help slow it down and relax the mind and body.

Your starting position is lying on your stomach on your yoga mat with your head turned to one side. Place the palms of each hand alongside each shoulder and lift your head to face forward. Inhale, and as you exhale, begin to lift the top of the body, the whole of the chest, off the yoga mat.

Do not force the body into this position, and only come up as far as you feel comfortable. Keep the arms slightly bent to support the weight of the upper torso and keep the bottom and legs still. There should be no straining of the lower back to lift the chest; instead, use the breathing to help the muscles relax enough for you to carry on lifting.

This is a tough posture for beginners so do not throw

yourself into it. Work slowly up to a full lift of the chest without straining any other part of the body, and hold for as long as comfortable.

Bhramari Pranayama (Humming Bee Breath)

This is a fantastically calming pranayama practice. Yes, you will sound silly doing it, but that should not stop you because the health benefits include relieving stress and cerebral tension, alleviating anxiety and, according to yoga scripts, accelerating tissue healing after accident trauma or surgery, suggesting it has a very positive benefit on the immune system. And it could not be more simple to do.

Sit comfortably, either on your yoga mat or on a chair, making sure you keep your head straight and your spine erect. In other words, do not slouch! Close your eyes and bring your awareness to your breath, which will help the whole body relax. Keep your lips gently closed and the teeth slightly separated, which will allow you to feel and hear the humming vibration once the practice begins.

Relax the jaw and raise the arms to plug each ear with your index finger and block out any external noise. Keep the arms raised and the elbows bent throughout the humming.

Keep the body absolutely still and breathe in. Exhale slowly and as you do, allow the voice to make a deep, low humming noise that you will experience as a vibration. This humming should be smooth and even and last the whole extent of the exhalation. As you breathe in, allow the humming vibration to continue but this time at a much higher pitch. Again, the high-pitch humming should be smooth and even and last the length of your inhalation. This high-pitch humming is often harder to master but do not fret; you will still get the health benefits if you simply breathe in slowly and deeply and only hum the lower-pitched hum when you breathe out again.

Bhramari bee humming is said to induce a calming meditative state and the best time to practise is late at night or early in the morning when there are fewer external noises and distractions.

CHAPTER SIX

Depression and Mood

Unlike other body tissues, the brain needs a constant supply of oxygen and glucose. This is relevant to anyone interested in natural remedies because it means you need to be looking at those natural agents that work to (a) boost or maintain oxygen uptake such as **ginkgo biloba** (see page 317), and (b) help the brain to better utilize glucose supplies, which is what **vinpocetine** (see page 319), a safer compound made from **periwinkle**, has been shown to do.

You can also use food, herbs and nutritional supplements to bolster levels of the brain chemicals that control everything you feel and do. **St John's wort,** for instance (see page 307), works as a natural antidepressant because it helps maintain levels of the feel-good chemical serotonin, which also plays a key role in maintaining good sleep patterns. **Rhodiola** (see page 252) is another herb that does the same.

Vitamin C is critical to optimum brain function. The amount of this antioxidant nutrient in the cerebral spinal fluid (CSF) is 3–5 times higher than that in the plasma, and in brain cells levels can be another 3–5 times higher than in the CFS. One of the first early warning signs of a vitamin C deficiency is fatigue, and this nutrient also has a key role to play in support for people withdrawing from addictive substances (see page 330).

The principal enzyme that works to make the mood-controlling neurotransmitter dopamine relies on both **calcium** and vitamin C to work, which is why both these nutrients have long been associated with having a calming action. Dopamine is eventually converted to another brain chemical, norepinephrine, which controls both mood and behaviour, low levels of which have been associated with both depression and an inability to think clearly.

> ### Tried and Applied
> The reason chocolate is such a powerful brain stimulant is that it contains another chemical, phenylalanine, that the body also uses to make norepinephrine – that explains why I find myself keeping a secret stash of dairy milk in the fridge to get me to the end of a new book!

Depression

Depression is, of course, a part of the human condition, but while for most people it will be triggered by an outside event, such as the death of a loved one, for some 5 per cent of the population it is a clinical disorder that will not go away simply because someone tells you to buck up.

Most common among younger adults (the average age of onset is twenty-something), it is also a widely reported psychiatric illness among the elderly. Women are two or three times more likely to suffer from depression than men, and rates increase when someone is coping with other health disorders, including heart disease, diabetes or recovering from a stroke (see Chapter 3).

Heredity plays a role too – both depression and suicide appear to cluster in families – and first-degree relatives of patients suffering from depression are up to three times more likely to experience the same disorder as normal controls. The symptoms reflect changes in levels of the brain chemicals, specifically norepinephrine (a chemical cousin of adrenaline), serotonin and dopamine, and insomnia is almost invariably a side effect.

Natural remedies that help to regulate mood usually work to increase levels of serotonin; this is what the popular supplement **St John's wort,** which has become known as nature's own Prozac, does. This plant is useful for the treatment of mild to moderate depression and helps maintain normal levels of serotonin by blocking its breakdown in the body.

Most of the research to date has concentrated on the use of hypericin, a single active agent from the plant, with researchers now recommending a daily dosage of 300mg, three times a day, using a supplement where this agent has been standardized to 0.3 per cent. That said, natural healers often argue that you should not select just one active agent but use the whole plant, which is why you will also find herbal supplements and tinctures on sale that have not been standardized in this way. The theory is that all the chemicals in a plant work together synergistically to produce its full therapeutic benefits, so this is something to discuss with your health carers when deciding which brand of supplement and what form to take.

This herb now comes with a warning on the packet for anyone taking anticoagulant medication and anyone who has been taking the contraceptive pill for a long time, which means lots of consumers have been looking for 'alternative' alternatives.

If you are looking, other natural agents that work the same way to counter depression include the powerful adaptogenic herb rhodiola (see page 252) which Russian researchers used to help make their athletes (and even their cosmonauts) the very best they could be, both physically and mentally.

This would be my first herb of choice for any mood disorder since it can also, simultaneously, help improve the body's resistance to stress and normalize other systems, including hormones and immunity. In animal studies, the active agents rosavin and salidroside, which come from the root of the plant, were shown to enhance the transport of the serotonin precursors, tryptophan and 5-hydroxytryptophan (5-HTP), into the brain, and to inhibit the action of the enzyme that degrades serotonin. This suggests that combining rhodiola with 5-HTP would make for a powerful natural antidepressant alternative to the conventional drugs. Rhodiola also works to increase dopamine levels, making it an important remedy for adults and children coping with attention deficit disorders and hyperactivity (see page 326).

The **B vitamins** are also important in tackling depression. **Vitamin B6**, for example, is needed to help convert tryptophan to serotonin, and since deficiency is often caused by taking prescription drugs, supplementing this nutrient is a good idea too. **Folic acid** has also found to be lacking in up to 38 per cent of depressed patients. In hospital trials, patients who were given folate supplementation for six months recovered from psychiatric illness faster than those who were given a placebo pill.

The food you eat plays a critical role as well. Depression and other common mood disorders are frequently linked with, for example, imbalances in the **essential fatty acids** (see pages 314–15 and 378) that protect the brain cell membranes, and **vitamin C** is important too since it helps maintain normal brain function.

One of the most widely investigated non-drug antidepressants is **S-adenosyl methionine (SAMe)**, a naturally occurring substance the body uses to make neurotransmitters. It is now sold in health stores but is an expensive supplement to use in a therapeutic dosage long-term, making the other remedies more attractive if cost is an issue.

The simplest antidote to depression is **exercise**, which can also help counter associated tiredness by raising levels of the feel-good brain chemical serotonin, and the good news, if you need more motivation, is that scientists now know that muscles respond at a molecular level to physical exercise programmes, such as weight training, within two to four weeks of starting, which is much sooner than previously thought. You may hate the thought of having to move your body and the idea of resistance training, but since depression and chronic tiredness are two of the major risk factors for mortality as we age, you will be investing in your health in a way that will pay significant dividends in the longevity stakes as you get older.

Tried and Applied

Use essential fatty acids with antidepressants to enhance their effects. In trials, patients taking antidepressants who were also given 1g of EFAs, twice daily, scored lower on scales of depression after a month than those given a placebo pill. Researchers concluded that either the fatty acids work to augment the action of the prescription medicine without adverse side effects, or they bring their own antidepressant properties to the party.

The One to Watch – Melissa Officinalis

Traditionally, herbalists have used lemon balm (Melissa officinalis) as a remedy for melancholia, and scientists have subsequently shown that it really does have both a calming and **mood-boosting** effect on the brain.

Even used as an **aromatherapy** oil, lemon balm can have a dramatic impact on the brain. In one double-blind, placebo-controlled trial, where 71 patients suffering from severe dementia were given four weeks of treatment, all were deemed to be less agitated, less withdrawn and more constructively active compared with the placebo control group.

In a recent study reported in the journal *Pharmacology, Biochemistry and Behaviour*, UK researchers investigating the use of lemon balm for both mood elevation and cognitive performance in healthy, young student volunteers aged between eighteen and twenty-two found it was *much more effective at a lower dose of 300mg a day* than at either 600mg or 900mg. They also suggested that splitting the dose throughout the day would be even more beneficial. Again, this confirms the traditional herbal adage that sometimes less is more.

In light of these findings, I suggest you use a brand that provides 100mg of standardized extract of **lemon balm** per tablet and take three a day. If you cannot find one locally, mail order from Revital (0800 252875; www.revital.com).

Mood Swings and Sugar Cravings

The brain needs a constant supply of glucose – a drop in levels can lead to low mood and feelings of weakness and fatigue in men, women and children – but sugary sweet foods are not the answer since these trigger blood-sugar highs followed by rapid blood-sugar lows, resulting in mood swings.

Everyone knows diabetics have to pay close attention to their blood-sugar levels (see Chapter 3, Syndrome X, page 122) but fewer of us realize we all need to do the same thing, especially to help maintain a good mood. The best way to maintain an even mood throughout the day is to eat more foods from the lower range of the **Glycaemic Index (GI**; see page 124).

The best herb for regulating blood-sugar levels is the Indian

Ayurvedic herb **Gymnema sylvestre.** The part of the plant used to control diabetes is the leaf, which contains gymnemic acids, which have been shown to reduce the rate of intestinal absorption of glucose and to stimulate the pancreas to increase insulin production.

In trials on gymnema, no adverse side effects have been reported to date, although some preparations can decrease the absorption of iron in the body. That said, the extract used in clinical studies is known as GS4, which does not include the constituents that can cause this problem, so make sure you use this preparation. The daily dose you need to be taking is 400mg. Mail order from the NutriCentre (0800 587 2290; www.NutriCentre.com).

Anxiety and Panic Attacks

These are more conditions, like stress, for which you will have greater sympathy once you have experienced them yourself. Panic attacks are, in effect, a manifestation of extreme anxiety, where symptoms can include shortness of breath, feeling smothered, heart palpitations, shaking, a fear of going mad or losing control, dizziness, sweating, sleep disturbance (see page 322) and chest pain. The chest pain is frightening to experience and it is not uncommon for sufferers to fear they have a serious medical condition to face. A panic attack will last around twenty minutes, with the symptoms peaking halfway through.

If you do suffer, see your doctor to rule out other causes and put your own mind at rest, then try to work out just what is triggering this extreme response.

A simple emergency measure is to rub calming lavender oil on the inside of both wrists and to add it to a soothing bath. You can also drop the oil onto a tissue and inhale the aroma to help calm yourself. The Australian Bush Flower Essences also work quickly to help restore an emotional equilibrium. Use **Emergency Essence** in the throes of an attack (take seven drops under the tongue) and switch to **Calm & Clear** until you have worked through the crisis. (For more on these essences, which work on an energetic level, making them safe to use as an adjunct to other medication, visit www.ancientroots.com.)

My favourite herb for helping lower levels of anxiety is cooling **cardamom**, which will also help counter sweating and the hot rush of an attack. In Ayurvedic medicine, it is considered a sattvic or pure food, which can promote deep, restful sleep, calmness, a good strong immune system and a relaxed, focused mind. No wonder, then, this herb has an important role to play in the prevention of anxiety-induced panic attacks. Take this herb either as a soothing tea or in tincture form. Crush the seeds and sprinkle over a glass of warm milk, which will also help lower anxiety levels, thanks to the presence of both calcium and tryptophan.

Researchers have also linked chronic anxiety with a higher risk of other health problems, including digestive disorders, especially constipation (see page 95). When they examined the lifestyles and attitudes of thirty-four female patients (average age of thirty-six) who had suffered from constipation for more than five years, and compared their findings with nineteen healthy women, they found that on-going anxiety and depression does have an adverse effect on intestinal function (see pages 254 and 256–8 for how mood can affect immunity which, in turn, can affect digestive functioning).

Magnesium works in the body as a muscle relaxant, and tension in the body has been linked with people who suffer panic disorders, so take a supplement of 250mg a day. You can also try **5-hydroxytryptophan (5-HTP)**, which the body uses to make feel-good serotonin, but not if you are already taking conventional anti-anxiety drugs.

Tyrosine is an amino acid that acts as a precursor to the neurotransmitters that help control mood and emotional state. The therapeutic dose is 500mg, three times a day, but do not use this supplement, without medical supervision, if you suffer from high blood pressure. In women, the contraceptive pill can lower levels of this nutrient, raising the risk of anxiety disorders and depression.

Avoiding stimulants, including caffeine, alcohol, sodas, chocolate, refined sugars and carbohydrates, can also help prevent anxiety attacks. You also need to take steps to reduce the stress in your life. See Chapter 5 and think about taking up a relaxation technique, such as yoga, meditation or pranayama (see page 137).

Remember, if you are an anxiety sufferer, you are anything but alone. This is the single most common mental disorder encountered in clinical practice – some 8 per cent of the population will experience at least one anxiety attack at some point in their lives – so there are thousands of others who know exactly what you are going through. To find them, contact the UK support group, No Panic at www.nopanic.co.uk or call freephone 0808 808 0545, and go back to Chapter 5 (Stress and Immunity) for details of a new anti-anxiety herbal supplement called **Calm & Calmer** (page 291).

Brain-protecting Fatty Acids

Your body burns fat for energy and sources its fat stores in two ways: either from the diet or from the breakdown of glycogen (the body's storage form of energy it has derived from foods, including fats). Fats are not bad, but act as the body's energy reserve and also serve other important functions, including insulating the body and cushioning vital organs. Every cell in the body needs fatty acids to make new cells, and they are critical for the transmission of nerve impulses and for healthy brain development and functioning.

All fats are a mixture of **fatty acids** composed of carbon molecules linked with attached hydrogen and oxygen atoms, but the molecular structure can vary, which is what marks the difference between so-called saturated and unsaturated fats. That said, all dietary fats and oils are a mix of all three different types of fatty acid – the one that predominates determines the overall classification.

Saturated fatty acids (SFAs) have carbon bonds that are saturated with hydrogen molecules, and while the body prefers these types of fats to burn as energy, they are generally regarded as the least healthy form of fat intake.

Monounsaturated fats (MUFAs) have a link in their carbon chain where two carbon molecules share not one but two bonds with each other. Body fat contains MUFAs, which the body can easily convert to energy.

Polyunsaturated fatty acids (PUFAs), which have two or more double bonds linking their carbon chains, are regarded as the healthiest option, and while the body can burn these for energy, too, they also have other vital functions in the body, including protection of the brain and its cell membranes.

There are two fat members of the PUFAs family that the body cannot make and it is these that are called the **essential fatty acids (EFAs)**, meaning you have to get them from the diet. These two fats are **linoleic acid (LA)** and **linolenic acid (LNA)**; names so similar they simply add to the confusion. People often know these better as **omega-6 (LA)** and the less common **omega-3 (LNA)** fatty acids.

The omega-3 essential fatty acids (see DHA, page 315) are important for protecting the nervous system and, particularly, the integrity of the brain cell membranes. They are less common in the diet than the omega-6 fatty acids, mostly because of the polyunsaturated oils we tend to use in both cooking and food processing. For foods that contain both types of EFAs, see A–Z of Brain-nourishing Foods, page 337.

In mood disorders, the right ratio of omega-3 to omega-6 fatty acids in the diet (currently thought to be 2:1 omega-3 to omega-6 – though our ancestors ingested even more omega-3 than this) has also been shown to help and, according to integrated practitioners, supplementing these nutrients can both improve mood and help relieve depression in as little as one to two weeks. Make sure your daily intake includes a good quality EFA supplement providing the right ratio of omega-6 and omega-3 fats. I recommend Green People's clever sprinkle sachet, which does just that. For more information, look at www.greenpeople.co.uk.

The Other One to Watch – DHA

Docosahexaenoic acid – thankfully shortened to DHA (and also known as one of the omega-3 fatty acids) – is used in hospitals to supplement the diet of premature infants, and added to baby formula to enhance brain development. It is present in breast milk and is probably the single most important supplement for supporting mental functioning and reducing the risk of dementia in senior life.

There is no typical dosage although 5g of fish oil contains between 72mg and 312mg of DHA. Levels of DHA and another fatty acid called arachidonic acid (AA) have been shown to be out of balance in people suffering from cystic fibrosis. DHA alone has also been used to help reduce aggressive behaviour in stressed-out individuals.

If you are pregnant, you should definitely be taking a DHA supplement in the last trimester. For more details on a safe range, formulated by a qualified midwife for both pre- and post-conception, check out the Pregnancy Planning supplementation at www.zitawest.com.

Alzheimer's and Sage

If the drug companies are excited enough to invest in research into a natural agent then you know there must be gold in them there pills. The hot herb currently under the microscope in the battle against Alzheimer's disease is **sage**, which has been more traditionally used to help alleviate hot flushes in menopause and for menstrual problems. The reason for all the excitement is that researchers now believe this everyday garden plant can work in the body to help restore an impaired vascular supply to the brain of sufferers.

It also has a calming action in the body, making it a key remedy to consider in geriatric medicine.

Alzheimer's disease is the most common form of dementia, responsible for some 60 per cent of all cognitive dysfunction in later life. Over half of all those people aged eighty-five and above have Alzheimer's disease, and while we still do not know the cause, there is a clear genetic link.

The long, slow and painful loss of intellectual function interferes, initially, with daily life and, after many years, death is usually the result of several factors, including compromised nutrition, complications associated with the immune system and trauma. Before then, memory and the ability to recognize people, places and even objects diminishes over time, making this one of the most distressing conditions for relatives to cope with.

Scientists remain unclear which of the brain lesions associated with this condition are the more damaging: the plaque deposits that increasingly develop in the spaces between the nerve cells or the neurofibrillary tangles that develop inside the nerve cells. Because we cannot examine the brain of an Alzheimer's patient before a postmortem, we do not know which appear first or whether they occur at the same time, or what triggers their formation.

Beta amyloid is a protein that is produced from enzymes called secretases, which are present on the surface of the brain. One leading theory is that the cells in the brains of Alzheimer's patients produce not only too much beta amyloid, but also a particularly 'sticky' version. In 1992, researchers discovered a gene that also increases the risk of Alzheimer's disease. APOE is a lipoprotein involved in the metabolism of cholesterol; APOE4 is a variant of this gene, already known to be a risk factor for heart disease, and scientists are now asking if the APOE4 version of this gene gives rise to a greater risk of Alzheimer's too.

What we do know is that people who take antioxidant supplements (**vitamins A, C, E and selenium**, for example) and those who take **anti-inflammatory medication** suffer less degeneration than matched (equivalent) counterparts who do not, making these steps an important consideration if you are looking for natural approaches to support conventional treatment.

According to laboratory studies, **SAMe** (see page 308), which has a positive effect on brain cells, is present in lower levels in the cerebrospinal fluid of patients with Alzheimer's disease and neurological complications than in non-sufferers. As well as supporting brain biochemistry to help prevent the deterioration of brain cells, this naturally occurring substance, which is now on sale in health stores in supplement form, boosts the production of **phosphatidylserine**, a lipid (fat) that is important in maintaining both memory and mood, and also increases levels of the antioxidant **glutathione**, which has an anti-inflammatory action too. The dosage used in most clinical trials is 1600mg a day, although a daily maintenance dose of 400–1600mg a day has proved effective in countering associated depression.

Ginkgo biloba, the circulation-boosting Chinese herb, has also been found to be helpful in the short-term in alleviating symptoms including memory loss and depression. A recent review of some fifty double-blind placebo-controlled trials, where patients with chronic cerebral arterial insufficiency were given ginkgo supplements, concluded that ginkgo extract could help delay and even reverse the mental deterioration associated with early Alzheimer's.

The reason it works is that, specifically, it supports circulation in the peripheral vessels (this is the reason it is also being investigated to help prevent deep vein thrombosis (DVT) caused by long-haul flying), and another theory is that it works to enhance the uptake of oxygen and utilization of glucose by the brain. This herb can also inhibit platelet-activating activity, so another idea is that it may be reducing the adhesive nature of those platelets that are clotting to help prevent the formation of plaque.

Ginkgo biloba also promotes the nerve transmission rate, improves synthesis of brain chemicals and normalizes acetylcholine receptors in the hippocampus – that part of the brain most affected by Alzheimer's disease. The dosage used in most clinical trials was 180mg of standardized extract providing 24 per cent of the active ginkgo flavonoids. For extra support, take this with sage in tea form. (Make this by steeping 1–2g of sage leaves in 150ml of boiling water for 5–10 minutes, three times a day. Allow to cool before giving it to anyone.)

Essential fatty acids (EFAs), which work to support normal brain functioning, are important too (see pages 314–15 and 378), and the critical thing to remember, whichever remedy you choose, is that the sooner you start, the better the outcome. If you have a family history of Alzheimer's or other dementia-type conditions involving poor memory, use these remedies before the first sign of symptoms to give the brain the best support you can.

Do not mix herbal remedies with prescription drugs without medical supervision and make sure you take a herbal medicine two hours apart from conventional medication; do not use ginkgo biloba if you are taking any blood-thinning medication, such as warfarin.

Memory and Periwinkle

Most adults retain a vocabulary of around 30,000 words, which is testament to the brain's astounding memory function. The idea that we can 'train the brain', just as we train other parts of the body, to stay healthy and alert is nothing new; remember the adage **use it or lose it** applies as much to your mental functioning as to your muscle tone.

One natural agent that is getting increasing attention for its ability to support brain health is periwinkle. It works to increase blood flow to the brain and thus boost mental productivity. It is said to help prevent loss of memory and concentration, reduce feebleness, improve thinking capacity and prevent premature ageing of brain cells.

So why isn't it already on your shelf?

The problem in using an extract of the plant itself is that it contains potentially toxic alkaloids, including one called vincristine, which may cause cell, nerve, liver and kidney damage, as well as skin-flushing and intestinal complaints.

People do still use this agent in tincture form but the supplement industry has come up with a solution to these adverse side effects by converting the active agent, vincamine, in the laboratory into a safer compound called **vinpocetine**, which is then marketed as a supplement.

No significant side effects were reported when vinpocetine was given in large doses (60mg a day) to Alzheimer's patients for a year. Although still unclear on the precise mechanism of action, preliminary evidence suggests vinpocetine stimulates cerebral metabolism and can help improve memory in both healthy people and those whose recall has been adversely affected by benzodiazepine anti-anxiety tranquillizer drugs. What we do know about this agent is that it can help the brain use more of the glucose supplies that are available.

The therapeutic dose if you plan to take this supplement is, typically, 10mg, three times a day, but you must take it with food, since this also enhances the bioavailability of the active agents.

Keeping the brain challenged should be a deliberate and conscious decision as we age and learning new skills such as playing a musical instrument or speaking a foreign language can help keep the brain sharp. In other words, intellectual exercise is as important to your long-term health and well-being as physical exercise.

Tried and Applied

Rats whose diets are supplemented with acetyl-L-carnitine and alpha lipoic acid perform better in memory tests and have better cellular metabolic activities and more energy according to researchers, who reported that every rodent given this diet looked and behaved more like a younger animal than those not given supplementation. Acetyl-L-carnitine is one of the more extensively researched nutrients that has been shown to help prevent brain ageing. The therapeutic dose is 3g a day.

Insomnia and Sleepless Nights

We spend a third of our lives asleep, which is, as it turns out, anything but an inactive biological state. Sleep is a dynamic and active process where the body carries out most of its repair and rejuvenation mechanisms, and when we do not get the rest we need, we are not able to perform either our physical or our mental tasks to the best of our ability when we wake.

The average person changes position between 80 and 100 times while asleep, and during the night you will pass through five distinct stages of the sleeping process. These five stages, outlined below, make up one full sleep cycle, which takes, again on average, between 90 and 110 minutes to complete.

The Five Stages of Sleep

Light Sleep

This is stage one, the point at which, unless you suffer from insomnia which affects about 40 per cent of women and 30 per cent of men, you begin to drift off. Your eyes move very slowly and your muscles start to slow down too. Some people experience sudden muscle contractions – known as hypnic myoclonia – which is often preceded by a sensation of falling. If you wake again during this initial sleep stage, you will probably remember fragmented visual dream-like images.

Spindle Sleep

In this second stage, all eye movement stops and brainwaves become slower, with occasional bursts of rapid waves known as sleep spindles.

Delta Sleep

In this third stage, very slow brainwaves called delta waves begin to appear, again interspersed with smaller, faster wave activity.

Slow-wave Deep Sleep

This is the sleep from which it is usually very difficult to wake the sleeper. During this fourth stage, the brain produces almost exclusively the slow, delta waves and there is no eye movement or muscle activity. If you are woken from this stage, you are likely to feel disorientated and take several minutes to adjust to the fact you are now awake again.

REM (Rapid Eye Movement) Dreaming Sleep

In this fifth stage, your breathing becomes more rapid, irregular and shallow. The eyes jerk in different directions and both the heart rate and blood pressure increase. This is the dream stage of sleep and to protect ourselves (and our bed partners) and stop us from lashing out, our legs and arms become temporarily paralysed.

The first few sleep cycles of the night contain relatively short REM periods and long periods of stage four deep sleep, but as the night progresses, the REM stages lengthen and the deep sleep stages shorten. By morning, we are spending almost all our sleep time in the first two stages and in REM dreaming sleep. In general, half of all non-elderly healthy adults spend half the night in stage two, spindle sleep, about 20 per cent in dreaming sleep and the rest in the other stages.

If you suffer from insomnia – you wish!

Disturbed, disrupted sleep can lead to serious health problems, including high blood pressure, heart disease, depression, lowered immunity, diabetes and chronic fatigue, and the main stressors that give rise to insomnia include worry, stress, side effects of medication, environmental noise, extreme temperatures and other changes in the surrounding environment.

If you have difficulty falling asleep, if you wake frequently during the night, if you wake too early in the morning and cannot get back to sleep, and if you wake feeling more tired than when you went to bed, you can consider yourself an insomniac and look forward to a day of increasing irritability, tiredness, lack of energy and difficulty in concentrating on tasks, which is the collective upshot of inadequate or poor quality sleep.

The good news is that you can use natural remedies that boost levels of those brain chemicals that control sleep, to reduce the time it takes to get off to sleep, reduce the number of night-time awakenings and help improve morning alertness. You could, of course, take sleeping pills, but the problem here is that they often cease to work after prolonged regular use and, if you have used them, you will know for yourself they do not produce good quality sleep. In other words, you may wake feeling no better for the fact you knocked yourself out for the night.

The other thing you must resist is the temptation to use alcohol to conk out with since, again, the upshot will be poor quality sleep and a depletion of, for example, the vital B vitamins which actually help the body cope better with the stress and anxiety that researchers have now identified as the real cause of chronic insomnia in the majority of cases.

The hormone that regulates our internal biological clock, and thus our sleep pattern, is **melatonin,** which is secreted by the pineal gland located in the brain in response to a complex pathway of internal signalling about levels of daylight.

We produce the highest levels of melatonin at night, when it is dark, and production gradually cuts back as dawn breaks. In healthy adults, levels of melatonin start to rise between 8 and 9 p.m., peak between 1 and 3 a.m. and then fall slowly back to daytime levels. As we age, we produce less melatonin, and by middle age we may have less than half the levels of a younger person, which might explain why sleep difficulties often accompany older age.

In a study of men and women with an average age of seventy-six, melatonin supplementation was shown to reduce movement during sleep, thus lowering the risk of awakening and improving the quality of sleep so that those taking part in this trial said they were waking up feeling more refreshed. Even better, their bodies did not 'adapt' to the higher levels of melatonin thanks to the supplementation, which meant they were still reporting the same benefits after two months of taking 2mg of melatonin every night.

Scientists have also found that melatonin can help reduce how long it takes to get to sleep in the first place and increase the number of hours participants to various trials were able to sleep, making it the first supplement to think about if you have sleep problems.

In America, you can still buy melatonin over the counter; in the UK, you have to ask your doctor for a prescription (since it is deemed too potent for self-prescribing); or take a clever step back in the biochemistry of the brain and instead use a supplement called 5-hydroxytryptophan (5-HTP), which the body uses as a precursor to making serotonin which, in turn, is used to make melatonin. Alternatively, get your melatonin from friends in America or the internet.

If you prefer a herbal remedy, **Siberian ginseng** (see page 280) also helps the body trigger the manufacture of melatonin, making it a good agent for short-term deficiency caused by jet lag (see below).

1, 2, 3 . . . Easy Steps to Overcoming Insomnia

Take a melatonin supplement or, if you cannot source it, use 5-HTP, and take as directed on the bottle. In the UK, mail order from Higher Nature (01435 882880) or another good quality supplier.

Take calcium (800mg a day, plus 400mg of magnesium, since these two are synergistic) because a deficiency in this mineral is often linked with sleep problems.

Have a small carbohydrate snack such as a banana or muffin just before bedtime, which has been shown to help the brain better utilize tryptophan in the diet or in supplement form (5-HTP).

Tried and Applied

Those weekend lie-ins may be doing you more harm than good because, according to research, sleeping for an additional two hours on Saturday and Sunday mornings can cause a 30-minute disruption to your melatonin 'rhythm'. Taking a single dose of melatonin on Sunday night after a lazy weekend can help stop the Monday morning lacklustre blues.

Jet Lag Remedies

If you have flown long-haul, then you have experienced jet lag, and you know just how much of a space cadet you can feel in those first few days of your arrival or return, while your body adjusts to a different time zone.

Siberian ginseng can help trigger increased production of melatonin to help cope with those time changes and the Ayurvedic herb **gotu kola** can help prevent water retention while flying.

A favourite among long-haul cabin crew fighting jet lag is **guarana,** a fantastic and exotic herbal energy booster which comes from the Amazon rainforest. Described as a 'tonic herb', it is not used for specific health properties, but rather as a general revitalizer. In South America, it is routinely incorporated in drinks, cereals and even sweets, and here you can now buy it as a breakfast cereal bar or energy-boosting chewing gum.

Guarana does contain caffeine, but a 500mg capsule provides just 15mg of this natural stimulant, which is low compared with the 80–120mg dose you'll get in just one cup of coffee. The key difference is that guarana also contains other compounds, which effectively slow down the assimilation of that caffeine by the body so that a single dose will provide a more sustained energy hit that can last up to six hours. Wily cabin crew will take their guarana supplements an hour or two before landing to keep them up all day and beat jet lag.

Ultimate Energy is a clever combination formulation, which includes the Asian mushroom codonopsis to boost physical stamina, and gotu kola, but the real coup is the inclusion of all three energy-boosting **ginsengs** (see Chapter 5, page 280), which help the body cope better with stress and fatigue.

Probably the most potent of these is panax (Asian) ginseng (see page 281). Athletes swear this is the supplement that gives them the competitive edge, and in double-blind, placebo-controlled, randomized clinical trials, participants given ginseng supplements were deemed to have improved concentration, faster reaction times and better abstract thinking abilities than the group given a placebo.

Ultimate Energy is available in the UK from Victoria Health (0800 389 8195; www.victoriahealth.com). Mail order guarana supplements and buzz bars from South American herb specialist Rio Trading (01273 570987; www.riohealth.com).

Tried and Applied

The sleep disturbances and dehydration caused by long-haul flying can impair the body's natural detoxification systems, which take place at night when you sleep, making the body more acidic. Restore alkalinity by taking either apple cider vinegar or freshly squeezed lemon juice in water but do not substitute normal vinegars since they are themselves acidic.

Hyperactivity – in Grown-ups and Kids

I have a question for anyone who cares to ponder it. What happens to hyperactive kids when they grow up? Do they magically turn into calm and controlled adults or do the same problems haunt them throughout their life?

According to American research, half of all ADHD (attention-deficit hyperactivity disorder) kids turn into ADHD adults, where behavioural problems are likely to include antisocial tendencies, substance abuse, low self-esteem and a lack of social skills.

Thankfully, we do not give adults Ritalin (yet) since this drug, which is prescribed to the majority of hyperactive kids, is a stimulant, which has similar chemical properties to cocaine.

To understand why this remains the conventional drug of choice for millions of children diagnosed as ADHD in the western world, you need to know how it works to act on the central nervous system in the same way, albeit more slowly, as cigarettes, alcohol and amphetamines to boost levels of dopamine, the brain chemical that is involved in reward-seeking behaviour, control of movement, sexual behaviour, memory and the regulation of pituitary-hormone secretion (see Chapter 8).

In young animals, dopamine exerts a protective effect against hyperactivity, and in children diagnosed as having ADHD, researchers have identified a deficiency in this neurotransmitter. The theory is that these children have too many other molecules that use up dopamine supplies before it can be used for its regulatory functions, and what Ritalin does is bind to these other molecules to leave the dopamine free to do its job.

The upshot for children who are given this medication is that their behaviour switches to the opposite, leaving parents and teachers with zombie-like children who feel emotionally blunted and detached. Physical side effects can include loss of appetite, retarded growth and weight loss. Some children may experience hallucinations and depression; others are triggered into a state of increased euphoria and cocaine-like responses including insomnia.

Researchers have also reported that Ritalin may cause liver cancer in mice. This is not something that has been brought to most parents' attention, but it would be enough, in itself, to prompt the question: is there an alternative?

Dopamine is made from the amino acids tyrosine and phenylalanine, which are converted in the body by enzymes into L-dopa. Another enzyme converts L-dopa into dopamine, but only if there is enough vitamin B6 present. Studies of plasma amino-acid levels in ADHD patients showed lower than normal amounts, suggesting problems with either transportation of amino acids or absorption or both.

One simple way to increase dopamine levels naturally is to use the herb **rhodiola** (see pages 252 and 335), which also works as a natural antidepressant. It works to protect both serotonin and dopamine levels in the brain and can prevent their destruction by enzymes and any decline triggered by an excessive release of the stress hormones (see Chapter 5).

Diet is also crucial to managing hyperactivity disorders. Children suffering ADHD are often lacking in **zinc,** and up to half of all those diagnosed with this disorder have been shown to be sensitive to food additives, including colourings, flavourings and preservatives. The yellow food dye tartrazine is thought to bind with zinc in the blood to reduce overall levels. That said, cutting these chemicals from the diet is a challenge, not least because in the US alone, the daily per capita consumption of food additives is a staggering 13–15 grams, so visit my website, www.whatreallyworks.co.uk, for additive-free alternatives targeted at kids.

Hyperactive children and adults may also be reacting to **salicylates,** substances that occur naturally in certain foods, including almonds, apples, blueberries, cherries, currants, curry powder, dates, liquorice, oranges, paprika, peppers, pineapple, prunes, raspberries and, for grown-ups, tea. So cut these from the diet and monitor any improvements in behaviour.

Elimination diets have shown food intolerances do play a role in hyperactive behaviour, the worst culprits being **chocolate, cow's milk, oranges, cow's cheese, wheat, other fruits, tomatoes** and **eggs.** Again, remove these from the diet and monitor for behavioural changes.

Essential fatty acids (EFAs) have now been shown by mainstream researchers to help moderate hyperactivity and lots of ADHD kids are lacking in the **omega-3 fats** (see page 314 and A–Z of Brain-nourishing Foods). Males need to take in three times more essential fatty acids than females to achieve normal neonatal and infant development, which is consistent with finding that more boys than girls suffer from hyperactivity.

If you are dealing with this problem, omega-3-rich foods you should be able to persuade kids to eat include: **soy beans, salmon, tuna** and **dark leafy greens,** and you should definitely be giving them a daily EFAs supplement.

Breast milk is an excellent source of a fatty acid called **DHA** (see page 315), which is critical for healthy brain development. Researchers have now reported that children who have been diagnosed with ADHD were less often breastfed as infants than children who are not deemed hyperactive, proving just what an important role the fatty acids play in brain function and behaviour in both infancy and later life.

One of the best new supplements on the market combines rhodiola with mood-boosting relora. Lifetime's **Calm & Calmer** (see page 291) is an American supplement (on sale in the UK from Victoria Health, 0800 389 8195; www.victoriahealth.com). Give children an age-appropriate dose; for guidance on safe nutritional and herbal dosages for kids, visit my website www.whatreallyworks.co.uk.

Aggression

There is simply no question that food has a direct effect on mood and that knowing what not to eat or feed your kids is probably even more important than being able to reel off endless lists of so-called healthy foods.

In a series of studies made at youth detention centres in the US, for instance, researchers removed chemical additives, sugar and refined flour from the diets of over 8000 youngsters. At the end of the study, aggressive and destructive behaviour was reduced by 47 per cent.

In another prison trial, this time in an adult prison, younger adult prisoners randomly assigned a good quality multi-supplement plus essential fatty acids for a period of twenty weeks committed 26.3 per cent fewer offences requiring disciplinary action than their prison colleagues who were given a placebo pill, suggesting that antisocial behaviour, including violence, can be reduced by this 'shotgun' method of supplementation, and thus even more effectively managed by individual nutritional profiling of inmates to ascertain which of the nutrients in the multi-supplement mix they may be lacking and responding to.

DHA (see page 315) has also been used to reduce aggressive behaviour in stressed-out individuals.

Addiction

Vitamin C can help lessen the misery of withdrawal from addictive drugs, including heroin. In trials where heroin addicts on detoxification programmes were given high doses of vitamin C, only 10–16 per cent of participants suffered major withdrawal symptoms, compared with 56 per cent of those being weaned off the drug without vitamin C supplementation, suggesting that all detoxification and rehab centres should consider nutritional advice and supplementation as part of the recovery programme.

Melatonin (see page 323) has also been successfully used to support patient withdrawal from the benzodiazepine drugs.

Top Ten Natural Remedies for Lifting Mood, Warding off Depression and Supporting Brain Function

Choline

This is a key nutrient in the production of acetylcholine, a neurotransmitter, low levels of which are often associated with ageing and memory loss. As long ago as the mid-1970s, researchers demonstrated how the brains of Alzheimer's patients showed drastically reduced levels of the enzyme the body needs to make the neurotransmitter acetylcholine from the choline it gets in the diet (see A–Z of Brain-nourishing Foods), but which is also made in the liver.

In trials, where patients were given drugs to interfere with this conversion process, they suffered from confusion and temporary loss of memory that were as drastic as that suffered by a patient with advanced Alzheimer's disease. You can get choline in single supplement form where it is sold as choline bicartrate, and it is also made available in supplements that provide phosphatidy-choline.

Therapeutic dose
The recommended daily intake is 500mg a day.

Contraindications
None reported, but large dosages (2g or more a day) can cause diarrhoea.

Brewer's yeast
More usually used as an excellent source of stress-busting B vitamins, brewer's yeast is also a natural source of lithium, the heavy-duty psychiatric drug prescribed for manic-depressive disorders. The theory, in natural health, is that using dosages that would be present in normal levels in the diet can also help control mood and alleviate depression, without the toxic side effects of the conventional pharmaceutical medication.

That does not mean a patient can come off their prescribed medication and take brewer's yeast instead, but research has shown that when violent offenders were given a minuscule daily supplement of just 400mcg of lithium from brewer's yeast for a month, they all reported better mood states, suggesting this supplement can play a significant role in maintaining optimum mood states for otherwise healthy individuals.

Therapeutic dosage
For mood: 3g a day of brewer's yeast.

Do not use this supplement if you have a yeast allergy.

Calm & Clear

This is one of the excellent Australian Bush Essences which, as with all flower essences, work on an emotional and energetic rather than a physical level. This also makes them safe to take with other medication. If you suffer from anxiety and/or panic attacks, take this remedy to help you stay calm under stress. Now on sale in lots of health stores around the world, if you have trouble finding this range locally, visit the UK supplier, www.ancientroots.com.

Therapeutic dose

Take seven drops under the tongue in the morning and again at night. Increase this dosage to seven drops as and when you feel you need it, during times of more anxiety and stress.

Contraindications

None.

Co-enzyme Q10

Every cell in the body contains this vitamin-like compound, which is present in higher levels in the energy-producing mitochondria (see page 357) than any other part of the cell structure. The reason we believe it is important to brain functioning and mood is that we know it works, alongside the all-important fatty acids, to stabilize cell membranes, and, in addition, it acts as a powerful tissue-protecting antioxidant.

There is a suggestion that CoQ10 sourced from soybean oil may have a superior bioavailability compared to other extracts so check this before you buy your supplement. CoQ10 is a key anti-ageing supplement, which will support all the body's systems, not just the brain.

Therapeutic dose

100–200mg a day.

Contraindications

Do not mix this supplement with prescription medication, including warfarin, or with medication for lowering blood pressure. Diabetics should not use CoQ10 without medical supervision.

DMAE

Known as 'IQ food', dimethylaminoethanol is similar to choline (see page 330) and is also involved in memory and learning. It has been used to help patients suffering from a variety of mental disorders, from autism to dementia, and for those suffering with impaired memory. It also works to improve mood and mental alertness and has been used to help manage the symptoms of attention-deficit hyperactivity disorder (ADHD; see page 326).

Therapeutic dose

This is not a supplement to take every day but only when you need to feel more alert and focused. In those cases, take 500mg a day.

Contraindications

Do not use with anticholinergic drugs.

Gotu kola

I travel frequently to India and have a huge bias towards the Ayurvedic herbs that we are only just beginning to learn more about in the west. Animal studies in the west suggest that, as well as working to support circulation, gotu kola, which is sometimes referred to as 'food for the brain', can also help improve memory and cognitive performance, hence its inclusion in some of the best cutting-edge combination formulas for brain support (see Top Three Combination Remedies . . . page 336).

The active brain-supporting agents, sourced from the above-the-ground parts of the plant, include compounds called sugar esters, known as asiaticosides, that are believed to help protect neurons from beta amyloid toxicity (see Alzheimer's Disease, page 316). It also contains other active ingredients which have a more sedative and even anticonvulsive effect in the body (see Seizures, page 351). Gotu kola is also a rich source of vitamin B5; see below.

Therapeutic dose
120mg a day.

Contraindications
Gotu kola can elevate blood-glucose levels in diabetics; it can also raise cholesterol levels in susceptible individuals.

5-HTP
Tryptophan is one of the amino acids the body uses to make the brain chemical serotonin that helps control mood. It is sold in supplement form as 5-hydroxytryptophan (5-HTP) which can be used to help alleviate several related conditions, including depression, anxiety, panic attacks and insomnia (see pages 306, 311 and 320).

This agent, which the body also needs to make vitamin B3 (niacin; see pages 12 and 338) is not found in foods but is made from the seeds of the African plant Griffonia simplicifolia. For maximum effect, take with vitamins B6 and C.

Therapeutic dose
100mg, 3 times a day.

Contraindications

Do not mix with antidepressants or carbidopa, which is prescribed for Parkinson's disease (see page 348).

Lifeflower

Formulated from the Chinese herb Erigeron breviscapinus, and sold as Breviscapini, Lifeflower is new to the west but now available in the UK and the US. In clinical trials in China, where it was administered intravenously to stroke patients, over 80 per cent of participants under investigation reported improved brain function (see Chapter 3).

The reason it is so effective is that, as well as having an 85 per cent bioavailability, Lifeflower can cross the blood–brain barrier to boost supplies of oxygen and glucose to the brain. There are no known contraindications for this herb but it would be wise to consult with your current health advisors before taking it.

Therapeutic dose

Take as directed on the bottle; available in the UK from www.victoriahealth.com.

Contraindications

None, but do not take without telling your health advisors.

Relora and rhodiola

Relora is the anti-anxiety dietary supplement made from an extract of the magnolia plant (see Stress and Immunity, page 282), and rhodiola has been shown to help beat depression by preventing the breakdown of serotonin, the brain's feel-good chemical, and works to increase dopamine levels too, making it an important remedy for adults and children coping with attention deficit disorders and hyperactivity (see page 326).

Don't waste your money on single supplements when you can

use a combination remedy (Calm & Calmer, see page 291) that combines both with an additional calming agent called theanine.

Vitamin B5

Often included in over-the-counter anti-anxiety supplements, vitamin B5 or pantothenic acid is present in every single cell in the body. It plays a key role in the conversion of both fats and sugar to energy and is needed for the body to utilize choline (see page 330).

It has been shown to help children with learning difficulties and is known to be involved in the transmission of nerve impulses in the brain and in helping the adrenal glands (see Stress and Immunity, page 248) respond to stress. It can help the body recover from a hangover, is useful in the treatment of Parkinson's disease (see page 348) and works to improve oxygenation to the brain.

Therapeutic dose

5mg a day (works best as part of a good quality B complex which combines all the B vitamins).

Contraindications

None at this recommended dosage.

Top Three Over-the-Counter Combination Remedies for Mood and Brain Support

You can get all these from specialist in US supplements Victoria Health (0800 389 8195; www.victoriahealth.com).

New Chapter's Supercritical Neurozyme

This has the lot: omega-3 fatty acids, sage, ginkgo biloba, gotu kola, lemon balm, ashwaganda, holy basil, vitamin E and club moss (huperzine A; see page 342). You take one soft-gel capsule twice a day with meals and a large glass of water.

Lifetime's Brain Support

This formula is excellent too. It includes DMAE (see page 333), which is known as 'IQ food'; plus DHA, periwinkle, ginkgo biloba and phosphatidylserine (see page 346).

Glutamine

If you only take one supplement, take glutamine (500mg, twice a day on an empty stomach). Probably the single most important antioxidant and anti-inflammatory agent in the natural supplement arsenal, people take it for moodiness and depression. Glutamine helps improve thinking by picking up excess ammonia from the brain and can be useful in clearing the brain fog caused by excess alcohol and tiredness. Use a good quality supplement such as Solgar's (www.solgar.com).

A–Z of Brain-nourishing Foods

If you're tempted to save money by ignoring organic foods, think again, because according to new preliminary evidence, organic fruits and vegetables really do offer many times more nutritional value than non-organic equivalents, including up to 20 times more calcium and manganese, 13 times more selenium and 4 times more of the important trace minerals the body needs. Organic food also contains up to 40 per cent less aluminium and other toxic metals, including lead (25 per cent less) and cadmium (29 per cent less). These figures come from an organization called Doctors' Data based in West Chicago.

A is for avocado, one of nature's superfoods and rich in vitamin B6, which the brain needs in relatively large amounts to make serotonin. This neurotransmitter increases the REM dreaming stage of sleep (see page 321), which could explain why a lack of vitamin B6 has been noticed in patients who report they do not dream at night.

B is for brewer's yeast, a natural source of dietary lithium (see page 331), and baked beans, which contain phenylalanine, a precursor of the brain chemical norepinephrine (see page 307). This amino acid is also found in meat, cheese and chocolate, and is now sold in health stores in supplement form.

C is for cabbage, a vegetable source of memory-boosting choline, and cauliflower, which provides the same nutrient. Also vitamin-C-rich foods such as acerola cherry and broccoli, which the brain also needs (see page 345).

D is for dairy products, which provide chromium, a trace element that plays an important role in maintaining blood-sugar levels. Chromium supplements may cause an unhealthy accumulation in the body's tissues so better to source it from the diet. A 200g/7oz serving of wholegrain rice will help meet your daily maintenance dose of 0.025mg of chromium.

E is for eggs, which provide tryptophan, another precursor for the feel-good brain chemical serotonin. Go To Work On An Egg was not just a clever advertising slogan, it also makes good sense healthwise to eat an egg for breakfast (though not every day, since when it comes to health, moderation is the key), since egg yolks also provide choline which the brain uses to make acetylcholine, the substance that is secreted at the ends of many nerve fibres to transmit nerve impulses, low levels of which have been linked with memory loss.

F is for oily fish such as salmon or mackerel, one of the best food sources of the polyunsaturated fats that are so critical to mood and brain development (see page 314); also dried figs, which provide calming calcium.

G is for grains, which provide vitamin B3 (niacin or nicotinic acid), which the brain needs to ward off senility. This nutrient has been prescribed in mega doses to help treat both alcoholism and schizophrenia. In the body, its natural form is nicotinamide dinucleotide (NAD), which acts in the same way in the brain as anti-anxiety benzodiazepine drugs.

H is for honey, which has a calming, natural sedative action on the brain, as do celery seeds, sage, onion, parsley, fennel, garlic and ginger. Dissolve a teaspoon of New Zealand manuka honey in a glass of warm milk at bedtime to boost calcium and tryptophan levels and get a good night's sleep.

I is for inhibitory neurotransmitters. Roughly a third of the brain's cells send inhibitory rather than acceleratory signals to protect you, and to do this, they rely on calming gamma-aminobutyric acid (GABA). This substance is made from glutamic acid and its sedative effects are enhanced by the presence of vitamin B6. Food sources of the latter include beans, dairy, crab, peas, potatoes, prunes, rice, spinach, sunflower seeds and soybeans.

J is for junk food, which will exacerbate mood and behavioural disorders, including hyperactivity in adults and kids. Switch to organic foods where you can, and try to avoid as many as possible of the 5000 or more chemical colourings, flavourings and preservatives that have been proven to disturb not only mood and behaviour but the nutritional balance of the body too.

K is for kale, an excellent source of brain-calming and sleep-inducing calcium, for those suffering either panic attacks, insomnia or both. Lightly steam and serve both the stem and the leaves if you are using younger leaves; cook for longer if the leaves are older. I often use this vegetable, after steaming, in my chillit pie (for the secret recipe, see O is for Oats, below).

L is for legumes (see page 81), which provide vitamin B6, a nutrient the body needs to convert L-dopa to mood and behaviour-controlling dopamine. Other good dietary sources include bananas, fish, potatoes, poultry, leafy green vegetables and brewer's yeast.

M is for magnesium, a muscle-relaxant that can help overcome a panic attack; foods rich in this mineral include nuts, wholegrains, beans, dark green vegetables, fish, meat, dairy products, molasses and kiwi fruit.

N is for niacin or vitamin B3 (see page 338), which helps calm the central nervous system; good food sources include dairy, fish, wholegrains, legumes, meat, peanuts and poultry.

O is for calming oats, which help maintain even blood-sugar levels and avoid mood swings. Here is my recipe for **chillit**: a simple, oat-based pie I make at least once a week, to serve hot or cold. The base is a brilliant alternative to the fag of making pastry and you can fill it with any roasted vegetables, herbs, feta cheese or other delicious and healthy combinations. Use a cup to measure – it's the ratio not the quantity that matters. In a bowl, mix together half a cup each of flour and oats. In a jug, mix together a quarter of a cup each of oil and water. Start pouring the water and oil into the flour and oats, mixing with a knife until you have a wettish but not too sticky mixture. Press it into the pie tin using the heel of your hand and your fingers. Chill for an hour and then fill with vegetables. Mix six eggs and a large pot of natural yoghurt with grated cheese, season with herbs, pour over the vegetables and bake until golden brown.

P is for pumpkin seeds, a good source of brain-protecting omega-3 fatty acids (see page 313), and pistachios, which provide monounsaturated fats for extra energy.

Q is for quercetin, a bioflavonoid that is synergistic with vitamin C (see page 289) and thus works to superboost its action in the brain. There is a suggestion that quercetin, when used with other antioxidants such as vitamin C, may be a useful adjunct to conventional treatment of schizophrenia, but this is still only a suggestion. Good dietary sources of this agent include red wine, onions, green apples, berries and brassica vegetables.

R is for riboflavin (vitamin B2), one of those nutrients now extensively used to 'fortify' breakfast cereals, especially for kids. Riboflavin, along with vitamin C, zinc, magnesium and tryrosine, can help support worn-out adrenal glands (see Chapter 5, page 248), which, if left unsupported, will cause depression and fatigue. Foods that are high in riboflavin include rice, salmon, spinach, eggs, cod, cheese, brazil nuts and beans.

S is for soy, an excellent source of brain-boosting phosphatidyl-choline, which not only enhances the availability of other nutrients but which is also a key component of the neurotransmitter acetylcholine, low levels of which have been linked to memory loss. Egg yolks and meat also provide this nutrient.

T is for tomatoes, which provide the antidepressant nutrient phenylalanine, which can also further enhance memory.

U is for unsaturated fats (see page 314), which help protect brain cells and their membranes. Monounsaturated fats are present in avocado, cashews, peanuts, pistachios, pumpkin seeds and walnuts. Polyunsaturated fats are present in fish, flaxseed oil, sesame seeds, soybeans and sunflower oil.

V is for vitamin E, which can help increase circulation – and thus the transportation of glucose and oxygen – to the brain. Since this nutrient is an important antioxidant, it can also protect brain cells from free-radical damage and destruction. Foods that are rich in vitamin E include eggs, mayonnaise, milk, salmon, sweet potato, peanuts, cold-pressed oils, dark leafy greens and lettuce.

W is for wheatgrass juice, a source of liquid oxygen and a natural antioxidant that is reported to promote 'clearer thinking'. You have to build up your tolerance to this supplement, which has a very unpleasant taste that is, unfortunately, hard to disguise. For details on a wheatgrass starter kit and accompanying manual, contact the UK specialists Wholistic Research (www.wholisticresearch.com).

X is for Xynergy (08456 585858; www.xynergy.co.uk), the UK-specialist supplier of green superfoods, including spirulina, which are rich in brain-supporting nutrients such as vitamin B5 (see page 336).

Y is for yoghurt, a good dietary source of tyrosine (see page 312), low levels of which have been linked with anxiety disorders and panic attacks. You find this same nutrient in avocados, eggs, cheese, bananas, spinach, watermelon, figs, cucumber and watercress.

Z is for zinc, low levels of which have been linked with hyperactivity and antisocial behaviour in adults and kids. The therapeutic daily dose for adults is 30mg but you can increase the amount of zinc in your diet by eating more shellfish, pumpkin seeds, eggs and red meats. Zinc deficiency has also been linked with autism.

Ancient Wisdom, 21st-century Healing

Traditional Chinese Medicine (TCM)

The herb of choice for the treatment of dementia-style conditions, including Alzheimer's disease (see page 316), in China is **huperzine A**, which, as well as being less toxic than the conventional medication, appears to be more effective in several different areas.

An extract from the plant club moss (Huperzia serrata), this compound, which can also be made synthetically in the laboratory, was traditionally used to treat fever and inflammation, and has now been used to treat over 100,000 patients in China where researchers at the Shanghai Institute of Materia Medica report that it works to improve memory better than Tacrine or other conventional drugs.

In one trial, where fifty Alzheimer's patients were given 200mcg of huperzine A supplementation for eight weeks, twenty-nine showed significant improvement in memory, cognitive and behavioural functioning, according to the Wechsler memory scale and the Hasegawa dementia scale, both internationally accepted standards of testing.

Huperzine A is thought to act in the same way as the conventional drugs to stop the breakdown of acetylcholine, which plays an important role in memory and learning, but as ever, in natural medicine, if you want the same reported results, you need to make sure you are using the same dosage: 200mcg.

Ayurvedic (Indian) Remedies

Uplifting and traditionally used in its native India by those on the spiritual path towards greater enlightenment, **holy basil** is said to have been found growing around Christ's tomb after the resurrection, thereby making the plant symbolic of new life. Described in the Ayurvedic texts as the 'Mother Medicine of Nature', it is also known as tulsi, which means the 'incomparable one'. Holy basil is also what is known in Ayurvedic medicine as a **rasayana**, meaning an extraordinary herb that works on its own to nourish a person's growth towards well-being and enlightenment.

Holy basil's active agents also include Cox-2 inhibiting anti-inflammatory molecules (making it helpful in managing joint pains and stiffness, see Chapter 4), plus anticancer chemicals, which have now been studied in both America and the Far East. (New Chapter's Supercritical Holy Basil is harvested at the company's organic farm in Costa Rica. Visit www.newchapter.info.)

Ancient Egyptian

Chamomile, widely used as a general tonic by the ancient Egyptians, is a safe and mild sedative that can help induce sleep in both adults and children. Rich in calcium, magnesium and the B vitamins, it works to strengthen the nervous system and promote restful sleep.

What is less well known is that this everyday herb also contains tryptophan (see 5-hydroxytryptophan, page 334), which can help counter low mood and depression too.

This is definitely one to keep in your emergency cupboard in both tea and tincture form. Get your supplies from Tree Harvest, 01452 849 123, or www.tree-harvest.com.

You can also get an excellent rose incense (sourced from Greece) from the same company which is helpful to burn in times of grief; see Relaxation Techniques, page 271, for more on burning incense to change your mood.

Native New Zealand Remedies

According to 19th-century botanists, the Maori were as prone to depression and low mood states as any person living today, and their herb of choice to counter the condition was a native relative of the **passionflower** plant.

This works as a mild sedative and nerve tonic, and is widely used across the world to alleviate nervous tension, insomnia, anxiety and hyperactivity. One of my favourite remedies is an alcohol-free tincture that combines passionflower with soothing valerian from the Eclectic range (www.victoriahealth.com). I give this to my young daughter when we fly long-haul to prevent overexcitement and restlessness.

Again, this is a plant that contains both calcium and magnesium; the former, as we have seen, is an important calming agent, and magnesium, which is commonly deficient in adults, especially women, works as a muscle relaxant, making it a good headache remedy to keep on standby.

What Really Works for Managing Mood and Brain Function

Cognitive Function

This is the term we use to describe a person's state of consciousness – not in the yogic sense of enlightenment, but in the sense of alertness and orientation, memory, attention span and insight.

Changes in cognitive functioning, such as confusion, lethargy and delirium, can be triggered by many medical conditions, including fever, trauma, circulatory problems and brain disease, and by environmental and dietary factors such as drugs or toxins. Cognitive tests also assess memory span, insight, command of language, fund of knowledge, abstract reasoning and judgement before a clinical diagnosis is made, but the single most common symptom of decreased cognitive function is memory loss (see Memory and Periwinkle, page 319).

Vitamin C is the first supplement to consider since many studies with elderly patients demonstrate that those whose diet includes higher amounts of vitamin C, plus supplementation, have better cognitive function. Cognitive impairment has also been linked with a deficiency in **vitamin B12**, which has been shown to improve brain function in patients suffering from mild dementia for less than two years, but which had no real effect in more serious and longer-lasting cases.

Phosphatidylserine is the most abundant phospholipid in the brain, where it plays a critical role in maintaining both the structure and functioning of brain cells. Numerous studies report that this agent can help improve memory, learning, concentration, word recall and mood in middle-aged and elderly patients suffering from dementia or age-related cognitive decline.

Vinpocetine (periwinkle) is another important brain-protecting compound (see page 319), which has been shown to protect brain cells from damage induced by drugs and which also has an anticonvulsant action in the body (see Seizures, below).

1, 2, 3 . . . Easy Steps for Protecting Cognitive Function

Take vitamin C along with DHA (see page 315).

Take phosphatidylserine (**www.solgar.com**).

Use Lifetime's Brain Support formula which includes vinpocetine (www.victoriahealth.com).

Headaches, Including Migraines

The new generation herb that is overtaking feverfew as the remedy of choice for headaches, especially migraines, is a plant called Peasites hybridus, sold under its more common name of **butterbur**.

The active agents, extracted from the root of the plant, have an anti-inflammatory and analgesic action, both of which appear to kick in faster than feverfew, which can require several weeks to take effect.

To produce this supplement, a patented manufacturing process is used which removes from the plant the pyrrolizidine alkaloids, which are both potentially hepatoxic and carcinogenic. In Germany, this extract is now licensed as a pharmacy medicine and the therapeutic daily dose, which has also been shown to be safe and effective when given to children over the age of six, is 50mg of the active agents.

Butterbur works as a painkiller by blocking the action of prostaglandins and leukotrienes, which cause inflammation, and in animal trials, the extract of this herb has been shown to prevent muscle contraction that is a result of the action of acetylcholine and histamine.

In controlled clinical trials, in 170 migraine patients who were given between 100mg and 150mg of butterbur extract daily, no adverse side effects were reported, although some participants complained about the unpleasant taste and smell of the product (unfortunately, most herbal remedies do not appeal to either the nose or the palate – but then neither do a lot of prescription drugs!). In trials in Germany, prescribing butterbur to migraine patients for eight weeks brought about a 60 per cent reduction in the frequency of migraine attacks.

Migraines tend to affect women more than men – three out of four sufferers are women – and some 18 per cent of females will suffer them at some time in their lives, compared with just 6 per cent of males. They occur most frequently first thing in the morning, reaching their peak of intensity and pain within an hour of the onset of symptoms. Food allergens, especially chocolate and caffeine, can trigger an attack so rule these out.

Other natural agents that can help manage headaches and migraines include **magnesium** (50 per cent of sufferers have lower levels of ionized magnesium during an acute attack), a mineral which is thought to affect serotonin receptors in the brain, and **vitamin B2 (riboflavin)**, which performed better in trials than a placebo pill to reduce both the number and the severity of attacks.

The **omega-6 fatty acids** (see page 314) help reduce inflammation, making **evening primrose oil** a useful adjunct to any painkilling remedy.

1, 2, 3 . . . Easy Steps to Help Prevent Migraines and Other Headaches
Take butterbur extract: 50mg–150mg a day.

Take magnesium: 250mg of a food-state supplement.

Take evening primrose oil every day.

You can get food-state magnesium and evening primrose oil from most good health stores; mail order butterbur from Victoria Health (0800 389 8195; www.victoriahealth.com) if you have problems finding it locally.

Parkinson's Disease

The Pope hit the headlines when it was revealed he used **papain**, a mix of enzymes sourced from the papaya fruit, to help manage the symptoms of this disease, but the single most important agent is a nutritional one called **nicotinamide dinucleotide hydrogen (NADH)**, which you take in liquid form.

The theory is that this substance, which is present in every cell in the body, helps the brain make dopamine (see page 327), which is important since this disease is characterized by the loss of dopaminergic neurons.

In hospital trials involving over 800 patients, half of whom were given NADH intravenously and half of whom received the medication in capsule form, only 20 per cent failed to report significant clinical improvement. The researchers also noted that the younger patients and those with shorter durations of the disease responded better than older patients who had been afflicted for longer.

Parkinson's disease is a condition of mid to later life, although some 30 per cent of patients report recognizable symptoms before the age of fifty. Classic symptoms include tremor at rest, rigidity, a stooped posture, a 'masked' face and urinary dysfunction.

Depression (see page 306) is often a feature of the early disease and between 15 and 40 per cent of all Parkinson's patients develop some form of dementia as the condition progresses.

Platelets taken from the mitochondria (see page 357) of

Parkinson's patients have been shown to have lower levels of **co-enzyme Q10** (CoQ10; see page 332) when compared with normal controls, and in animal studies this agent has been shown to protect the dopaminergic neurons of mice injected with a chemical that would otherwise damage these cells. In variable dosage trials with humans, researchers concluded that Parkinson's patients given 1200mg a day of CoQ10 developed less disability than those taking a placebo pill. These higher doses were also deemed to be well tolerated.

Grapeseed extract is a powerful anti-inflammatory agent that works synergistically with **vitamin C** (see page 305) to protect brain tissue from oxidative damage.

1, 2, 3 . . . Easy Steps to Help Manage Parkinson's Disease

Take NADH but make sure you use the FSC brand (widely available in health stores) since this is the one that has been used in the clinical research. Take as directed on the bottle.

Take 1200mg a day of co-enzyme Q10; find a supplement sourced from soybean oil for better bioavailability. If you are not sure, write to the manufacturer and ask before you buy.

Take grapeseed extract with 1g of vitamin C a day to prevent oxidative damage.

Seasonal Affective Disorder (SAD)

Twice as common in women than men and most likely to start in your thirties, seasonal affective disorder (SAD) is now said to affect up to 20 per cent of the adult population, making the winter months miserable for many of the sufferers.

The main symptom is depression (see page 306), but other tell-tale signs of this condition include developing an increased appetite with strong cravings for carbohydrates and sweets, weight gain, fatigue, wanting to sleep for longer and get up later, plus an energy slump in the afternoons.

SAD has now been linked by researchers with a decrease in the levels of those hormones and brain chemicals that control both mood and sleeping patterns, which means that you can use a number of alternative remedies which trigger an increase in production of these substances to try to redress this imbalance.

The most important hormone the body relies on to regulate the body clock is **melatonin.** In animals, it controls seasonal behaviour, including hibernation. The chemical precursor used to make melatonin, as we have seen, is serotonin, and you can use **St John's wort** or **rhodiola** to increase production of this neurotransmitter naturally.

One of the most important triggers for the production of serotonin is natural daylight but, since 90 per cent of us spend 90 per cent of our time indoors, especially in winter climes, you will need to make a special effort to get outside to benefit from it. Those suffering with full-blown SAD symptoms tend instead to compensate with the use of specially developed light boxes and even light bulbs that simulate natural daylight indoors.

Another natural winter mood-booster is an amino acid called **tryptophan,** sold as **5-HTP,** a precursor to serotonin. Present in foods as diverse as roasted pumpkin seeds and baked potatoes with their skins on, it is also one of the active agents in a seaweed called kelp (see Sea Vegetables, page 72). To make serotonin, the body also needs a good supply of **vitamin B6,** which is found in carrots, fish, lentils, peas, potato, spinach and sunflower seeds, so it is a good idea, if you are a SAD sufferer, to increase your dietary intake of all these.

1, 2, 3 Easy Steps to Ward Off SAD

Use St John's wort or rhodiola (see pages 307 and 252).

Supplement your diet with kelp (see page 220).

Take a good quality vitamin B complex.

Seizures

Epilepsy – or seizure disorder – is a neurological condition with symptoms ranging from a momentary lapse of attention to full-blown convulsions. It is one of the first brain disorders ever to be described (it was first mentioned in ancient Babylon more than 3000 years ago) and the word 'epilepsy' comes from the Greek word meaning 'attack'.

Seizure disorder affects an estimated 0.5 per cent of the population and can affect people of any age. It may be the result of a head injury, brain tumour or infection, but in many cases the cause is unknown.

Antioxidants play a key protective role – plasma levels of vitamins A, C and E are normal in patients who have been seizure-free for a year, but among those with active seizures, levels are lower than among healthy controls.

The key remedy to investigate is the neuro-protective herb **vinpocetine (periwinkle)**, which has anticonvulsant as well as memory-boosting attributes (see page 319).

A high-fat, low-carbohydrate diet may also help. In a survey of 150 children diagnosed with seizure disorders, researchers at the John Hopkins Medical Center in Baltimore reported that those who were placed on a high-fat diet and followed it for three to six years suffered a 90–99 per cent reduction in the frequency of their seizures, and were able to reduce their medication to either just a single dose or none at all.

1, 2, 3 . . . Easy Steps to Supporting the Brain When Seizure Disorder Has Been Diagnosed

Use vinpocetine or Lifetime's Brain Support formula (see page 337), which includes this herb.

Take a good quality antioxidant supplement.

Switch to a high-fat, low-carbohydrate diet but take a supplement such as Perfectly Balanced (see page 298) to make sure the body is still getting all the nutrients it needs.

Roll Out Your Yoga Mat

The aim, with meditation, is to stop the ceaseless chatter of the mind (easier said than done for most of us) but there are additional techniques, including the yoga mudras, you can employ to help achieve this state where the brainwaves actually slow down.

Mudra translates roughly as 'gesture' or 'attitude', and mudras work to change the flow of energy or prana through the body. They are very subtle and work at a deep level to alter mood. I like them because they are the yogic 'short-cut' to better mood and well-being.

They may look simple but, if you are serious about them, they form part of a more advanced yoga practice. There are five groups of yoga mudra but here we will concentrate on the simpler, starter mudras, which, despite the fact they do not look much like active postures, are said to change energy flow and mood.

Here are my **1, 2, 3 easy mudras** to improve mood and brain function.

Hridaya Mudra (Heart Gesture)

This, my favourite of all the hand mudras, acknowledges that the seat of the emotions is not the brain but the heart. It helps to release pent-up emotions and is especially useful during times of emotional conflict, crisis and rollercoasting mood.

Adopt a comfortable sitting position that you can maintain for twenty or thirty minutes without feeling stiff or sore. Use a chair if you need to but do not slouch, since slumping will affect the flow of the pranic energy to the heart centre.

Keep your head and spine straight and place the tips of each index finger at the base of each thumb. Now join the middle and ring fingers on each hand to the tip of the thumb. Keep the little finger outstretched. This is the mudra.

Place your hands on your knees, palms facing towards the ceiling, close your eyes, relax the whole body and stay as still as you can.

Bring your awareness to your breathing, which will begin to slow down. Don't think about anything. Forget 'Am I doing this right or wrong?' Just allow your body to settle into the mudra and build up to sitting for twenty or thirty minutes at a time.

That's it. The mudra does the work for you and it couldn't be more simple or effective. Anyway, don't take my word for it. Try it yourself and see just how calming each practice can be.

Nasikagra Drishti (Nose-gazing)

It sounds silly but bringing your awareness to the tip of your nose and keeping your attention there is an excellent way to dispel tension and built-up emotions, especially anger. This mudra also works to develop your powers of concentration, and if you can build up to a longer practice of, say, twenty or thirty minutes, it will also induce a calming meditative state. In a more advanced practice, this mudra allows the yogi to 'transcend' normal awareness.

Again, adopt any sitting position that is comfortable but allows you to maintain a straight head and spine. Although you are keeping your eyes open – to gaze at the tip of your nose – the purpose of this mudra is to bring about intro-spection so practise somewhere calm and quiet, preferably later at night when the kids are in bed and you are not likely to be disturbed.

Rest your hands on your knees with the index finger curled into the inside of the thumb in another hand mudra known as the psychic gesture of knowledge. What this signifies is you are 'open' to increasing your awareness as you practise your yoga. In the morning, you rest your hands with the palms turned upwards in this mudra; in the evening, reverse the position so the palms are facing down on your lap.

Keep your eyes open and focus them on the tip of your nose. Do not strain to do this. When they are correctly focused, you will see a double outline of your nose, which converges at the tip to form a V-shape. Concentrate your gaze on the apex of this V (i.e. the very end of your nose).

Concentrate only on your gazing and try not to think of anything else. After a few minutes, close your eyes and repeat the practice again. Try to build up so you can practise nose-gazing for five minutes at a time.

Shanmukhi Mudra (Closing the Seven Gates)

The aim of this mudra is to balance internal and external awareness, but because it can be a very powerful experience it should not be practised by anyone suffering from depression.

It is one of my all-time favourite yoga practices. Once you have mastered it, you will not need me to tell you why.

Again, adopt a seated position that allows you to sit comfortably while keeping the spine and head erect. If you need cushions for extra padding, use them. The important thing is not to be distracted by aching limbs once you start the practice.

Close your eyes, place your hands on your knees and concentrate on slowing the breath as you begin to relax the whole body.

Now raise the arms in front of the face, with the elbows pointing sideways. You will be keeping the arms in this position.

Close the ears with the thumbs.

Close the eyes with the index fingers.

Close the nostrils with the middle fingers.

Close the mouth by placing the ring and little fingers above and below the lips.

Release the hold of the middle fingers to breathe in through the nostrils. Inhale slowly and deeply. At the end of breathing in, replace the middle fingers to firmly close the nostrils again.

Hold your breath only for as long as you are comfortable doing so. As you sit with all the external senses blocked, become aware of anything you hear or see in your mind.

Keep your awareness on the area in the middle of your brow, just above your eyes. This is the area called anhata chakra, or the mystical third eye. This is the seat of your extrasensory powers of perception, and just like the muscles you can see and train and tone, you can practise this mudra to develop more instinctual, even psychic awareness.

When you are done holding your breath, release the nostrils again and breathe out through the nose.

This counts as one round. Practise this mudra for just five minutes at first, building up to thirty minutes as you become more experienced.

At the end of your session, do not jolt yourself back into the real world but slowly lower your arms, keep your hands resting on your lap and bring your awareness back to your physical body, sitting in a quiet room. In other words, don't suddenly leap into action but give yourself time to adjust.

Again, don't take it from me. Try it, make a note of anything you feel in this area and decide for yourself if it works for you.

CHAPTER SEVEN

Energy and Fatigue

The single most common health complaint in the stressed-out western world is fatigue and lack of energy, which is deemed chronic when it is not rectified by a good night's sleep. In fact, this has become the single most common complaint of patients seeking some form of medical treatment.

The Real Root of the Problem – Mitochondrial Dysfunction

It is, of course, related to ageing, although the ageing I am talking about here has nothing to do with how many birthdays you have celebrated or the number of lines on your face but the ageing of those biological systems responsible for energy production – the mitochondria.

There are between 500 and 2000 mitochondria present in every cell, except red blood cells and the lens of the eye. You will find more in the organs that work the hardest – the heart, the kidney and the brain – and almost all your mitochondria (99.9 per cent) come from your mother. It is here that food is converted to energy.

Known as the powerhouse of the cells, the tiny mitochondrial organelles produce a substance called adenosine triphosphate (ATP). When you use your muscles, ATP is broken down into two other compounds: adenosine diphosphate (ADP) and inorganic phosphate, and it is this process that produces cellular energy, which, among other things, powers the muscles making this a cyclical process.

As we age, the mitochondria age too. They produce less and less ATP so you become like a car that is slowly running out of petrol. And since, to make ATP the body has to use ATP, if you don't have enough energy in the first place, it is inevitable that you start to run out of steam.

As far back as the mid-1950s, scientists began to investigate the idea that ageing and its associated gradual loss of energy begins with damage to the mitochondria, which are even more suscepti-ble to free-radical attack (see page 259) than other cellular structures.

The reason for this is that while mitochondria have their own DNA, unlike the genetic material in the nucleus of the cell, mito-chondrial DNA has no protection and no in-built repair mechanism. DNA in the nucleus of the cell, for instance, is pro-tected by histones. These are positively charged, protective 'storage' proteins around which nuclear DNA is wound, like a thread around a spool, but these are not present in the mitochon-dria. All those complex repair mechanisms that exist in the nucleus of the cell to protect DNA are also missing, and to make matters worse, mitochondrial DNA is located in the mitochon-drial matrix, near the inner mitochondrial membrane, where both energy and damaging free radicals are produced, making this genetic material even more vulnerable to free-radical attack.

In young, healthy adults, the mitochondria adapt to increased energy demands by replicating rapidly to produce more ATP. As we age, this replication process slows down, which means we have fewer mitochondria to meet the same energy demand. They will attempt to do this by increasing in size (as opposed to number) but larger mitochondria are less efficient and produce more damaging free radicals than their more youthful, more numerous and smaller progenitors.

Protecting the Body's Energy-making Organelles

The single most important supplement to take to help prevent further damage to the mitochondrial organelles is a good quality **antioxidant** combining **vitamins A, C, E** and **selenium**. Many herbs, including **ginkgo biloba** have antioxidant properties too and other important nutrients include **co-enzyme Q10** (see page 332), **N-acetyl cysteine** (NAC; see page 147), **L-carnitine** (see page 360), the **B vitamins** and the cell membrane-protecting **omega-3 fatty acids** (see page 314).

Co-enzyme Q10, for example, has been shown in trials to increase production of ATP, reduce levels of lactic acid, improve muscle strength, decrease muscle fatigue and act as a potent antioxidant in its own right to mop up scavenging and damaging free radical molecules. It is even more effective when taken with **L-carnitine** and **essential fatty acids**, which will all work together to boost flagging energy levels.

Exercise is important too and we are not talking an amble round the park with the dog. As we age, the body tends to use more glucose and less fat during exercise, so what you need is resistance or weight training, which will compensate for this biological change by decreasing glucose production and increasing the oxidation of fat.

If you have heard that exercise is bad for you because it also generates more free radicals (which it does), which would surely cause more damage to the mitochondrial organelles, you cannot use this as an excuse for slouching on the couch, because **the right kind of endurance exercise** will counter this.

Scientists at the Guang-zhou Institute of Physical Education in Canton, China, have now shown how weight-training works to increase the production of mitochondrial manganese superoxide dismutase and glutathione peroxidase: two powerful antioxidants which help counter any increase in the production of free radicals.

Tried and Applied

. . . with fruit flies! Australian researchers at the National Ageing Research Institute in that country extended the lifespan of fruit flies by 15 per cent using nicotinamide (see page 364) to re-energize their energy-producing systems. The flies were given a therapeutic dose of 250mcg (micrograms) in 1ml of water.

The One to Watch – L-Carnitine

Known as 'the energizer', **carnitine** plays many roles in the body, including preventing the mitochondria from shutting down when the body's energy-producing system backs up. It does this by stopping another substance, called acetyl co-enzyme A, from building up and shutting down the energy cycle.

The body makes carnitine naturally, but only when there is enough of the amino acid **lysine** (see Top Ten Remedies, page 379) available. In supplement form, it is sold as L-carnitine. For maximum energy-boosting effect, take **L-carnitine** with **co-enzyme**

Q10 (known as the capsule of youth), **magnesium, lysine** and **essential fatty acids.**

Fatigue and Brain Fog

Both classic symptoms of energy-deficient syndromes such as chronic fatigue and fibromyalgia, tiredness and brain fog are also common complaints in otherwise healthy people. For more ideas on how to support healthy brain function, go back to Chapter 6, Depression and Mood.

To clear brain fog, take **NADH (nicotinamide dinucleotide hydrogen)**, which is also known as co-enzyme 1. It works to boost energy levels and helps clear thinking by increasing dopamine levels in the brain (see page 306). Studies show NADH – which increases the production of dopamine by stimulating the enzyme tyrosine hydroxylase (TH), the key enzyme involved in production of this neurotransmitter – can boost levels of both dopamine and norepinephrine by up to 40 per cent. Dopamine also works to lower levels of prolactin, a hormone that is often elevated in people with chronic fatigue syndrome and fibromyalgia, due to the suppression of the hypothalamus (see page 363).

Vitamin C . . . for Kicks

The reason you can't get going without that first latte or double-shot macchiato of the day is that your body has come to depend on this first hit of caffeine to kick-start it into all-systems-go.

Ever wondered how this works?

Coffee is a natural stimulant belonging to a family of chemicals known as methylxanthines. What these chemicals do is disable one of the enzymes (phosphodieterase) that would otherwise destroy another substance, cyclic adenosine monophosphate (cAMP), which is in fact the agent that activates the neurotransmitters in the brain. In other words, drinking coffee gives your brain a jolt into action. Give up coffee for a week, and if you've been relying on regular hits to boost your energy levels enough to get you through the day, you'll soon have a crippling detox headache.

What you may not know is that **vitamin C**, in the form of ascorbic acid, works in exactly the same way! It too blocks this same enzyme and so raises levels of cAMP to give the brain a good jumpstart without the side effects of caffeine.

Chronic Fatigue Syndrome

By definition, a syndrome is a group of symptoms that occur together and characterize a specific condition. In both chronic fatigue syndrome (CFS) and fibromyalgia (FM), these symptoms include:
- Fatigue
- Diffuse achiness
- Poor sleep
- Brain fog
- Increased thirst
- Weight gain (the average weight gain with these conditions is 32lb/14.5kg)
- Digestive disorders
- Poor libido
- Frequent infections
- Multiple food/chemical sensitivities

The clinical diagnostic criteria for CFS are now so stringent that many natural healers believe they exclude a staggering 90 per cent of those who actually have the syndrome. What all these patients have in common, despite a diverse range of symptoms, is depression of the **hypothalamus,** the master gland that controls sleep, hormone function, temperature regulation and the autonomic nervous system, which regulates blood pressure, blood flow and movement of food through the bowel.

Suppression of the hypothalamus, which has been linked back to mitochondrial dysfunction (see page 357), would explain why CFS and FM patients experience weight gain and repeated infections, which are a sign of a struggling immune system that has become compromised due to impaired sleep. They are also often lacking in key nutrients because digestive problems mean they are not absorbing all the nutrients the body needs.

At any given time, an estimated 12 per cent of the adult population is suffering some form of severe, disabling fatigue, which has been present for at least a month. For a natural approach which takes into account all the above factors and which claims a 90 per cent improvement in the quality of life of such patients, visit www.endfatigue.com.

Dietary changes to help manage these symptoms need to include cutting down on coffee and alcohol and drinking more filtered, pure water to avoid dehydration, which can exacerbate symptoms.

Top Six Remedies to Counter Chronic Fatigue Syndrome (CFS) and Fibromyalgia

Elderberry

What we do now know is that in 40 per cent of cases, there is a proven link between CFS and an infection by the **Epstein-Barr virus (EBV).** Although still the minority, 40 per cent remains significant, not least because researchers know that, depending on the tests being used, a significant number of individuals – up to 15 per cent – who have had the EBV infection will still test negatively for it. And if you add the two together, then in the majority of sufferers there could be a link.

EBV is responsible for the typically teenage infection we know as glandular fever – also known as 'kissing disease' since in healthy people it is shed in their oral secretions. As a member of the herpes family of viruses, it has the same ability to remain dormant in the body long after the primary infection. It 'hides' in the salivary glands and the B-cells of the immune system where, unless something goes wrong, it can usually be kept in check by the other immune system cells.

The humble hedgerow **elderberry** has antiviral properties and will act specifically against the herpes viruses, especially the Epstein-Barr relative. The way it works is that the active ingredients inhibit or block the virus's replication mechanism. It too has strong antioxidant properties to protect the body from free-radical damage and is used as an immune system tonic to return the immune system to optimum functioning, so even if you don't know if your child has had a viral infection, giving this herb will still help.

Solgar (**www.solgar.com**) makes a supplement that combines a standardized elderberry extract (150mg) with the equivalent dosage of powdered raw herb.

Nicotinamide

The first enzyme involved in energy production in the body is nicotinamide dinucleotide hydrogen – NADH – which is also known as co-enzyme 1. Enzymes are proteins that trigger chemical changes in the body, and NADH, which is a derivative of nicotine, is so important it is found in all living cells. The only supplement brand that has undergone clinical trials in the US or here is FSC's NADH, which is on sale in GNC high street health stores.

Athletes report that NADH makes them feel stronger and more

energized. You need to take this supplement, which can also boost concentration levels, half an hour before eating, and limit your dosage to no more than two tablets a day.

Co-enzyme Q10

This nutrient has been shown in trials to increase production of ATP, reduce levels of lactic acid, improve muscle strength, decrease muscle fatigue and act as a potent antioxidant in its own right to mop up scavenging and damaging free radical molecules. It is even more effective when taken with **L-carnitine** and **essential fatty acids**, which will all work together to boost flagging energy levels.

You can adjust the doses of carnitine and co-enzyme Q10, but to start off, take 500mg of carnitine and 30mg of CoQ10 twice a day, with breakfast and with lunch. With extra stress, step up the carnitine to 3g and increase the co-enzyme Q10 to 90mg a day.

Malic Acid

This agent occurs naturally in foods and fruits, especially apples, but when levels are low, the body has to shift to a more inefficient (anaerobic) way of producing energy. This shift can contribute to the build-up of lactic acid that can cause the typical muscle pain and achiness reported by fatigue patients.

Vitamin B12

This is another key nutrient in helping manage fatigue, and even if blood levels are normal, research has now shown that levels in the brain and nervous system, which make a huge demand on this vitamin, may not be.

The theory is that metabolic dysfunction associated with fatigue conditions means the nutrient is not getting through the blood–brain barrier into the brain where it is needed to counter higher levels of the neurotransmitter nitric oxide, which is often too high in such patients and may be contributing to the disease. Speak to your natural health advisor about taking a course of vitamin B12 injections, which will be more effective than oral medication.

You will not benefit from any of the supplements you take if your digestive system is impaired and you are not able to assimilate these agents, so include a **digestive enzyme** (see page 85) in your daily supplementation regimen.

Betaine Hydrochloride

Again, you will be wasting your money if you cannot absorb the additional nutrients you need. Low levels of stomach acid have been linked with fatigue-type conditions. Remedy this with a betaine hydrochloride supplement (see page 55).

Tried and Applied

Kombucha tea: This is a living yeast culture that you ferment with sweetened tea to produce a health drink that is packed with vitamins, enzymes, minerals and organic acids, and said to be very effective for fatigue conditions including CFS. Contact the UK's Kombucha Tea Network, based in Bath, for a starter culture and book which explains how Kombucha tea works to strengthen the whole body, detoxify the system and help manage immune-related conditions including arthritis, digestive disorders, psoriasis and even cancer. The recommended daily dose, once you are up and running, is 150ml or a wineglassful, three times a day.

Fibromyalgia (FM)

Thought to affect between 2 and 4 per cent of the adult population, fibromyalgia is a rheumatic autoimmune condition, which is also closely linked with CFS (page 362).

Although symptoms such as disturbed sleep, fatigue and stiffness can vary from patient to patient, the key characteristic symptom is widespread musculo-skeletal pain. Indeed, the only real difference between those meeting the clinical criteria for a diagnosis of fibromyalgia and chronic fatigue is the degree of musculo-skeletal pain that FM patients report; Substance P, a pain neurotransmitter, has been found at levels up to 300 per cent higher in FM patients than normal controls.

The current clinical definition of FM is widespread musculo-skeletal pain in all four quadrants of the body which has been present for at least three months, and tenderness at eleven of eighteen specific designated points on the body. Some 90 per cent of FM sufferers are female (see Women and Autoimmune Conditions, page 372) and the average age of onset is slightly less than fifty years.

Again, medical science has not come up with either a cause or a cure, leaving sufferers with a range of theories to decipher and an element of 'pot luck' to take in deciding how best to manage symptoms using natural adjuncts to the conventional therapies.

One thing that FM patients do have is changes in metabolism, energy production and the regulation of neurotransmitters including serotonin, dopamine and norepinephrine, so make sure you read the chapter on Stress and Immunity (Chapter 5) and my recommendations for boosting energy to counter chronic fatigue in this chapter. There is also often an overlap between patients with FM and gastrointestinal disorders, including irritable bowel syndrome (IBS) – some 70 per cent of FM patients have IBS as well as food sensitivities – so you will need to read the chapter on digestive disorders too.

S-adenosylmethionine (SAMe) is a useful natural remedy to consider but, unfortunately, an expensive one for longer term use (see page 308). In double-blind trials, patients taking 800mg a day for six weeks reported less depression, less pain and less fatigue, prompting researchers to conclude that this agent would seem to be an effective and safe therapy in the management of primary FM – if the patient can afford it.

Magnesium and **malic acid** (see page 365) will help bolster low energy levels and you can use **5-hydroxytryptophan** supplements (see page 334) to help re-regulate sleep patterns and mood. A good quality probiotic, such as **lactobacillus acidophilus** (see page 10), can help counter gut disorders, and **digestive enzymes** (see page 85) will help too.

Turmeric can help relieve rheumatic-type conditions, and **astragalus** (see page 276) is an excellent tonic that can help the body to better cope with the stress of all the associated symptoms of FM to increase overall stamina and endurance. That said, it has immune-stimulating properties too, so do not take it without consulting your health advisors.

One of the new generation combination supplements designed specifically to help counter energy depletion associated with FM is **Fibro-My-DMG** (available from Victoria Health: 0800 389 8195; www.victoriahealth.com) which includes several of the energy-boosting agents on pages 312, 363–5 and 369, including malic acid, magnesium and NADH, plus dimethylglycine (DMG), which is included to help reduce overall stress on the body and promote better quality sleep.

Multiple Sclerosis (MS)

This is one of the demyelinating diseases where the protective myelin sheath that surrounds the nerve cells of the central nervous system (CNS) is stripped away. Although first described 130 years ago, the exact cause remains a mystery and there is still no known cure.

The term multiple sclerosis refers to the two primary characteristics of the disease: the plaques or sclerosed areas that are a hallmark of MS, and the numerous affected areas of the brain and spinal cord that are producing multiple neurologic symptoms that accrue over time.

Rare in Japan and among black Africans, this is a disease predominantly of temperate climates, but it can run in families too with siblings being the most commonly reported relationship.

Nobody knows precisely what part of the body is activated to attack the myelin sheaths but those parts of the immune system that appear to be implicated include macrophages, T-killer cells, lymphokines, antibodies or any combination of these elements. These cells are activated in the periphery, possibly after viral infection, and recognize the myelin proteins as antigens, which they then attack. Demyelination causes a disruption of the nerve impulses triggering neurological symptoms, which reflect those parts of the brain most affected.

In the early stages of this disease, the patient suffers unpredictable, recurrent attacks of neurological dysfunction with no set time lapse between attacks and a range of partial to complete recovery in between. In the secondary stage, there is more progression of the damage and disease between attacks, causing a gradual increase in disability that can be drawn out over years, even decades.

A significant number of MS patients have been found to be lacking in **vitamin B12** (see page 365), which is likely to be more than a passing coincidence. Oral supplementation will not be as effective as IV supplementation so you will need to find a qualified health practitioner who can offer these jabs at their clinic.

Magnesium levels are also often lower in the CNS tissues of MS patients. The body needs extracellular magnesium to release nitric oxide from its cells and so one theory is that excess levels of trapped nitric oxide in the cells combine with superoxide to form peroxynitrite, a powerful free radical that can cause damage to the myelin sheath.

Zinc is also deficient in those demyelinated areas in MS patients, which means the first step towards supporting any treatment of this condition should include a good quality multimineral supplement.

In studies of MS patients instructed to increase their dietary intake of the **omega-3** and **omega-6 fatty acids**, those who complied with the higher fat intake guidelines survived longer than those who ignored them. In fact, only 5 per cent of those increasing their fatty acid intake failed to survive the 34-year duration of the study, compared with 80 per cent of those who did not follow these dietary recommendations. Researchers in this study concluded those who stepped up their EFA intake sooner, rather than later, did best of all, and further studies have suggested it is the **omega-3 fatty acids**, more than the omega-6, that are most critical (see Essential Fatty Acids, page 378).

Reishi is one of the medicinal mushrooms that have been shown to confer both antioxidant and immune-normalizing properties, and to help inhibit intracellular superoxide (see Magnesium, above) activities. For more on this agent, which has the most active polysaccharides in the whole plant kingdom, see Traditional Chinese Medicine (page 387). New Chapter (www.newchapter.info) make reishi supplements. You can also use **phosphatidycholine** to help repair myelin damage. Use a single supplement from Solgar (www.solgar.com).

Schisandra is another herb that can help the body better resist both viral infection and antioxidant damage. It is one of the super-boosting adaptogens (see page 251) and so is another useful adjunct to conventional management of MS.

More bizarrely, some patients have reported improved symptoms when submitting themselves to the unusual therapy of . . . **bee stings**. Calling themselves 'stingers', these patients report that after the very first stinging session, much of the debilitating pain they experience disappears. Ice packs are used to first numb the stinging areas and patients then use honey as a salve to alleviate the itching and bruising that inevitably follows a stinging session.

This therapy, which, as you can imagine, has its critics, should only ever be investigated with an experienced practitioner. There is no clinical evidence to tell us how it works and none of the MS support groups or societies are fans. It must also, of course, be avoided by anyone already allergic to bee stings. For more on how it is being successfully used with MS patients in America, Europe and Asia, visit www.apitherapy.org and make up your own mind.

Following the same homeopathic principle of 'treating like with like', some doctors have been researching the idea of tackling MS by giving patients oral doses of replacement myelin protein, the protein that the body itself is attacking. The idea is to encourage the body to build a 'tolerance' to this substance, which, due to an immune dysfunction, it has started to treat as an antigen. You can read more on this quest for a cure in Susan Quinn's fascinating book, *Human Trials: Scientists, Investors and Patients in the Quest for a Cure* (Perseus Publishing).

Finally, another pioneering treatment for MS, which remains outside the mainstream, is the idea of injecting histamine, the very substance implicated in adverse allergic reactions. As with so many of the ideas we investigate in natural health circles, this is another that is anything but new – one of the first doctors to try it out on patients was running his clinic in 1946. There is, again, a fascinating story surrounding this theory, why it works for some MS patients and the obstacles that have blocked its journey into the mainstream, and you can check all this out for yourself by visiting www.tahoma-clinic.com.

I am not endorsing any of these more 'alternative' treatments here. I am simply reporting that they exist, because if they really can work for hundreds of patients, that would be something I would want to know about if one of my relatives, or indeed I myself, were a sufferer from MS.

Women and Autoimmune Conditions

Around eight different conditions, ranging from arthritis to MS and gout to Crohn's disease, have been linked with an abnormal immune response, but what has baffled researchers to date is why women should be so much more susceptible than men. Some 75 per cent of cases are female, and while genetics and family history play a role, the new theory is that the female hormones, oestrogen, progesterone and prolactin, are also contributing in some way.

Women and men differ not only on the outside, but on the inside too. They have different physiology, psychology, immunity and even cellular and molecular activities, and in those differences must lie the explanation as to why females are more prone to autoimmune disease.

For example, women have a generally lower metabolic rate than men, and in investigations of metabolic types, researchers have found that females tend to be what is classified in neuroendocrine circles as the Slow Metabolic Type 1.

This is relevant because with this type of profile, that part of the immune system that is the body's primary defence against invading organisms and toxins does not function as well as in other metabolic types. In perfect health, all parts of the immune system work together and are balanced but some 80 per cent of women (and only 50 per cent of men) exhibit dominance of the cellular immune response over what is called the humoral (primary) immune response. In other words, the immune system only really kicks in once a virus, bacteria or infection has invaded the cell.

Hair-tissue mineral analysis (HTMA) studies of both sexes show those falling into the slow metabolic type categories are often lacking in essential minerals including zinc, which is critical to immune function, calcium and magnesium. If you suffer from an autoimmune condition, take a good quality multisupplement to address this and tackle any underlying digestive disorders (see Chapter 2) that will otherwise inhibit assimilation of the nutrients your body needs.

Pain Management

Our experience of pain may be subjective but the one thing we all agree on is that our instinct, when we feel pain, is to find relief and make it stop; making pain, and its alleviation, the number-one reason any of us seek medical advice. Since the body cannot communicate with us in any other way, it is, of course, also the single most important symptom, since it signals the presence of disease, trauma, tissue injury and the fact something is not right.

There are two categories of pain: **acute**, which is generally easily treated and short-lived, and **chronic**, which is a more widespread problem and which is so debilitating it usually results in low mood and even more serious psychological disorders, including depression. A chronic pain is any pain that lasts longer than the normal expected healing time, and generally describes a pain that has persisted for three months or more. There may be pain-free intervals, or the pain may be constant but the severity waxes and wanes.

If you are in acute pain, get to your doctor and get a painkiller. As I was writing this book, my dog fell sick and was rushed into emergency surgery, followed by complications, which meant she had to be operated on again. She was very sick and in enormous acute pain from the surgery, and I was not on the phone to the homeopathic vet asking for assistance, nor was I reaching for the herbal remedies, but I was at the animal hospital, making sure she was getting her daily painkilling shots.

In other words, there is a time and a place to use pharmaceuticals, and, as ever with complementary medicine, it is not a question of either/or. The painkillers I am going to talk about here are for chronic conditions, and not for emergencies or acute pain.

The truth is, we still know very little about the complex mechanism of pain in the body. The first step is the stimulation of receptors known as nociceptors, which are sensitized by numerous agents including serotonin, prostaglandins, histamine, potassium and hydrogen ions, bradykinins and leukotriene. What marks the difference between different pain sensations is the pathway they travel from the spinal cord to the brain. Pain sensations sent along the A-delta nerves are perceived as sharp, localized pain. Those sent along the C afferent nerves result in a dull, aching pain that is more typical of the chronic pain we are addressing here.

Doctors use three terms to further describe pain. **Somatic pain,** which can be mild or severe, is generally characterized as a dull, sharp or aching pain. **Visceral pain** is described as diffuse or gnawing. Both types respond well to conventional opioid medications. **Neuropathic pain,** which is the result of a peripheral nerve injury and which can be burning, shooting, tingling or numbing, is more typical of chronic conditions, including fibromyalgia (see page 366), and can be relieved with more non-traditional analgesics.

Glucosamine (see Chapter 4, The Spine and Joints) is an effective painkiller for arthritic-type conditions and is even more effective when combined with **chondroitin** (see page 211) and the Indian herb **turmeric** (see page 214).

Another excellent but less well-known painkilling agent is **methylsulphonylmethane** (**MSM**), a form of organic sulphur which some surgeons now use to accelerate tissue healing after surgery, and which integrated clinicians working with multiple sclerosis (see page 368) often use to help reduce pain and muscle soreness.

In one study, arthritic patients taking MSM for a month reported a 60 per cent reduction in pain, and those who continued taking the supplement for another fortnight reported an 80 per cent reduction.

Aspirin is actually a synthetic copy of anti-inflammatory painkilling salicyates found in the bark of the white willow tree, and lots of painkilling supplements include white willow, but **turmeric,** another anti-inflammatory agent, is a better option for anyone with increased risk of thrombosis since it also works to inhibit platelet aggregation. In Ayurvedic medicine, turmeric is prescribed both for general pain relief and, specifically, to help manage chronic pain associated with shoulder injuries. It works because it inhibits enzymes that would otherwise help make those inflammatory substances, including leukotrienes and prostaglandins, which send pain signals to the brain.

Boswellia is a powerful anti-inflammatory and vascular-supporting herb produced from the gum of the Indian Boswellia serrata tree. The key active ingredient is boswellic acid, which is as powerful as the over-the-counter painkiller Ibuprofen, and which is extracted from the resin of the trunk of the tree.

Top Ten Natural Agents to Boost Energy and Stop Fatigue

Ashwaganda

Also known as Indian ginseng, my favourite description of this anti-ageing Ayurvedic herb is that it 'makes a man potent as a horse'. The name is a Sanskrit one: 'ashva' means 'horse'.

This is one of the adaptogens (see page 251) that works to bolster all the body's systems, including energy levels. The parts of the plant used in supplements include the root and berries, and while nobody knows the mechanism of how it works, scientists believe this tonic can increase bone-marrow-cell and white-blood-cell counts to bolster immune functioning.

Therapeutic dose

2–4ml, 3 times a day if using in tincture form; 1–6g if using capsules.

Contraindications

Do not use this herb with immunosuppressant drugs, antidepressants or thyroid medications.

Aspartates

These are compounds based on the amino acid aspartic acid, and, like malic acid (see below), they work to support the energy cycle. Low levels of aspartates (and malic acid) mean the body will shift to a more inefficient, anaerobic means of energy production, which can then cause an abnormal build-up of lactic acid, resulting in muscle pain, achiness and fatigue after exertion.

These supplements are safe, effective and cheap to take, but to work they should be combined with potassium and magnesium in a formula where these minerals are chemically attached to the aspartate (clinical trials have shown that taking them separately does not have the desired effect).

When taken in the correct form, up to 85 per cent of fatigue patients reported significant improvement (compared with 25 per cent given a placebo pill), and said symptoms began to improve within ten days.

Therapeutic dose

1g, taken twice a day after meals, or you can split the dosage into 4 x 250mg. Take for 12 months then stop. If fatigue recurs, take for 6- to 8-week periods with breaks of 2 weeks in between.

Contraindications

None.

B Complex

The B vitamins are described as the 'backbone' of energy production so any daily supplement regime needs to include a good B complex to provide them all in a therapeutic dosage. They work in the body to produce more energy from carbohydrates in the diet, and have become known as nature's own stress-busters. When they are lacking, you will feel more listless, irritable, edgy and depressed.

They can also help address the underlying digestive disorders linked with fatigue-type conditions that will otherwise prevent absorption of nutrients. See vitamin B12 (page 365) for more details on how this particular nutrient is crucial for the management of fatigue-type conditions.

Therapeutic dose

Take as directed on the bottle.

Contraindications

None.

Essential Fatty Acids

Involved in both energy production and maintaining healthy cell membranes, the essential fatty acids are those the body cannot make but must glean from the diet (see Depression and Mood, page 314). One of the most potent sources of these fats is flaxseed oil, which is described as providing a rich source of health-boosting phytomedicines (plant chemicals) for the 21st century. This is also a good alternative for vegetarians who do not wish to take fish oil capsules.

Therapeutic dose

1 tablespoon of liquid oil on your breakfast cereal; if you prefer capsules, take as directed on the bottle.

Contraindications

None.

Glutathione

This is one of the proteins produced in the liver that works in the body to stop the destruction of natural killer cells (see page 261). Repeated infections suggest a glutathione deficiency among fatigue patients and all the amino acids that make up glutathione – cysteine, lysine and glutamine – are found in lower levels in post-viral conditions, including chronic fatigue. Take a good quality combined amino-acid supplement to remedy this or a combination remedy that includes glutathione itself.

Therapeutic dose

250mg a day.

Contraindications

Do not take with asthma drugs.

Guarana

Providing a healthier buzz than coffee, guarana does contain caffeine, but a 500mg capsule provides just 15mg of this natural stimulant, which is low compared with the 80–120mg dose you get in just one cup of coffee. The key difference is that guarana also contains other compounds which effectively slow down the assimilation of the caffeine, so that a single dose will provide a more sustained energy hit that can last up to six hours.

This is an especially useful agent for shift-workers and frequent travellers whose sleep patterns have become disturbed leading to low energy levels when they are awake.

Therapeutic dose

200–800mg a day.

Contraindications

Do not mix with any prescription drugs without consulting your health advisors.

Lysine

This amino acid can inhibit viral replication and so is especially useful in patients suffering low energy following viral infection (see Epstein-Barr virus, page 363).

This agent, which some people use to help improve athletic performance, also bonds with heavy metals in the body to reduce detoxification and lessen the overall burden on the immune system.

Therapeutic dose
Up to 6g a day.

Contraindications
Avoid arginine-rich foods, including fish, chocolate and peanuts, and do not take if you have osteoporosis (since it can affect calcium absorption) or kidney problems.

Malic Acid

This agent is used to 'rescue' the body's energy-producing cycle when it is struggling, especially in patients suffering from chronic fatigue or fibromyalgia. This is often the case when levels of another nutrient, called thiamine pyrophosphate (TPP), are low. For maximum effect, malic acid needs to be combined with **magnesium** (see page 369), so check out the over-the-counter combination remedies below.

Therapeutic dose
Sold as magnesium malate, providing 200mg of malic acid.

Contraindications
None.

NADH (Nicotinamide Dinucleotide Hydrogen)

Also known as co-enzyme 1, this substance is needed to carry the energy made by burning the carbohydrates, proteins and fats in the diet to the mitochondria (see page 357), where it can be converted to ATP (see page 358).

In people with both chronic fatigue syndrome (page 362) and fibromyalgia (page 366), the body does not produce enough NADH, making supplementation a key part of any treatment. NADH also works to stimulate the production of the brain chemicals serotonin and dopamine (see Chapter 6, Depression and

Mood) to help relieve brain fog. In trials, one in four CFS/FM patients improved when taking a daily dose of 10mg for a month. That said, it can take two months to gain the full benefits.

Therapeutic dose
The brand to use is ENADA, since this is the one that has been used in clinical trials.

Contraindications
None.

Spirulina
One of the energy-boosting 'superfoods' reported to protect against DNA damage and other ravages of ageing, spirulina is an energy-booster too. It is rich in chlorophyll, protein, vitamin B12 (see above) and soothing vitamin B5 (pantothenic acid), and so can help counter low moods and depression, which are a common side effect of fatigue disorders.

Spirulina is a microalga that thrives in hot sunny climates; it can also help boost mineral absorption, which is helpful in chronic fatigue where levels of calcium and zinc are often lower.

Therapeutic dose
None specified, take as directed on the bottle.

Contraindications
None.

Top Three Over-the-Counter Combination Remedies to Boost Energy

Ultimate Energy
This American supplement from Nature's Secret combines

energy-boosting ginsengs (see Stress and Immunity, page 280) with astragalus, liquorice and gotu kola to help keep you on your feet. Mail order from specialists in US supplements Victoria Health (0800 389 8195; www.victoriahealth.com).

ENADA

This tablet supplement form of NADH (see pages 364 and 380) is the one that has been used in clinical trials in the UK and the US. The tincture to use is the FSC brand. Order Springfield's ENADA capsules from the NutriCentre (0800 587 2290; www.NutriCentre.com).

Guarana

Now available in tablets, buzz bars and chewing gum, this natural stimulant provides all the same energy-boosting benefits as a cup of coffee, without the side effects. In the UK, mail order from rainforest herbal specialists Rio Trading (01273 570987; www.riohealth.com).

A–Z of Energy-boosting Foods

The single biggest drain on the body's energy reserves is the digestion of food, which naturopaths reckon uses some 70 per cent of all the available energy. Overeating taxes the digestion and depletes the body of energy, which is why it is better to eat little and often.

To stabilize energy levels throughout the day, avoid refined sugar and carbohydrates, and eat more fruit, vegetables and wholegrain foods. Also try to eat more foods from the lower ranks of the **glycaemic index** (see pages 124–5), and avoid snacking on chocolate and cakes which *will* give you a high-energy hit, but for which you will pay the price with an equally rapid low-energy slump.

A is for apples, which are especially high in malic acid (see pages 365 and 380), which can support the body's energy-producing cycles when levels of another nutrient, called thiamine pyrophosphate (TPP), are low, which is often the case in low-energy syndromes including chronic fatigue.

B is for beef and other red meats, which provide energy-boosting carnitine (see page 360), which the body can better use in the presence of an amino acid called lysine (see page 379). Lysine is present in potatoes, dairy products and brewer's yeast.

C is for vitamin C, which can jump-start a sluggish brain in the same way as a cup of coffee (see pages 256 and 361) but without the side effects. Kiwi fruits and acerola cherries are better sources of vitamin C than oranges. C is also for cod, which is rich in the B vitamins that help the body convert the carbohydrates you eat into even more energy, so when reserves are low, make a delicious fish pie.

D is for magnesium-rich dark-green leafy vegetables, which can help counter fatigue and aching muscles. Other good dietary sources of magnesium include sesame seeds, nuts, fish, meat, beans and kiwi fruit.

E is for essential fatty acids, which the body needs to make energy. Cold-water oily fish such as salmon are a good source, but for a plant alternative, use flaxseed oil (see page 378). Add one tablespoon a day to your breakfast cereal, or if you dislike the taste take it in capsule form.

F is for fennel, another herb that is high in the energy-producing B vitamins and also in calcium, which can help remedy poor sleep patterns and is often lacking in patients with low-energy, autoimmune conditions. Traditionally used to aid digestive disorders, it can also bolster the immune system, making it a good all-round tonic for fatigue sufferers.

G is for green tea, another powerful antioxidant. It contains epigallocatechin gallate (EGCG), a type of polyphenol that has been shown to penetrate cells to protect DNA from hydrogen peroxide, a potent free radical. Green tea encourages the body to burn more fat, and is a better antioxidant than black tea since it has not been left to ferment, a process which destroys most of the polyphenols in normal tea.

H is for hypothalamus, the master gland that controls appetite. According to traditional Chinese medicine, this gland is programmed to make the body seek a certain amount of every different flavour in a meal, making it difficult not to overeat. Foods that can help suppress overeating include green tea (see page 89 and above).

I is for antioxidant immune-boosting nutrients in everyday foods, including vitamins A, C, E and the trace minerals selenium and zinc. Eat more crab, kelp, mushrooms, pumpkin seeds and soybeans to increase dietary zinc, as well as more antioxidant foods, including oats, spinach, sweet potatoes, green leafy vegetables and berries.

J is for juicing, which is the fastest way to get energy-boosting nutrients into the bloodstream. Juice apples (see **A is for**) and cabbage then stir in cinnamon to make a get-up-and-go tonic that is rich in calcium, potassium and vitamins B6, C and A.

K is for kale, which is a good dietary source of antioxidants, and kelp, which can help boost flagging energy levels. Kelp can help flush out toxins that place extra stress on the immune and cellular systems, and is rich in all the B-complex vitamins, which are critical for managing energy-related conditions.

L is for liquorice, used in Chinese medicine to boost energy levels and increase both strength and endurance. Lots of the Ayurvedic herbal teas include this herb, which is another good source of the B-complex vitamins.

M is for malic acid (see apples and other fruits), which plays an important role in the energy cycle. All fruits supply this nutrient but apples are an especially good dietary source. The body also needs magnesium to make energy so eat more nuts, dark-green leafy vegetables, dairy products and kiwi fruits.

N is for nicotinamide dinucleotide hydrogen (NADH; see pages 364 and 380) which plays a key role in both DNA repair and cellular immune functioning. A form of vitamin B3 or niacin, good food sources of this nutrient include fish, meat, dairy products, legumes, leafy green vegetables and potatoes.

O is for oats and olive oil, both of which contain nutrients that confer extra antioxidant protection and so can help counter the effects of ageing mitochondria (see page 357). Broccoli and brazil nuts are excellent antioxidant foods, as too are sweet potatoes and watermelons.

P is for peppermint, which can help soothe digestive disorders linked to chronic fatigue, and which has a painkilling analgesic action in the body to help relieve tired or aching muscles. Other analgesic foods include cinnamon, clove, garlic, ginger, liquorice, onions and chilli peppers.

Q is for quercetin, another anti-inflammatory agent that can help counter pain and boost the antioxidant action of vitamin C (see page 277) to keep energy levels high. Onions and apples are both good dietary sources of this agent.

R is for rose hips, which, like quercetin, are synergistic with vitamin C. These fruits contain calcium, which autoimmune patients often have low levels of (see page 179), and are also rich in the B-complex vitamins that support the nervous system and are described as 'the backbone' of energy production. If you need an energy boost, drink rose-hip tea (or take it in supplement form).

S is for spinach, an excellent source of mitochondria-protecting antioxidant vitamin A, which can help prevent loss of energy caused by free-radical damage. Also selenium, another important antioxidant, found in garlic and wholegrain bread, which the body uses to make glutathione peroxidase, an enzyme which destroys the free radical hydrogen peroxide.

T is for taurine, another nutrient that can boost the biosynthesis of energy, hence its inclusion in so many sports drinks. Food sources include eggs, fish, meat and milk. The body can make taurine from cysteine (in the liver) and methionine (elsewhere in the body) but only when levels of vitamin B6 are high enough.

U is for unrefreshing sleep, which is a symptom of low energy levels and fatigue; eat more calcium-rich tofu, broccoli, hazelnuts, wholegrains and soybeans, plus a carbohydrate-rich snack such as a banana at bedtime to raise levels of serotonin, which can help re-regulate the body clock.

V is for vitamin B12, which can help clear fatigue-related brain fog. Good food sources of this nutrient include dairy products, fish, meat and eggs. The latter also contain cysteine (see page 162), which the body uses to make glutathione, the single most important tissue-protecting antioxidant, which can help slow down mitochondrial damage and ageing.

W is for selenium-rich wholegrains, which can help protect cells from oxidative damage and ageing. These are complex carbohydrates, which help keep blood sugar and energy levels even throughout the day. They include wheat, rye, oats, rice, millet, buckwheat, bulgur wheat, barley, couscous and quinoa.

X is for Xynergy (08456 585858; www.xynergy.co.uk), the UK specialist company that sells energy-boosting superfoods, including spirulina (see page 381) and blue-green algae.

Y is for yams or sweet potatoes, a natural source of glutamic acid, which the body will use to make the superantioxidant glutathione. These are also one of the best food sources of potassium, which helps regulate the transfer of nutrients through cell membranes, a function that can deteriorate with age, causing lower energy levels.

Z is for zinc, critical for healthy immune functioning. Repeated infections increase the body's demand for this mineral so zinc deficiency is common in fatigue-type conditions.

�֍

Ancient Wisdom, 21st-century Healing

Traditional Chinese Medicine (TCM)

Reported to have the most active polysaccharides in the whole plant kingdom, **reishi mushroom** or **ling-zhi** is known in China as 'the plant of immortality'.

In Japan, 99 per cent of reishi growing in the wild are found on old plum trees but they are still so rare that only a few reishi are generally found for every 100,000 plum trees.

In laboratory studies, the polysaccharides in this plant have been shown to increase DNA synthesis in the bone marrow of mice, and in test-tube trials to increase DNA synthesis of spleen cells in mixed lymphocyte cultures.

Reishi mushrooms also contain oleic acid, which is known to inhibit the release of histamine to prevent allergic reactions and inflammations. That said, some people may be allergic to the mushroom itself so if you plan to use this agent in supplement form and think you might be at risk, start with a low dosage, monitor yourself for any adverse reactions and stop taking it if you have any.

Ayurvedic (Indian) Remedies

The Indian herb **gotu kola** is described as 'food for the brain' and is often combined with Siberian ginseng, bee pollen and capsicum by traditional herbalists to make an energy-boosting tonic. In Ayurvedic medicine, this plant, which also contains quercetin (see page 385), is used to support brain and nerve functioning and prevent mental fatigue.

It is rich in energy-boosting magnesium and immune-boosting, cell-protecting antioxidant nutrients, including vitamins A and C and zinc. Gotu kola, which can help the body better resist disease, is an excellent herb to use when you need to re-energize the body and brain, especially after travelling (see Jet Lag Remedies, page 324) or periods of extreme stress and tiredness. It is also being investigated for its painkilling analgesic action in the body.

To order in tincture or capsule form, call Pukka Herbs (08456 585858; www.pukkaherbs.com).

Ancient Egyptian

Chamomile contains a natural hormone that is very similar to the thyroid hormone thyroxine, which can help boost energy levels, especially when the thyroid is sluggish or underactive (hypothyroidism). That said, you should never try to self-treat thyroid problems or mix herbs with medication since you may risk overdosing on your hormone intake. Instead, find a qualified practitioner who can monitor levels and work with you to better support thyroid functioning.

The herb is high in magnesium, which the body needs for energy-production, and in the B-complex vitamins which support nerve functioning (see page 377).

In animal studies, chamomile has been shown to have antihistaminic effects, which could make it a useful adjunct to conventional and natural therapies for autoimmune conditions, including multiple sclerosis (see page 368).

Native New Zealand Remedies

Still the best-selling herbal immune-booster worldwide, **echinacea** is nature's protection against viral infections. In New Zealand, the company NZ VitaLife (www.nzvitalife.co.nz) is currently working on the North Island in partnership with land-owning Maori to develop ever more potent strains of this herb for worldwide export in tincture form.

The award-winning organic range currently includes an alcohol-free echinacea tincture and even echinacea tea bags, plus an inspired echinacea and kiwifruit 'smoothie' milkshake-based tincture that will have everyone in the family clamouring for more.

Clinical trials suggest echinacea can be safely used for up to twelve weeks at a time, after which you need to take a break. **Do not use this herb without medical supervision if you suffer from autoimmune conditions, since its immuno-stimulating activities may exacerbate your symptoms.**

Tried and Applied

The tingle factor: Test the potency and efficacy of a herbal tincture with your tongue. The stronger the 'tingling' sensation, the more potent the remedy. This simple, foolproof tingle test has long been used by medical herbalists to ascertain efficacy. If there is no tingle sensation with the remedy you are using, you may need to switch to a more potent brand.

Roll Out Your Yoga Mat

A stressed body will be a tired body because your energy is being squandered in tight, tense muscles. Mental tensions manifest in the body as a constant, partial contraction of the muscles, which will not only deplete energy reserves but disrupt breathing too. You may be so fatigued you feel you simply don't have the energy to move any part of your body, but unless you learn how to release that muscular (and mental) tension, your body will not be able to rest, even when you are inactive.

I am not suggesting you hurl yourself into Astanga (power) yoga but the Vini yoga (www.viniyoga.co.uk) that I am such a fan of will help you release tensions and recover some of that much-needed energy you have lost.

In the meantime, here are my **1, 2, 3 top yoga asanas** for getting tension out of an already tired body.

Tadasana (Mountain Pose)

Hard to imagine how simply standing tall can release tension and fatigue, I know, but it really does work. In fact, standing properly, and staying in that position, is more difficult than you might think.

To practise this posture, stand on your yoga mat with your feet hip-width apart. Check you have not imagined your hips to be wider than a bus – we are talking the distance from one hip joint to the other, not from the outside of one thigh to the other.

Lift the toes and spread them out, one by one on the mat, to relax them. It will be counterproductive if you are standing and gripping the mat with tense toes.

Bring your awareness to your knees and make sure you are not hyperextending them. Again, tension in the knees will be counterproductive.

Now take your hands and place your little fingers on your hipbones. Spread the hand to its full span, and as you do so lift the middle section of your body. Your thumbs should be tucked under your ribcage and lifting this part of your torso as you stretch the hands.

Circle the shoulders in their joints and allow them to fall back so that the arms now dangle at the side of the body. Remember, with yoga, it may look as if the body is doing no work, but you should be holding your arms at the side, with the fingers stretched straight and pointing downwards.

Now bring your awareness to the back of your neck and the small axis bone on which the head rotates. This is at the top of the neck and if you cannot locate it, circle the head so you can feel this joint working.

Do not jut out your chin but imagine a string coming out from the middle top of your head, pulling it up towards the ceiling. This will bring the head and the neck into the correct alignment.

You are now standing in the mountain pose, which is an active posture. Concentrate on slowing down your breathing and maintain this posture for as long as you feel comfortable.

Bhujangasana (Cobra Pose)

This is another posture that is harder than it looks but which works to get tension out of the back and keep the spine supple. It's also wonderful for the immune system, and is described in that chapter (Chapter 5; see page 301). Hold the pose for a few seconds and then return the body to lying flat on the mat, head turned to one side, to allow the heartbeat to return to normal.

Shakti Bhandi

Go back to Chapter 4, page 237, where I have given a detailed account of how to release tension from the feet, ankles, knees, hips, hands, wrists, shoulders and neck to improve energy flow throughout the body.

CHAPTER EIGHT

Love, Sex and Hormones

If you accept the premise that the root of all disease is the **interaction of chemical toxins, oxidative stress and hormones**, then not only can you see how, even if you had a perfect genetic blueprint, you would still fall sick, but you can also see what a crucial role the body's hormones play in our everyday health and well-being.

Of course, it is one thing when your hormones are working with you to maintain good health, and quite another when you feel, thanks to mood swings, heavy periods or a disappearing libido, you are at their mercy.

In this chapter, I have concentrated on those subjects that tend to crop up the most in my postbag from queries about natural alternatives to viagra to advice on improving your chances of pregnancy.

First, though, we will take a quick look at those glands and organs that make up the body's hormone-controlling endocrine system and, again, we will see, as in every other chapter, that you cannot take an isolated approach to your health because the workings of one part of the body, say, the thyroid gland, will always affect the workings of other parts too, such as weight control and metabolism.

The Endocrine System

All glands are secretory organs, and those glands that secrete hormones directly into the bloodstream and make up the endocrine system include the following:

- pineal
- pituitary
- thyroid
- parathyroid
- thymus
- adrenals
- pancreas
- gonads (ovaries and testes)

Hormones are, in effect, highly sensitive chemical messengers, which is why natural healers prefer the use of plant hormones (phytoestrogens) to synthetic ones, since the natural version have only one-thousandth of the potency, and thus a much weaker and more subtle action in the body.

Red clover, for instance, contains at least a hundred different chemicals, including isoflavones, those substances that are chemically similar to oestrogen, albeit much weaker, and are thus known as phytoestrogens.

The Thyroid

Lots of people know that **iodine** plays a key role in supporting the thyroid, but it is less well known that the body can better utilize iodine, from either the diet or supplements, if you take it with an amino acid called **tyrosine**. This is because both nutrients are needed to make the thyroid hormones.

Tyrosine is more usually used to help counter depression and as an appetite suppressant. It is also the nutrient that is used to help support cocaine addicts through the withdrawal period.

Thyro-Vital, made by Ethical Nutrients, combines iodine and tyrosine with panax ginseng and other minerals in supplement form. (Ginseng is one of the adaptogenic herbs that work to normalize all the body's functions, including thyroid functioning.) You can get this supplement from Victoria Health (0800 389 8195; www.victoriahealth.com) but do not use this or any other tyrosine supplement if you are already taking thyroid medication. Instead, support the thyroid further by increasing your intake of iodine-rich foods, especially alfalfa and kelp.

If you suspect you have thyroid problems, you must get your doctor to test you. For the rest of us, there is growing concern among nutritional experts that we are no longer getting enough iodine from the 'normal' daily diet, so if you are feeling sluggish or struggling with unexpected weight gain, get checked and think about adding a seaweed supplement or sea vegetable (see page 71) to your diet.

Fertility

The single most important thing to say about fertility problems is that you will not get pregnant if you do not have enough sex. Once a week is simply not enough!

Even if you are a supersexy 25-year-old, who is firing on all cylinders, brimming with glowing good health and having sex five times a night during your fertile period in order to get pregnant, you still have only a 25 per cent chance of conceiving.

This, coupled with the fact that researchers now suspect a woman's fertility starts to decline in her twenties and not her thirties, is depressing news for the growing number of women who delay having their first child until their thirties and whose chances of conceiving at the drop of a hat then are even slimmer.

An estimated one in six couples will experience fertility problems at some point and in a third of all cases where couples are having trouble getting pregnant doctors will reach a diagnosis of 'unexplained' infertility – leaving both parties to obsess about what is going wrong and who is to blame.

What then happens, in far too many cases, is the couple gets bounced from the GP's surgery to the IVF fertility clinic with no time to catch their breath, let alone think about the relatively simple and inexpensive lifestyle and dietary changes which those of us working in the so-called 'alternative' field of natural health know really can make a difference and swing the odds in favour of a successful pregnancy and a live baby to take home.

Getting NHS funding in the UK for fertility treatment is a lottery and will depend not only on your age but where you live. No wonder then that 85 per cent of couples with fertility problems end up in private clinics paying around £3000 for a single treatment cycle.

All of them are hoping to be among the lucky 25 per cent who will, ten months later, walk out of hospital with a bundle of joy, but pretty soon they will learn it usually takes more than one cycle to succeed and that it is not unusual to end up paying for three or even four treatments. None of them will want to know that in order to get pregnant, the woman must take drugs which in effect send her body spinning into an early menopause and back out again with a wallop.

If it sounds brutal, that's because it is.

Far less of a shock to the system is the idea of natural fertility, and an increasing number of couples are beginning to understand that they can do a lot more to enhance their chances of success by, say, improving the quality of the eggs and the sperms beforehand and by supporting the body through the shock of the fertility treatments.

Many women who are having trouble conceiving have no idea, for example, that the over-the-counter painkillers they may be taking to cope with painful periods can adversely affect ovulation and fertility, or that lubricant jellies kill off 70 per cent of sperm, or that cold decongestant medication can significantly alter the body's own secretions.

Women who have already embarked on IVF and other fertility treatments may not have been told that losing weight can improve the chances of a successful implantation or that detoxifying the liver before a cycle can make the fertility drugs more effective. Studies from China, for example, also show how a weekly acupuncture treatment can improve the chances of success by boosting the quality of the growing follicles from which the mature eggs will be released.

Where a fertility doctor will start an investigation with a scan of the ovaries and uterus, a TCM practitioner will start by treating the kidneys which, again, in Chinese medicine, control reproduction and which in many cases of unexplained infertility simply need strengthening through acupuncture and better nutrition.

Most couples already know to cut out alcohol and smoking to improve the chances of conception but few will know that both the man and the woman should take folic acid before conception – her to prevent neural tube defects in the foetus and him to improve the quality of sperm.

The woman will likely be asked to refrain from using tampons, which can alter the mucus in the vaginal tract, to avoid swimming when she has a period, and also to keep out of the gym during menstruation when, according to Chinese medicine, the body should be rested not strained.

Most sensible practitioners specializing in this area are not against IVF treatments and assisted conception, but if there is one message for couples coping with the disappointment of infertility it is that they should do their homework. According to Zita West (www.zitawest.com), the UK's leading practitioner in the field and author of *Natural Pregnancy – Complementary Therapies for Preconception, Pregnancy and Postnatal Care*, too many couples facing unexplained infertility ignore this simple advice.

'These treatments are big guns using big drugs and I am always amazed by the fact that some people will put more effort into researching a holiday than they do into researching fertility treatments and the clinics that offer them,' she says.

The UK fertility organization Foresight – formerly the Association for Pre-conception Care – can boast a high rate of success in helping many couples conceive. For details of testing for nutritional deficiencies, and complementary health practitioners who specialize in this field in your area, write to the charity at 28 The Paddock, Godalming, Surrey GU7 1XD, enclosing a 1st-class SAE.

Tried and Applied

Prayer & IVF: Prayer and meditation can help increase your chances of success if you are undergoing fertility treatments. In a small pilot study, where 219 IVF women, aged between twenty-six and forty-six, were randomly assigned to intercessory prayer, those who were being prayed for had almost twice the chance of getting pregnant than those who were not. This study was shared between researchers in Korea and the United States who enlisted the help of prayer groups in America, Australia and Canada. You may think it is all in the mind but so what? There are no adverse side effects, it costs nothing to try, and doubling your chance of success with a treatment that is as expensive as it is uncomfortable has to be worth a try.

PCOS

The problem with polycystic ovary syndrome (PCOS) is that not every woman who has this condition has the exact same symptoms. Excess facial hair, fertility problems, acne and unexplained weight gain are telltale signs in some sufferers, but others may have very few and very minor symptoms. The only way to confirm this diagnosis is to book an ultrasound scan of the ovaries where the cysts will show up looking like a string of pearls on the surface of these glands.

PCOS, which can be an underlying cause of unexplained infertility, is much more common than you might think. Now thought to affect up to one in ten women, the true figure could be as high as one in five. And since sufferers have a significantly increased risk of both diabetes and heart disease, it is worth getting a diagnosis so you can begin to tackle the problem and these associated risks.

This is a genetic condition for which there is no cure so the best you can hope for is to manage the troubling symptoms, which go right to the heart of a woman's self-esteem. Losing weight if you have gained it is important, since this will help reduce the other symptoms. To do this most effectively, switch to a higher protein and lower carbohydrate diet and read up on Syndrome X (see page 122), which I have a hunch may be linked in some way.

Many PCOS sufferers take the prescription drug Dianette to control the acne (one of the more common symptoms of this condition), which is a sign that the body has too much testosterone. What you need, if you want to stop taking this drug and stop the acne coming straight back, is a herbal alternative that will do the same job.

I have been searching, with no luck, for a specific PCOS remedy ever since I started writing about natural health six years ago, and not least because I also suffer mildly from this condition. The best I can suggest at this stage is to use the anti-androgenic herb **saw palmetto,** which is more usually recommended to help manage prostate problems.

Nobody really knows how saw palmetto works with the sex hormones to stop the conversion of testosterone to a more potent form called dihydrotestosterone (which can trigger the acne), but one theory is that it disables an enzyme called 5-alpha-reductase, which is key to this process. What we do know is that saw palmetto is relatively free from unwanted side effects. In a three-year study, only 34 of 435 people taking this herb complained of mild gastrointestinal disturbances. The therapeutic daily dose is between 250mg and 500mg.

Sperm – How to Get More of Them and Better Swimmers

Sickly sperm will not be able to fertilize an egg, so when it comes to male reproductive health, a man needs strong, healthy sperm that can swim. **Zinc** plays a key role in reproductive health in both sexes and men with fertility problems should take a daily dose of 30mg, plus 1mg of **copper,** to maintain the proper mineral balance.

The other nutrient that has been shown to help improve sperm count and mobility is **vitamin B12.** Again, men with poor sperm counts or motility should take 1000 mcg (micrograms) a day.

Carnitine is useful in men seeking specifically to improve sperm motility, and **vitamin** E is important too. In one placebo-controlled trial of men whose sperm showed impaired activity, a daily dose of 100 IUs of vitamin E resulted in healthier sperm and an increased rate of pregnancy. Research now shows that naturally sourced vitamin E is more effective than synthetic forms so check this with any brand you buy.

One of the herbal remedies recommended for male fertility problems is **ashwaganda,** which is often called the Indian ginseng. In his book *Essentials of Ayurveda*, Professor Priya Vrat Sharma says this is the herb that makes a man 'potent as a horse'. There is no clinical evidence for its potency with male fertility but it is an adaptogen (see page 251), which can help normalize the body's systems and increase its resistance to stress that would otherwise adversely affect sperm health. The therapeutic daily dose is 120mg, or it can be brewed into a tea made from the powdered herb, which should be drunk three times a day.

If you want to take the nutritional route, Male Source from UK specialist supplier Revital (0800 252875; www.revital.com) includes natural-source vitamin E, carnitine, zinc, arginine, taurine and selenium. Trojan for Men, from the same company, includes the herbs ashwaganda, ginkgo, nutmeg and tribulus terrestris (see page 416).

Pre-conception tests show that in nine of every fifteen infertile couples the male has a genito-urinary infection. If one partner is infected, the other partner may be too. The main offenders are herpes and chlamydia, so visit your nearest GU clinic for a free and confidential check-up. Don't be shy – this can make the difference between having a baby or not. If you know your lifestyle is grubby, clean it up. Smoking tobacco and cannabis and drinking alcohol do more damage to sperm than anything else, so stop.

Eggs

Women are born with all the 400,000 eggs they will ever have. These are present in the ovaries at birth, after which the number will start to decline. Prescription drugs, injury and infection, both in childhood and in adult life, can all take their toll on the number of healthy ova.

Sadly, we know very little about the use of herbs or nutrients to support healthy ova. Research has shown that regular acupuncture sessions can help; the theory, as I mentioned before, is that a weekly treatment can improve chances of conception by boosting the quality of the growing follicles from which the mature eggs will be released.

Double-blind trials have shown that simply improving the quality of your nutrition by taking a multivitamin/multimineral supplement does improve female fertility but nobody has identified precisely which nutrients work to support the ova.

Hot Flushes

Hot flushes are often among the first signs a woman has that her ovaries, which are effectively starting to shut down, are producing less oestrogen. Conventional hormone replacement therapy (HRT) works by rebuilding levels of the female hormones, but since it can also increase the risk of breast cancer, more and more women aged fifty and over are asking about alternatives.

One of my all-time favourite quotes came from a doctor who, with apologies to all cat-lovers for the analogy, told me: 'Using HRT to treat hot flushes is like using a steam roller to crush a cat.' His point, in case you are not sure, is that there are lots of excellent herbal remedies that will do the job without the risk of the side effects now associated with the long-term use of hormone replacement therapy.

The single most effective natural agent to use for this problem is **sage,** and Italian researchers have now shown how a combined supplement of sage with alfalfa worked to reduce the number of hot flushes women were having from ten a day to just two, over the course of three months.

These trials were double-blind (i.e. nobody, neither the researcher nor the participants, knew who was getting a placebo or an active pill) and the supplement used provided 120mg of sage and 60mg of alfalfa. Both plants have an oestrogenic action in the body, but since the dosage of the alfalfa used was not high enough to bring about such a dramatic improvement in symptoms, the scientists concluded it must be the sage that was the more important agent.

UK herbal supplement company Bioforce now makes a simple sage herbal tincture to help tackle hot flushes. To get the right dosage (the equivalent of 120mg a day), take 20 drops in water or fruit juice, three times a day. (For stockists call 01294 277344; or visit www.bioforce.co.uk.)

Perimenopause – the Changes Before Menopause

Never heard of it? You're not alone. Most females aged thirty-five and over will have experienced some of the symptoms of perimenopause – even if they have never heard the name. (When I went to my doctor at thirty-five and said something's wrong, she told me I was simply getting old!) In fact, sudden weight gain, erratic periods, mood swings, hot flushes and insomnia are all signs of the hormonal changes that can start some fifteen years before menopause.

To tackle these symptoms, you need to link the same three remedies – Meno-Herb, Woman Essence and the Barlean's mix of organic oils in The Essential Woman – that I recommend for the menopause (see below).

Menopause – the HRT Debate

I have heard natural healers describe HRT as the 'single biggest medical bungle' of the 21st century and with researchers themselves now warning of the increased risks, including breast cancer, hundreds of thousands of women have been panicked into seeking an alternative.

If you missed the headlines, you may not know that scientists have now abandoned a major research programme into the benefits of HRT after a new study showed that taking hormone replacements in the longer term not only increases the risk of breast cancer by 26 per cent but also the risk of blood clots.

The single most effective natural regimen that many women are now successfully using as an alternative is a three-pronged approach that combines phyto (plant) oestrogens in the form of herbs, essential fatty acids in oil form and one of the powerful Australian Bush essences that works on an emotional level. Phytoestrogens work to rebalance hormones but are much weaker than the synthetic versions. Do not ask me for clinical references to prove the efficacy of this approach because there aren't any. That doesn't mean it doesn't work – hundreds of women are reporting it works for them – but what it does mean is nobody has researched it.

Meno-Herb is a herbal combination of natural plant oestrogens from red clover, dong quai and black cohosh, plus wild yam (natural progesterone), raspberry leaf, squaw vine and nettles – in short, every herb you would have on your wishlist in trying to control the symptoms of perimenopause and the menopause that will follow. Mail order from Victoria Health (0800 389 8195; www.victoriahealth.com) and take two tablets a day.

Support hormone functioning by taking **The Essential Woman**, an organic mix of flax and evening primrose oil with isoflavones from soy. This is part of the excellent Barlean's range and is available from Healthy and Essential (08700 536000; www.healthyandessential.co.uk).

Finally, **Woman Essence** is one of the powerful Australian Bush Essence combinations, which comes in tincture form. It includes She Oak, which works to help regulate the ovaries, and Mulla Mulla, which, like sage, can control hot flushes. As with all flower remedies, these essences address the underlying emotional and psychological changes that accompany rites of passage such as perimenopause or menopause.

What to Use If You Want to Stay On HRT

If you are still taking HRT and do not want to stop, you should consider using another supplement which can help lower the associated risks of long-term usage. Several months ago, I was tipped off about a new oestrogen-boosting supplement called **DIM** (**diindolylmethane**), which anyone already taking HRT should consider since it can help reduce the risk of associated cancers – the reason for all the adverse publicity.

Made from extracts of cruciferous vegetables, DIM works to change how oestrogen is metabolized in the body. There are two different pathways, one of which generates more of the potentially damaging free radicals, and unfortunately this is the pathway through which the synthetic hormones are metabolized.

A proportion of the oestrogen in your body will always be metabolized along this pathway but what DIM is reported to do is shift the balance so that the majority is metabolized via the less harmful route. If you take DIM alongside your HRT, you are, in effect, protecting yourself more from any adverse side effects.

DIM is also widely used in America to protect against prostate problems (see page 434) and for premenstrual symptoms (see page 411). Tyler's Indolplex supplement, which provides a therapeutic dose of DIM, is now available in the UK from Victoria Health (0800 389 8195; www.victoriahealth.com). Take two a day.

Natural Progesterone – It's Not Natural At All

The first point of confusion to clear up is the fact that 'natural progesterone' does not mean natural at all. It is only called this because it is *chemically identical* to the progesterone that is produced naturally by the ovaries during the second half of the menstrual cycle and throughout pregnancy.

Natural progesterone is a hormone, which means, in this country, you can only get it on prescription. Initially extracted from human placentas, but now made from soy plant sterols, it was first promoted in the 1960s as a cure for PMT. In America, it has been sold as a skin wrinkle cream but without FDA approval. There is no conclusive evidence it can protect against osteoporosis but clinical trials are underway now. You also need to remember that if you take it you are in effect embarking on HRT but using progesterone instead of oestrogen.

Wild yam is a herb that works to support progesterone levels. It can also be very useful for treating PMT and menopausal symptoms (although according to Dr Marilyn Glenville, author of

Natural Alternatives to HRT, **agnus castus** is better). You cannot take progesterone orally because it is destroyed in the liver, so the theory is that you can get round this problem by using wild yam since it contains a sterol called diosgenin, which the body can then convert to progesterone. This, though, is where the real confusion starts because on this point the experts do not agree. Some swear blind this cannot happen and the only time you get progesterone from wild yam is in the laboratory. Others say even if it did work, you have no guarantee about the dose you are getting.

To help you decide, I am going to quote from a book that is my own health bible, *The Natural Pharmacy* (www.primahealth.com) 'Contrary to popular belief, wild yam is not a natural source of progesterone, nor has it been shown to reduce the symptoms of menopause. Although a pharmaceutical conversion process can produce progesterone from wild yam, the body cannot duplicate this conversion.'

The other problem is that you might not be getting what it promises on the label. In a UK investigation of 'natural progesterone' creams, researchers reported that the 2oz jars of Progest cream being used in clinical trials contained just 100mg of progesterone per ounce and not 465mg as claimed by the maker.

Side effects of using progesterone can include weight gain, breast discomfort or enlargement, acne, fatigue, headaches, insomnia, fluid retention and skin rashes – all of which most women in their right minds would want to avoid. Factor in the additional problem there is still little or no evidence about its use topically (which can cause vaginal spotting) and you might want to take Dr Glenville's advice and stick with agnus castus, or chasteberry (see page 412), as it is sometimes called.

Tried and Applied

Ginkgo, sex and depression: The circulatory-boosting herb ginkgo

biloba can help improve sexual dysfunction caused by taking antidepressants, but you will need to take a therapeutic dose of 120mg a day
for six weeks and give it time to kick in. That said, do not use this herb
with blood-thinning medications such as aspirin or warfarin.

Andropause – Putting the Power Back into Manpower

It may not be an accepted medical condition but that does not
stop lots of middle-aged men from feeling that they hit the male
equivalent of the menopause in their early fifties when levels of
testosterone decline. I get lots of letters from men asking what
they can use to regain the energy, vitality and sexual functioning
they enjoyed in their twenties.

The single most effective natural agent that works to raise
testosterone levels in the body is the Eastern European herb **tribulus terrestris** (see page 416). In clinical trials, healthy males who
took 750mg a day for five days were found to have a 40 per cent
increase in testosterone, the key anti-stress and performance-
boosting hormone in men.

This is one of the vitality-boosting adaptogenic herbs that help
the body normalize its various systems, including hormones,
without adverse side effects. That said, at a therapeutic dosage it
will have an action in the body (there'd be no point taking it otherwise), which means you should not mix it ad hoc with any other
medication.

What you can safely mix adaptogens with is other adaptogens
since these herbs have now been found to be synergistic with each
other – in other words, they work together to maximize the therapeutic effects (see Synergy, page 203). So you could take both
tribulus terrestris and, for example, **Siberian ginseng** together. The
latter, which is often added to skincare products, can help boost

the immune system and is widely used as a general tonic for both sexes throughout the world.

Lifetime's **Manpower II** is a second-generation formula that provides not only a therapeutic daily dose of 500mg of tribulus terrestris from Bulgaria but the aptly named sex-boosting herb **horny goatweed** too. (Mail order from Victoria Health on 0800 389 8195; www.victoriahealth.com.)

Flagging Libido – Natural Viagra

Since the makers of natural health products cannot make medical claims unless their supplements have been licensed, you are not going to find any responsible manufacturer or distributor marketing their formulations as a herbal alternative to Viagra. That doesn't mean these products do not exist. It just means nobody will say this is what they do.

Currently the best-selling one (and the one that gets the highest number of repeat orders) is a formulation called **Veromax**, which is made for men. In trials, almost 80 per cent of participants aged between thirty-five and seventy reported improved sexual function when taking this supplement for three months. The study was placebo-controlled, and of those taking the placebo, some 47 per cent also reported better functioning, which would suggest that mind-over-matter plays an important role too.

Newer to the market is the female version of this supplement. Sold as **Vivace**, this too has been shown to increase levels of arousal and frequency of orgasm. One of the active agents in both formulations is **zizphi fructus** (derived from the jujube date), which works in the body to support those mechanisms that increase blood flow in both sexes during arousal.

In brand-new placebo-controlled clinical trials in America, 86 per cent of women taking part in the study reported increased levels of desire, compared with 25 per cent who were taking the placebo, and 81 per cent reported increased overall satisfaction with their sex life.

Veromax/Vivace are both available from NutriCentre in the UK (0800 587 2290; www.NutriCentre.com). **Do not take with prescription medication without seeking proper medical advice.**

Men seeking to boost libido should also check out **Manpower II** (see Andropause, above), while women should consider a South American herbal supplement called **Maca**, a sexual tonic and traditional Peruvian aphrodisiac that is rich in essential fatty acids and essential amino acids which the body cannot make but must source from the diet. This is another of those traditional remedies that has been used for thousands of years but which has not yet been put to the test in the laboratory or in clinical trials on humans. The typical dosage is 1500mg a day, split into three equal dosages.

Tried and Applied

Vitamin C and Sex: When forty-two healthy young adults in their mid-twenties with a current sexual partner were randomly assigned to receive either 3g a day of vitamin C or a placebo pill, researchers reported that those females in the group given the anti-stress antioxidant had more intercourse than those given a sugar pill. In fact, on average, the females taking vitamin C had sex ten times a month, compared with the control group who had sex just three times a month. Vitamin C, which can reduce anxiety and improve vascular function to enhance enjoyment of sex, had no impact on the males taking part. However, if you are tempted to try it, 3g is a high dosage which could lead to temporary stomach upset in more susceptible individuals.

PMS . . .

. . . better known to men around the world as Please Murder Someone else.

Although lots of women take vitamin B6 to help alleviate the very worst symptoms of premenstrual tension, I prefer the herbal remedy **agnus castus** or chasteberry, which has been shown in trials to relieve all the symptoms of PMS, including breast tenderness. This herb is so effective at tackling these symptoms, it has been shown to be helpful in 90 per cent of those women taking part in trials.

PMS sufferers should also supplement their diets with **calcium**. Again, this mineral has been shown to help reduce all the symptoms of PMS, but is often lacking in the diets of women, especially those who may be weight-watching.

In trials at the Columbia University Medical Center, some 500 women took 300mg of calcium (in the form of calcium carbonate) four times a day and reported a significant relief from mood swings, bloating, depression, headaches and food cravings. This supplement will have the added advantage of building and maintaining strong bone density that will be of benefit to women in later life.

To tackle PMS, take **agnolyt**, a liquid tincture standardized to provide the equivalent of 45mg of agnus castus per ten drops. Take ten drops in the morning and ten again at night. If you prefer capsules, take 100mg a day from Lamberts. Solgar's calcium carbonate supplement provides 600mg capsules: take two a day. (Mail order all these from the NutriCentre on 0800 587 2290.)

Tried and Applied

In trials where fifty-eight women aged between sixteen and fifty used the new Pain Ease Patch for a month to help relieve period pains, 76

Dear Susan – Natural Health Advice for the Lovelorn

If you've ever wondered why chocolate makes you feel almost as good as being in love, it's because it contains an amino acid called **phenylalanine**. When you fall in love, your brain makes more of a neurotransmitter called phenylethylalanine. To do this, it needs the precursor agent, phenylalanine, which is also found in less romantic foods, including apples, eggs, chicken, carrots and herrings.

When neurophysiologists at the University of Columbia in New York studied the brain biochemistry of love, they found that once an affair stops or turns sour, the brain drastically reduces its production of phenylethylalanine, and the lovelorn subjects being studied suffered serious withdrawal symptoms as a result.

Since a bar of chocolate encourages the brain to go back into increased production of phenylethylalanine, you can see why, when a relationship breaks down, people reach for the chocolate box and just keep eating.

Top Ten Natural Remedies for Fertility and Hormones

Agnus Castus (Chasteberry)

This clever hormone-balancing herb is often used for the symptoms of PMS, perimenopause and menopause (see page 404), but since it can have uterine-stimulating properties, it should not be used in pregnancy. It has also been used by men with benign prostatic hyperplasia (BPH) and can help boost libido. It is especially helpful for women who suffer from heavy periods accompanied by breast tenderness (see page 431).

The active agents come from the fruit of the chasteberry tree and include flavonoids and a glycoside called agnoside. Most standardized supplements provide 6 per cent agnoside.

Therapeutic dose

Take agnolyt (see page 411). If using a non-standardized extract, take up to 250mg a day.

Contraindications

Do not use in pregnancy or alongside HRT or the contraceptive pill, since it can interfere with their efficacy; stop taking it if you suffer from nausea, headache or gastrointestinal irritation.

Arginine

Sold as L-arginine, this is an amino acid found naturally in red meat, dairy, fish and poultry, which is often included in combination supplements designed to address erectile dysfunction, sexual dysfunction in both sexes and poor sperm health.

It is converted by enzymes in the blood vessels into nitric oxide, which has been shown to improve circulation and blood flow to the sex organs to enhance enjoyment of intercourse.

Therapeutic dose

For erectile dysfunction, clinical trials used 5mg a day.

Contraindications

Do not mix with prescription drugs, including HRT or the contraceptive pill. Stop taking if you suffer any nausea, flushing or vomiting.

Essential Fatty Acids (EFAs)

These are the fats that the body cannot make but must source from the diet (see pages 314 and 378). They have an anti-inflammatory action in the body, making them a useful adjunct to treatments for sex-related conditions, including sexually transmitted diseases and pelvic inflammatory disease (see pages 437 and 433).

Although some researchers claim the body can more easily utilize the EFAs from fish oils, vegetarians can successfully use supplements sourced from flax or linseeds, and my top-rated range, Barlean's from America, does just that with organic oils (in the UK, mail order from Healthy and Essential on 08700 536000; www.healthyandessential.com).

Therapeutic dose

Take the equivalent of at least 1g a day; you cannot overdose unless you start drinking oil by the bucketful.

Contraindications

Do not use fish or flax oils with anticoagulant medication since they can increase the risk of bleeding; do not use with high blood pressure medication and do not exceed a daily dose of 6g if you are diabetic.

Ginkgo biloba

An increasingly popular circulatory and memory-boosting supplement (see page 317), ginkgo has now been shown to help improve sexual dysfunction caused by taking antidepressants – a commonly reported side effect. That said, you need to take a therapeutic dose of 120mg a day for six weeks and give this time to kick in.

There is also some evidence that ginkgo can help relieve the breast tenderness associated with menstruation, and if you plan to use it this way, you need to start taking it on the sixteenth day of your menstrual cycle (day 1 is the first day of your last period) and continue until the fifth day of your next cycle. Interestingly, lower dosages of 120mg a day appear as effective, if not more, than higher dosages of up to 600mg.

Therapeutic dose
120mg a day.

Contraindications
Do not use this herb alongside blood-thinning medications, including aspirin.

Red clover

One of the key active agents in Meno-Herb (see page 405), red clover, also known as daidzen or genistein, can help reduce the loss of bone density associated with both perimenopause and menopause in women (osteoporosis is associated with declining oestrogen levels – see page 232). This is because the herb itself is rich in calcium, and for this specific health benefit you need to take the equivalent of 40mg a day for at least a year.

The flower tops of this plant contain at least a hundred different chemicals, which is why it crops up in so many different supplements claiming so many different benefits, from hormone-rebalancing to improved skin condition. It also contains isoflavones, those substances that are chemically similar to oestrogen, albeit much weaker, and are thus known as phytoestrogens.

Therapeutic dose
Take as directed on the bottle. If you are making a tea, steep 4g of the dried herb in 150ml of boiling water for 15 minutes. Cool, strain and drink 3 cups a day.

Women with hormone-sensitive conditions should avoid this herb.

Tribulus terrestris

This, one of the vitality-boosting adaptogenic herbs, is the single most effective natural agent that works to raise testosterone levels – for maximum potency you must make sure any supplement you use is made from the leaves of the plant, harvested in Bulgaria. In clinical trials healthy males who took 750mg a day for five days were found to have a 40 per cent increase in testosterone, the hormone that is key in lowering stress and boosting performance.

Therapeutic dose

750mg a day.

Contraindications

Do not mix with prescription medicines.

Saw palmetto

The herb of choice for both prostate problems (see page 434) and polycystic ovary syndrome (PCOS; see page 399), saw palmetto has also been used, traditionally, to help increase breast size and improve sexual vigour.

It has an anti-androgen activity and so is a useful agent for anyone suffering from adult acne, which is the result of an over-production of the male hormone testosterone. It has an oestrogenic action, too, which means you must not use it if you are likely to be pregnant.

The part of the plant used is the ripe fruit. Look for products that are prepared from the whole berries using lipophilic non-polar solvents, since these appear to be the most effective at extracting the fat-soluble active agents.

Therapeutic dose

160mg, 2 times a day, of a lipophilic extract (see above) that provides 80–90 per cent fatty acids.

Contraindications

Do not use this herb if you are taking the contraceptive pill or using HRT.

Vitamin C

This is the nutrient that has been shown in a recent study to enhance sexual activity among women in their early twenties (who did not live with their partners). The theory is that since vitamin C works to ward off stress, the women taking part in the study were more relaxed and more receptive to their partners' advances. That said, it had no impact on the males taking part in the study, and further research would be needed to make any definitive claim.

In any event, vitamin C is one of the best antioxidant, tissue-protecting agents we know of and taking 1g a day can not only help beat stress but will ward off winter ailments that would make you feel less like jumping into the sack (with a runny nose) anyway.

Therapeutic dose

1g a day.

Contraindications

Do not supplement vitamin C in one single dose if you have kidney stones. Instead, split the dose into 4 x 250mg so the body can flush out any excess between doses.

Vitamin E

Key to sperm health, researchers report that giving men 100 IUs a day improved not only sperm counts but motility too and resulted in a higher rate of pregnancy among couples struggling with unexplained infertility (see page 395).

Vitamin E may also be useful in protecting against prostate cancer (see page 435) and has been used in higher dosages (up to 800 IUs) alongside vitamin C to reduce the risk of pre-eclampsia in high-risk pregnant women. Research now shows that naturally sourced vitamin E is 100 per cent more bioavailable than synthetic versions, so check the brand before you buy.

Therapeutic dose

To improve sperm health and the chance of pregnancy, take 100 IUs daily.

Contraindications

Do not take this nutrient if you are using anticoagulant medication or having chemotherapy since it may interfere with their effectiveness.

Zinc

This is the single most important nutrient involved in reproductive health in both sexes and one of the most common deficiencies in adult men and women (white flecks across the fingernails are a telltale sign that you need supplementation).

Zinc, which is also an immune booster, can also help address impotence and sexual dysfunction in men. It can be depleted by the long-term use of antibiotics (and by heavy drinking), so anyone using these for acne should consider supplementation. Zinc levels are also adversely affected by rheumatoid arthritis (see page 233).

Therapeutic dose
30mg a day.

Contraindications

Avoid supplementation if you suffer from glaucoma; also avoid it if you have been diagnosed as HIV positive since there is some evidence linking higher zinc intakes and reduced survival time.

Top Three Over-the-Counter Combination Remedies for Fertility and Hormones

Native Woman

Mycomedicinal's Native Woman by New Chapter combines agarikon – a herb known as the 'elixir of life' and said, by traditional healers, to connect a woman with her deepest sexuality – with performance-enhancing medicinal mushrooms, including maitake, shiitake and reishi (see pages 288). For more, visit www.wisofnature.com.

Manpower II

Lifetime's Manpower II combines the testosterone-boosting male tonic tribulus terrestris with the aptly named herb horny goatweed to boost sexual performance. Mail order from Victoria Health (0800 389 8195; www.victoriahealth.com).

Damiana

This is a traditional aphrodisiac used for both sexes that can help address sexual dysfunction. The parts of the plant used are the leaf and the stem. For speedy results, use this herb in tincture form. Mail order from Revital (0800 252875; www.revital.com) and take the equivalent of 2–4ml a day.

A–Z of Food to Support Hormones

A is for apples which contain the mood-boosting amino acid phenylalanine, which the body uses to make phenylethylalanine, the same neurotransmitter the brain makes more of when we fall in love. Chocolate contains this same agent too so if you have been dumped or plan to break off a relationship, invest in a box of good quality chocolates to help you (or your soon-to-be-ex) get over withdrawal symptoms when production of this brain chemical slows down.

B is for broccoli and beans, both of which provide folic acid, which researchers believe can help prevent cancerous changes to the cervix (see page 426) caused by the human papilloma virus (HPV; see page 426).

C is for vitamin C, which has been shown in trials to increase sexual activity in women, even among healthy young non cohabiting partners (see page 410). Vitamin-C-rich foods include kiwi fruits, acerola cherries, citrus fruits, broccoli, papaya, peppers, rose hips, squash, tomatoes and strawberries.

D is for iron-rich dried fruits, which can improve fertility in both sexes, but especially women who lose iron when they menstruate (see Heavy Periods, page 431). The sea vegetable dulse is another excellent source (see Sea Vegetables, page 71).

E is for vitamin E, another nutrient that is critical to reproductive and hormone health. Avocados and eggs, nuts and seeds, leafy green vegetables and meat are all excellent dietary sources. If you plan to supplement this nutrient, make sure you use a naturally sourced brand, which will be more effective than a synthetic one.

F is for fertility-boosting foods rich in the B vitamins that may be lacking; these include eggs, fish, wholegrains, legumes, poultry, meats, dark leafy greens, bananas, salmon, asparagus, sunflower seeds and citrus fruits. Folic acid is also important if you have a history of recurrent miscarriage (see page 432). Good dietary sources include root vegetables and raspberries.

G is for wholegrains, which, again, provide the hormone-supporting B vitamins (see above) and which are an important alternative to refined carbohydrate foods for women with hormone-sensitive conditions, including polycystic ovary syndrome (PCOS; see page 399).

H is for homocysteine, a normal by-product of metabolism (see page 120), which has been found in higher levels in women who suffer recurrent and unexplained miscarriages (see page 432). Foods that help to lower levels naturally are those rich in vitamins B6 and folic acid, including bananas, fish, legumes, avocado, meat, oysters, green vegetables and raspberries.

I is for iron which is important to hormone health in both sexes. Best food sources include dried fruits, apricots, raisins, eggs, dark leafy greens, sea vegetables (see page 71), fish, poultry and organ meats.

J is for juicing, the single fastest way to get health-boosting live enzymes into the bloodstream. Blend your favourite vitamin-C- and enzyme-rich citrus fruits, especially kiwi and papaya, to make an energy-boosting tonic that will also support your hormones and sexual functioning.

K is for kale, another of the iron-rich 'super greens' that help support reproduction and sexual functioning in men and women. Just 67g will also provide almost 6000 IUs of vitamin A, plus other essential minerals including potassium and zinc.

L is for love and if you've lost that loving feeling, treat yourself to a bar of chocolate. It contains an amino acid called phenylalanine, which the brain uses to make a neurotransmitter called phenylethylalanine, levels of which are higher when you are in love. Phenylalanine is also found in less romantic foods including apples, eggs, chicken, carrots and herrings.

M is for menstruation, a time when Native American cultures believed a woman became so powerful she could kill a rattlesnake just by spitting on it. Support the body at this time by stepping up your intake of foods rich in the omega-fatty acids that the body cannot make, including dark leafy greens, soybeans, salmon, tuna, sesame and sunflower seeds.

N is for nitric oxide, a substance that plays a key role in male sexual health since it works to maintain dilation of blood vessels and blood flow to the penis. Its action is enhanced and supported by vitamin C, so if you have a problem, eat more of these foods, including red and green peppers, fruits, squash, tomatoes and berries.

O is for orgasm, which trial participants report is enhanced by supplements that include zizphi fructus, derived from the Chinese jujube date, which works in the body to support those mechanisms that increase blood flow in both sexes during arousal (see page 409). Start the day with a nourishing Chinese herbal porridge made from oats plus jujube dates (see page 15 for more and where to get this herb).

P is for pecan nuts, a delicious source of endocrine-supporting zinc, and, for me, a fond reminder of one of my favourite places for researching into Native American healing traditions: Arizona. A serving of around 100g will also provide 6.48 mcg (micrograms) of selenium, which is critical for prostate health (see page 434).

Q is for quince, another somewhat unexpectedly good source of folic acid (see above) plus vitamin C and potassium. If you just don't have the energy for sex, you may be lacking this mineral, which is also wiped out by heavy drinking and too much coffee. Persistent fatigue and having a 'sweet tooth' can both be signs of potassium deficiency.

R is for raspberries – this humble fruit is an excellent source of vitamin C and an even better provider of folic acid, which is crucial to reproductive health both pre- and post-pregnancy. Raspberries also provide a small hit of the B vitamins, selenium and zinc.

S is for selenium, a mineral sorely lacking in the typical diet, despite the fact it's crucial to prostate health in men. Good dietary sources include brazil nuts and sesame seeds, dried fruits and dairy products, wholegrain breads, tuna, clams and organ meats.

T is for taurine, another antioxidant amino acid, which, alongside arginine, is frequently included in combination formulations for male sexual and hormone health. Naturally present in human breast milk (I am not suggesting you have to drink this), it is also found in high levels in meat and fish.

U is for umeboshi, the fermented plums the Japanese and other cultures use as seasoning to replace less healthy salt and vinegar condiments. Fermented foods, including miso and natto (see page 146), encourage repopulation of the gut with healthy bacteria to resist infection such as candida and sexually transmitted bacteria (see pages 94 and 437).

V is for the vitamins in your food, but remember, when it comes to supplementation, there are two kinds: those that are fat-soluble and those that are water-soluble. The water-soluble vitamins include the B-complex family, vitamin C, the bioflavonoids and betacarotenes, which are easily flushed from the system. The fat-soluble vitamins, A, D, K and E, need more careful handling since any excess will accumulate in the body's fatty tissues. A rich and varied diet that includes fresh fruits, vegetables, legumes, wholegrains, nuts, seeds, fish and low-fat animal products will provide an excellent basis on which to build super nutrition with the more specific supplements recommended throughout this chapter, which are designed to promote your sexual health and well-being.

W is for enriched white breads, which are an excellent source of the selenium that may be lacking in the rest of your diet. This trace mineral is especially important to male sexual health and prostate functioning. Rye bread is an even better source since, slice for slice, it provides almost 10mcg (micrograms) per 32g slice, compared with the 6.4mcg from an enriched white loaf.

X is for Xynergy, the UK supplier of the super greens and sea green supplements recommended throughout this book, which can further support the endocrine system and boost fertility and energy levels in those facing mid-life hormonal changes, thus helping maintain well-being and normal sexual functioning. For a catalogue, call 08456 585858, or visit www.xynergy.co.uk.

Y is for yoghurt and other probiotic foods, which can help the body rebuild levels of good gut bacteria both during and after infection (see PID/STD, pages 433 and 437). Bananas are another good natural probiotic, but for best results you need a supplement that tells you which strain of bacteria you will be getting and in what dosages.

Z is for zinc, probably the single most important nutrient in the reproductive health of both sexes and the most commonly lacking mineral found in nutritional profiling. Increase your intake by eating more seafoods, especially crab, sea vegetables (see page 71), meat, mushrooms and poultry. Nuts and seeds are another good natural source.

Ancient Wisdom, 21st-century Healing

Traditional Chinese Medicine (TCM)

The hormone-balancing herb **dong quai** has been used by TCM practitioners for thousands of years and is described in ancient Chinese medical texts as a tonic for all female problems.

Today, we know this herb works to stimulate, as well as inhibit, uterine muscles, meaning this is one of the adapto-genic herbs (see page 203) that works to normalize the body's systems and do what needs to be done.

The herb itself is a good source of iron, plus zinc and vitamins C, E and B12 (see Top Ten Natural Remedies, page 412), which might explain why it is still a popular addition to combi-nation supplements for sexual and hormone health. That said, it has an oestrogenic action in the body and so should not be used without supervision by women with hormone-sensitive conditions such as fibroids or endometriosis. It is, however, excellent for tackling menstrual cramps, menopause and hormone-related skin problems.

Ayurvedic (Indian) Remedies

Anything that is said to make a man 'potent as a horse' deserves more than one mention in this chapter and, according to Ayurvedic practitioners, **ashwaganda** does not disappoint.

Also known as 'Indian ginseng', it is a popular anti-ageing tonic in India, where it is also prescribed for infertility prob-lems in both sexes and menstrual problems in women.

A healing tea is made by boiling the roots of the plant in hot water for fifteen minutes, but if this is too much fuss for you, you can now mail order organic capsules and tinctures of the more popular Ayurvedic herbs, including ashwaganda, from Pukka Herbs (08456 585858; www.pukkaherbs.com).

Native American Remedies

Although the Native American Indians were the first to use **lady's slipper** for 'female problems', early settlers soon cot-toned on to its usefulness too. It was listed in the US

Pharmacopoeia from 1863 to 1916 as an antispasmodic and nervine (nerve) medicine and was often used to help women cope with afterbirth pains.

Lady's slipper works, we now know, because it is rich in both magnesium and the B-complex vitamins, which can help reduce muscle spasm, including menstrual and uterine cramps. It is also high in calcium, giving it antistress and calming properties too.

Native New Zealand Remedies

If you are tackling a herpes infection or indeed any of the sexually transmitted diseases, including human papilloma virus (HPV), then you should take the new immune-boosting, antiviral combined olive-leaf and kiwi-fruit tincture Olive-Gold, from Vitalife (www.nzvitalife.co.nz), a company set up by English-trained doctor Caroline Fowler and her New Zealand husband Andrew (who has a background in agriculture).

The couple work in partnership with the Maori to produce their award-winning range on the North Island. Kiwi fruit is a better source of immune-boosting vitamin C than oranges, and olive leaf is one of the best antiviral agents in the natural weapons armoury. The Olive-Gold herbal tincture is alcohol-free; available from NutriCentre (0800 587 2290).

What Really Works for Sex, Hormone and Fertility-related Conditions

Cervical Cancer and Human Papilloma Virus

Controlled clinical trials are currently underway in London testing the efficacy of a natural treatment combining **folic acid** with a little-known Asian mushroom supplement called **coriolus versicolor.**

As ever with such trials, it follows highly encouraging preliminary findings which suggest the combination of these two remedies will work to trigger the body's own immune system to eradicate the human papilloma virus (HPV), which is responsible for a range of conditions, from cervical cancer to warts, both genital and the everyday ones people get elsewhere on the body.

An estimated 80 per cent of all women are infected by HPV within four years of becoming sexually active, and while only some strains of this virus have been linked with cervical cancer, 90 per cent of all cervical carcinomas are now believed to be caused by it. The theory, as yet unproven, is that this combination of folic acid and coriolus may not only help prevent cancerous changes to the cells of the cervix, it could even reverse them too.

Folic acid, of course, is better known as the supplement pregnant women take to help prevent neural tube defects in the developing embryo. It is present in foods, including broccoli, beans and meat, but in this natural form it is 40 per cent less bioavailable than when sourced from supplements. The typical therapeutic dosage is 400mcg a day.

The good news is that if coriolus can wipe out the more virulent HPV strains that do cause cervical cancer, it should also be able to wipe out the less harmful ones responsible for genital and other warts, making this a supplement you should certainly be aware of.

1, 2, 3 . . . Easy Steps for Managing Cancerous Changes to the Cervix

Please remember, that while early trials show promising results with this combination, it is by no means a cure or an alternative to conventional treatments for cervical cancer. If you are being monitored for changes to the cervix, take these remedies as an adjunct and do not simply cancel your next colposcopy examination.

Take Lambert's folic acid (400mcg a day).

Take coriolus supplements. In their preliminary trials, researchers used six 500mg tablets a day for the first fifteen days, and then cut back to three tablets a day, all taken with food. To mail order coriolus, call Stewart Distribution on 01273 558112 or visit www.lemonburst.net.

Eat broccoli three times a week (see B is for Broccoli, page 420).

The Contraceptive Pill

Taking the contraceptive pill wipes out levels of both **folic acid** and **vitamin C** and may also increase your risk of gum disease – the leading cause of tooth loss in adults.

One study, which showed that levels of gum-disease-causing bacteria in the mouth increased among women once they started to take the pill, suggests it might be wise to take precautions and use additional supplements which help protect the gums (see **gingigel,** page 198).

Taking potluck with supplementation is a waste of money and a better long-term investment is to have a nutritional status analysis which will show what nutrients you need and why. What you need to remember is that the pill, like HRT, is a synthetic hormone and may have other less welcome effects in the body that, to date, we know nothing about because nobody has investigated them.

Endometriosis

Endometriosis is a very painful condition where the same sort of cells that grow normally in the lining of the womb begin to grow outside the uterus. One theory is that these cells migrate from the uterus. Another is that they are different types of cells that have mutated due to an error in their genetic programming. The most likely sites for endometriosis to occur are the ovaries, the Fallopian tubes, the bladder and the bowel. Symptoms range from painful periods to infertility, and in many cases major surgery is undertaken.

The reason it is so painful is that it is an inflammatory condition. **Essential fatty acids** (see menopause and perimenopause on page 403) can counter this by producing substances called prostaglandins, which have a natural anti-inflammatory action. The best source of the omega fatty acids is an unpolluted fish oil or, if you are vegetarian, flaxseed oil. Aim for the equivalent of 1g a day. Many sufferers also have low levels of **zinc**, which has a potent inflammatory action too. Compensate for this by taking at least 15mg a day.

DL-phenylalanine (DLPA)* is a natural painkiller, which you can buy in your local health store. It works in 60 per cent of those who take it but needs several weeks to kick in. If there is no improvement after three weeks, it is not the solution for you. When it does work, the theory is that it promotes the production of endorphins – the body's own natural painkillers – and interferes with the brain's perception of pain by altering the action of the neurotransmitters or chemical messengers.

Saw palmetto, which is more traditionally used to support the prostate gland in men, can block the action of the sex hormone called follicle-stimulating hormone (FSH), which is known to increase endometrial tissue. However, with a condition this serious, do not try to self-treat. Instead, find a practitioner who has treated it successfully before (see Useful Contacts, page 447) and join a support group. Visit www.endometriosis.co.uk for more support.

1, 2, 3 . . . Easy Steps for Managing Endometriosis
Use saw palmetto. The daily therapeutic dose is 250–300mg.

Use a good quality EFA such as Barlean's. The Essential

---

* Avoid this supplement if you are pregnant, breastfeeding, taking antidepressants or have high blood pressure.

Woman includes anti-inflammatory evening primrose and flax oil, plus organic isoflavones from soy. Mail order from Healthy and Essential (08700 536000; www.healthyandessential.com).

Use DLPA* to help control the pain; mail order from Revital (0800 252875; www.revital.com) and take with vitamin B6 for better absorption.

Fibroids

Fibroids, which occur in around 20 per cent of women over the age of thirty, are the most common form of slow-growing and benign tumours. They are the result of an abnormal response to the sex hormone oestrogen, and while half of the women who have them have no symptoms at all, for others, severe PMS, low blood-sugar levels, painful periods, fertility problems and bleeding between periods are all common.

In most cases, fibroids shrink after the menopause, but if you have not reached that stage, a combination of the amino acid L-arginine (500mg on an empty stomach) together with 50mg of vitamin B6 daily and up to 10g of vitamin C can help retard their growth. Vitamin A (25,000 IUs daily) is also helpful since it works to restore the body's connective tissue to normal functioning.

1, 2, 3 . . . Easy Steps for Managing Fibroids

All these supplements are widely on sale in good health stores but do not take vitamin A if you might be pregnant, and expect to experience some stomach upset if you take more than 2g of vitamin C daily. Women with fibroids should also avoid the stress-busting adaptogens such as Siberian ginseng (see page 280), since these can have an unhelpful oestrogenic effect in the body.

Take 500mg a day of L-arginine on an empty stomach.

To retard the growth of fibroids, take 50mg of vitamin B6 plus 2g of vitamin C.

To help restore the connective tissue to normal functioning, take a therapeutic daily dose of 25,000 IUs of vitamin A.

Genital Herpes and Warts

Check out the new Asian medicinal mushroom **coriolus** (see Cervical Cancer, page 426). For topical treatments, see herpes (page 44).

Heavy Periods

Vitamin C can not only help women to enjoy sex more (see page 417), it can also be used to help reduce bleeding among those suffering from heavier periods. Even a borderline deficiency of this nutrient promotes capillary fragility and researchers have successfully combined vitamin C with **citrus-derived flavonoids** to treat heavy menstrual bleeding. This works because vitamin C and flavonoids have a synergistic action and enhance each other in the body, which can then use this combination, with the help of the female hormone oestrogen, to maintain the integrity of the lining of the womb.

The medical term for excessive uterine bleeding is menorrhagia, which, in turn, is the most common reason for **iron deficiency** among women. This then becomes a catch-22 because, when other causes such as endometriosis and fibroids have been ruled out, chronic iron deficiency is often itself a cause of heavier periods.

I know none of us ever measures it, but women who lose more than 60–80ml of blood per menses tend to become progressively iron-deficient without knowing it, and in trials 75 per cent of chronically iron-deficient women who took supplementation suffered less heavy bleeding compared with 33 per cent of those given a placebo pill, which is statistically enough of a difference to be significant.

You can mail order all these from the NutriCentre (0800 587 2290; www.NutriCentre.com).

Take a combined vitamin C plus flavonoid supplement such as C Plus by Vitamin Research Products (VRP).

Supplement the diet with Iron EAP2 by Biocare, which is not only highly absorbable but more suited to people sensitive to iron supplementation.

Take a good quality multisupplement such as Ultra One by Nature's Plus to provide additional zinc, manganese and copper, all of which are lost in menstrual fluid.

Miscarriages

If you are pregnant or hoping to be, you should not be self-treating with natural remedies but instead should seek the advice of a qualified naturopath, nutritionist or medical herbalist to help increase your chances of taking your pregnancy to term. See page 447 for a useful list of organizations that can refer you to specialists in your locality.

When you find a good practitioner, tell them researchers have now made a link between high homocysteine levels (see page 120) and a negative pregnancy outcome.

In a small pilot trial, where twenty-five women with high homocysteine levels and a history of recurrent miscarriages were given 15mg a day of **folic acid** and 750mg a day of **vitamin B6** to remedy the problem, twenty-two women became pregnant within three months of normalizing homocysteine levels and, of those, twenty went on to have a successful pregnancy with no evidence of fetal malformation.

Do not simply embark on this regimen without supervision; these are high dosages and taking them has implications for levels of other nutrients, especially zinc (see Synergy, page 203). But if you have a history of recurrent and unexplained miscarriage, get someone at least to check your homocysteine levels and rule this out as a possible underlying cause.

What I want to say here is that if you have a history of unexplained miscarriage (i.e. there are no structural problems), do not ignore it but seek advice and treatment before getting pregnant again. Lots of the hands-on bodywork therapies can help the body recover from the shock of a miscarriage and prepare for another pregnancy when you are ready to try again.

Weekly acupuncture sessions, for example, will help in both instances, and if you want the best, check out Zita West's new clinic in London's Harley Street (www.zitawest.com). A former NHS midwife, Zita has done more to bring awareness of the critical role of natural remedies and treatments in both pre- and post-pregnancy than any other UK practitioner and really knows her stuff. She has a celebrity client list – including royalty – as long as your arm, and while not everyone can afford a consultation, if a baby is what you want it will be an investment you will never regret. The clinic also runs a programme of free lectures throughout the year.

For details of the Zita West Clinic and Zita's specialist pregnancy-planning range of nutritional supplements, call 020 7224 6091. An initial consultation costs £140. Subsequent appointments are £95.

Pelvic Inflammatory Disease (PID)

This term is used to describe an ascending infection of the endometrium and/or Fallopian tubes and can cause fertility problems later on if not dealt with promptly. In fact, it has become the leading cause of infertility worldwide and is now considered responsible for the increase in ectopic pregnancies (the risk is eight times higher after just one episode of PID), where the fertilized embryo cannot travel to the womb for implantation but becomes trapped in a blocked Fallopian tube that has been damaged by infection. You are also more at risk if you have a contraceptive IUD or coil fitted.

In the early stages, symptoms include painful intercourse, a malodorous vaginal discharge and recurrent pain in the lower back and abdomen. If not treated, the acute symptoms include abdominal pain occurring soon after a period, increased vaginal discharge, uterine tenderness and heavy bleeding.

Since you must seek medical treatment, you will be likely to be taking antibiotics, which means you need to take a good quality **probiotic** too (see page 65). To rebalance and normalize the microflora of the vagina, make a douche by dissolving the probiotic **lactobacillus acidophilus** in powder form in a cup of lukewarm water.

The anti-inflammatory agent **bromelain** (see page 208), which is derived from the stems of pineapples, is another useful adjunct to the conventional treatment of PID since it also works to reduce soft tissue swellings caused by infection and to potentiate the use of antibiotics.

1, 2, 3 . . . Easy Steps to Help Tackle PIDs

Take lactobacillus acidophilus probiotic in capsule or powder form.

Use bromelain supplements to help counter inflammation and to potentiate your antibiotic treatment.

Use an organic flax oil from the Barlean's range; mail order from Healthy and Essential (08700 536000; www.healthyandessential.com).

Prostate

The only time newspaper editors (mostly middle-aged and male) get excited about natural health and think it might be more than some terrible snake-oil con on the public is when the subject of the antioxidant lycopene in tomatoes raises its head again.

When this happens, you can confidently expect the breaking news to push the page-three girl off her page, and a splash story with a big happy headline to tell you that tomato sauce (which the editors like on their chips) is good for you. Better than raw tomatoes even.

If this doesn't tell you that the mainstream media has its own agenda – and giving natural health a fair hearing is not on that agenda – I don't know what will.

The reason cooked tomatoes get column inches is that they are rich in the prostate-protecting antioxidant lycopene. Plants have developed their own protective substances called phytochemicals and lycopene is one of these. It is twice as potent as the cancer-protecting betacarotenes and 100 per cent more bioavailable if you cook it, which is the only reason why tomato ketchup gets a recommendation on the health pages.

The research underpinning the role of lycopene in prostate protection was reported in the journal of the National Cancer Institute of America after scientists found that men who ate ten or more servings of tomatoes and tomato-based foods on a regular basis had a 45 per cent lower risk of prostate cancer than those who did not. For the record, nobody defined the word 'regular', so you will have to work out for yourself how much is enough. And although lycopene is better known for its action on the prostate, it can also protect women against osteoporosis.

Israeli researchers, who have bred a hybrid tomato that contains four times the normal dose of lycopene, also report that its action is enhanced in the body by the presence of vitamin E, so take the two together but avoid vitamin E if you are on blood-thinning heart medication such as warfarin.

Doctors warn that all men, if they live long enough, will develop some kind of problem with the prostate gland, and that while it may not be the condition that eventually kills you, by the age of eighty prostate problems affect some 80 per cent of men.

The key herb for supporting the prostate is **saw palmetto** (see page 416).

Nobody has yet managed to pinpoint its precise action but the active ingredient, which has an anti-inflammatory action, also appears to stop a particularly damaging form of testosterone called dihydrotestosterone (DHT) from binding to hormone receptor sites in the prostate gland.

The trouble with clinical trials, though, is that few last for longer than three or six months, which means nobody, to date, can tell you what the long-term effects of taking a herb like this will be. There are adverse reactions if the dosage is too high and these include abdominal pain, back pain, constipation, diarrhoea, headaches, high blood pressure and decreased libido, so if you do suffer from any of these, then consult a qualified health practitioner to adjust your dosage.

One thing you should do, if you are going to take this herb in the long term, is to ask your doctor to test your PSA (prostate-specific antigen) levels. This can be done with a simple blood test and is now a routine health check for men over forty in America. It gives an indication of a man's risk of developing prostate cancer, and the reason you need to monitor it, if you do take saw palmetto, is because there is some suggestion the herb can produce false-negative PSA readings. In other words, the herb may mask the development of a prostate cancer condition.

1, 2, 3 . . . Easy Steps to Help Prevent Prostate Problems

Increase your dietary intake of cooked tomatoes and take a lycopene supplement such as Lyco-mato (0800 083 7040), alongside naturally sourced vitamin E (see page 417).

Ask your doctor for a PSA test to assess and monitor your risk.

Use saw palmetto. Clinical trials used 160mg, twice daily, of a supplement made from whole berry extract (see page 416). To help treat benign prostatic hyperplasia, take 1–2 a day of whole berries.

Sexually Transmitted Diseases (STD)

In the last decade, the incidence of sexually transmitted diseases and the number of infected people seeking specialist help has doubled. Since 1995, for example, the infection rate of **chlamydia** has increased by an appalling 76 per cent, and if you think the word **gonorrhoea** got left behind in the trenches of World War I by your great-grandparents, think again, because in 2001 the number of cases reported to the UK Public Health Laboratory Service (PHLS) rose by 27 per cent.

The age group most affected is both sexes in their late teens and early twenties, and in females under the age of nineteen infection rates for both diseases have now rocketed to *six times* that of the national average. Since both conditions are easily cured with antibiotics in the early stages, screening is important, and if you think you may have contracted an STD, visit your local genitourinary clinic *and* pluck up the courage to tell the person you have been sleeping with.

You will be prescribed antibiotics, which means you will need to take a good quality **lactobacillus acidophilus probiotic** (see page 10) to rebuild levels of the good gut bacteria that help the body resist infection. If you are taking antibiotics, take **bromelain** too (see page 208), since it has been shown to make their action in the body more effective. **Essential fatty acids** (see pages 190 and 378) can help reduce inflammation.

Check out the top-selling Barlean's range from America, which includes The Essential Woman: an organic oil combining flax oil, isoflavones from soy and evening primrose oil. (Source from the UK supplier Healthy and Essential at www.healthyandessential.com; 08700 536000.) Your natural therapy regimen to help tackle PID should also include 400 IUs of naturally sourced **vitamin E**.

Doctors estimate that 75 per cent of all women will experience at least one **yeast infection** during their lifetime. Symptoms include itching or irritation, a white clumped or curd-like discharge but no odour. Check the diagnosis with your doctor, and for advice on using natural remedies to cope with vaginal candidiasis, see Candida, page 94.

Normal discharge is generally non-odorous, white, highly viscous and acidic. It can become more profuse mid-cycle, at the time of ovulation, but any unusual vaginal discharge must be checked since it can also be a sign of other infections including **pelvic inflammatory disease (PID)** and **genital herpes**. It may be the result of an allergic reaction to spermicide creams, or a clue to a more insidious bacterial infection, such as chlamydia.

There is a suggestion, as yet unproven, that since the microflora in the reproductive organs are controlled by the balance of natural hormones, taking synthetic hormones can have an adverse effect on this mechanism. You might want to temporarily stop taking the contraceptive pill until the condition has cleared, and, if you are using HRT, to look for an alternative (see page 404).

1, 2, 3 . . . Easy Steps to Help Tackle STDs

Take lactobacillus acidophilus probiotic in capsule or powder form.

Use bromelain supplements to help counter inflammation and to potentiate your antibiotic treatment.

Use an organic flax oil from the Barlean's range; mail order from Healthy and Essential (08700 536000; www.healthyandessential.com).

Vaginal Dryness

When a group of women suffering from this problem were given a treatment plan which increased the amount of soya in their diet and which supplemented their intake of flax (linseed) oil and red clover, doctors noticed that the vaginal tissues changed, for the better, in just ten weeks. The results were reported in the *British Medical Journal*.

Flax oil is an important source of essential fatty acids, which lubricate the skin, joints and vaginal tissues. You can take this in liquid form but you can also get it from nuts, seeds and oily fish. Vitamin E will also help. You need to take 300 IUs daily. For more direct action, you can even insert the capsules into the vagina where the body heat will melt the outer casing allowing the nutrient to act where it is needed. If you do this, make sure you use a yeast-free preparation. The flax oil I recommend you use is Barlean's Essential Woman: an organic mix that combines flax with isoflavones from soy and evening primrose oil (see page 437).

You also need to be eating more of the plant phytoestrogens, which have been found to help rebalance hormones in both sexes. Check out Meno-Herb (page 405), which combines several of these important herbs and includes red clover.

1, 2, 3 . . . Easy Steps to Managing Vaginal Dryness
Take Meno-Herb from Victoria Health (0800 389 8195; www.victoriahealth.com). Take two capsules a day.

Use The Essential Woman organic oils from the Barlean's range. Mail order from Healthy and Essential (08700 536000; www.healthyandessential.com).

Take 300 IUs of naturally sourced vitamin E.

Roll Out Your Yoga Mat

Too many of us live more in our heads than in our bodies and, if nothing else, yoga works to bring more awareness of the physical body as well as more awareness of how we are. In fact, unlike analysis or therapy, yoga concerns itself solely with 'how we are' in any given moment and does not focus on why we are in this state but only on how to correct it and rebalance ourselves.

Here are my **1, 2, 3 top asanas** for increasing that all-important awareness and, at the same time, sending more energy (prana) to the reproductive organs.

For Both Sexes: Trikonasana (Triangle Pose)

You will already have seen this posture in countless yoga adverts and magazines since it is the one most often used to illustrate the active practice of yoga. It will be almost impossible to get the correct alignment without a teacher on hand to help, but for those of you who have some basic yoga knowledge, here is how you do it.

Stand with your feet about 1 metre apart and turn the right foot to the right side.

Raise your arms to shoulder height and stretch them out fully to the sides.

Bend slowly to the right, taking care not to bend forwards but to keep the correct alignment. As you do this, bend the right knee slightly.

Keeping your arms in the outstretched position, gently touch your right foot with your right hand. Turn the left palm forward and look up towards the left hand.

You have now made a triangle with your body.

Repeat this posture on the opposite side and, as you bend, concentrate on the long deep stretch you are giving the side of your body. This posture tones the pelvic area and the reproductive organs and, if you practise it regularly, can help trim fat from the waist too, which should leave you feeling more like a sex kitten and less like spending the night in front of the television with a bucket of ice cream.

For Her: The Butterfly

This simple asana also works to tone the pelvic region and its organs.

Sit on your yoga mat, keeping the spine erect, and draw the soles of the feet together, allowing your knees to fall out to the sides.

Clasp your feet with both hands and gently move your knees up and down. Do not strain in this posture – allow the body to move gently.

Keeping your back straight, gently lower the body forwards, stretching from the lower torso. Hold this stretch for a few minutes and notice how you are also stretching the top of the back of the legs.

With each breath you exhale, allow the body to move forwards and down. Hold the position each time you inhale, and only move again as you breathe out.

This posture can help alleviate PMS and menstrual cramping.

For Him: The Lying Down (Supine) Butterfly

Lie on your back on your yoga mat with your arms out to the side and raise your knees so you bring your feet as close in to your buttocks as you can.

Put the soles of your feet together (as above for the Butterfly) and allow the knees to fall out to the sides. If this is too uncomfortable to begin with, align the insides of the soles and prop your knees up with the support of pillows or cushions.

The point is to allow the body to relax in this position for at least five minutes, which it will not do if you are uncomfortable.

Again, the butterfly posture tones the pelvic region and its organs and sends more healing prana (energy) to this part of the body.

Close your eyes, or, if you cannot get that still, read a book, but try to stay in the posture, which sends more blood to the prostate and surrounding tissues, for as long as you can.

Acknowledgements

With thanks and love to the behind-the-scenes team, now and then, including Declan O'Mahony, who has more faith in me than anyone; Ellie, who reminds me every day of what is important in life; Yvonne Harkin, who told me (quite rightly) I'd make a better writer and journalist than a doctor; Yvonne Ferrell; Dr Neil Slade; Rory Kinahan, Megan May, Melissa Clark and Harriet Griffey, whose dedication keeps the website (www.whatreallyworks.co.uk) going when I want to give up and retreat back up the Amazon; Carol Golcher, for always being there; my editor Brenda Kimber, who understands the loneliness of writing; my agent Teresa Chris, for her endless enthusiasm; Tiffanie Darke, for her support and being a breath of fresh air at the *Sunday Times Style* magazine, and Sedona's Earth Wisdom guide David, for showing up when I most needed to sit with my feet in Oak Creek at the foot of Cathedral Rock and hear about the White Buffalo. Thank you, too, to the readers who send letters of thanks and encouragement telling me how remedies have worked for them, and to the critics and establishment organizations for the challenges that make me a better researcher and writer.

The Goose

Keynote: The Call of the Quest

Travels to Legendary Places

The V-formation of the goose flight indicates we are about to fix
ourselves to a new path.

The Goose Manifesto

In autumn, when you see geese heading south for winter, flying
along in V-formation, you might consider what science has discovered as to why they fly that way.

As each bird flaps its wings, it creates an uplift for the bird immediately following. By flying in V-formation, the whole flock adds at
least 71 per cent greater flying range than if each bird flew alone.

People who share a common direction and sense of community can get where they are going more quickly and easily if they are travelling on the thrust of one another.

When a goose falls out of formation it suddenly feels the drag and resistance of trying to go it alone and quickly gets back into formation to take advantage of the lifting power of the bird in front.

If we have as much sense as a goose, we will stay in formation with those who are heading the same way we are.

When the head goose (point) gets tired, it drops to the back of the V and another goose flies point. It is sensible to take turns in doing demanding jobs, whether with people or with geese flying south.

Geese honk from behind to encourage those up front to keep up their speed. What message do we give when we honk from behind?

Finally, and this is important, when a goose falls sick or is wounded by gunshot and falls out of formation, two other geese fall out with that goose and follow it down to lend help and protection.

They stay with the fallen goose until it is able to fly or until it dies and only then do they launch out on their own or with another formation to catch up with their own group.

If we have the sense of a goose, we will stand by each other like that!

Useful Contacts

Useful UK contact numbers for referral bodies and specialist suppliers.

For all the latest news on natural health, and to save money on supplements; join The Natural Health Club (0800 0281385; www.thenaturalhealthclub.com).

Nutrition

The British Association of Nutritional Therapists (0870 606 1284). You will be charged £2 for a referral list. The Institute of Optimum Nutrition in London trains more UK practitioners than anywhere else. Call 020 8877 9993 for a list of graduates and their specialisms.

Herbalism

The National Institute of Medical Herbalists (01392 426022), or try the British Herbal Medicine Association (01453 751389), whose members have different qualifications.
The Register of Chinese Herbalists (01603 623994).

Homeopathy

To find a doctor who is also a qualified homeopath, call the British Homeopathic Association (020 7935 2163). For other qualified and classically trained homeopaths, call the Society of Homeopaths (01604 621400).

Naturopathy

The British Naturopathic Association (01458 840072) holds a list of qualified naturopaths who combine nutrition, herbalism and homeopathy in their treatment programmes. Referrals are free. For courses in naturopathy – naturopaths treat illness without using drugs and rely instead on herbs, homeopathy or nutrition – write to the College of Naturopathic and Complementary Medicine at 73 Gardenwood Road, East Grinstead, West Sussex RH19 1RX, or call 01342 410505.

UK mail order and internet suppliers

Victoria Health (0800 389 8195; www.victoriahealth.com) specializes in US-imported, cutting-edge supplements, as well as UK brands.

The NutriCentre (0800 587 2290; www.NutriCentre.com) is the UK's largest supplier of natural health products and books.

Revital (0800 252875; www.revital.com) specializes in African and European supplements, as well as UK brands; plus foods.

Index

reticuloendothelial system (RES) 265
retinal 42
retinal implant 39
retinitis pigmentosa 39
retinoids 275–76
rheumatism 72, 76, 213, 221, 225, 233
    see also arthritis, rheumatoid
rhodiola 252–53, 291, 305, 308, 327,
    329, 335–36, 350
rhodiola rosea 203
rhododendron caucasicum 191
rhubarb 127
rhubarb greens 150
riboflavin 341
rice 154, 339, 341, 386
    brown 219
    wholegrain 338
rice bran 125, 262
Ritalin 326, 327
rooibos tea 79
rosa mosqueta 27
rosavin 308
rose incense 344
rose oil 269
rosehips 164, 222, 278, 385, 420
royal jelly 286
Rubin, Dr Jordan 188, 191
rue 212–13
rutin 112, 143, 291
rye 79, 152, 153, 220, 221, 386
    bread 424

S-adenosyl methionine (SAMe) 308–9,
    317, 367–68
sage 154, 316, 318, 336, 339, 402–3, 405
St John's wort 45, 143, 305, 307, 350
salads 218
salicylates 328
salidroside 308
saliva 54–55
salmon 154, 219, 286, 289, 328, 338,
    341, 383, 420, 422
salt 30, 117
salts 111
San people 87
sanitarywear 404
Saraswati, Swami Satyananda, Asana
    Pranayama Mudra Bandha 108
sarcoidosis 167
sardines 155, 219
SARS virus 296–97
sarsaparilla 8
sattvic herbs 157, 312
saw palmetto 8, 31, 42, 43, 400, 416–17,
    429, 436
schisandra 82, 252, 266, 276, 283–84,
    298, 370
schizophrenia 208, 341
sciatic pain 228–29

scopoletin 144
sea vegetables 70–73, 289, 395, 420, 421,
    424
seafood 212, 218, 219, 424
seasonal affective disorder (SAD) 349–50
seaweeds 70–73, 151, 395
secretases 317
sedatives, natural 344
seeds 151, 152, 219, 290, 420, 423, 424
seizures 351
selenium 154, 288, 290, 317, 337, 359,
    384, 386, 401, 422, 423, 424
senna 85
serotonin 253, 269, 287, 305, 307, 308,
    309, 312, 324, 327, 334, 335, 337, 347,
    350, 367, 374, 380, 386
sesame oil 219, 225
sesame seeds 152, 288, 341, 383, 422,
    423
sex 395–96
sexual dysfunction 408, 413, 418, 419
sexual tonics 409–10, 416
sexually transmitted diseases (STD) 414,
    437
Seyle, Dr Hans, Stress Without Distress
    248
shakti bhandi 227, 237–43
shallots 153, 289
Shanghai Institute of Materia Medica 343
shark cartilage 49
Sharma, Professor Priya Vrat, Essentials of
    Ayurveda 401
she oak 405
sheep sorrel 294
shellfish 155, 231, 291, 342
Sher, Helen 23
shiitake 283, 288, 299, 419
shingles 11, 45–46
shoulders
    exercises 241
    injuries 233–34
silica 27, 41, 67, 158, 166, 181, 218, 219,
    221, 222, 233
silicon 79, 225
silymarin 5
sinuses 143, 144
sinusitis 144, 153, 168–69
skin 3, 3–4, 53, 73, 218, 223
    ageing 25–27
    brushing 8
    disorders 22, 63, 281, 425
    feeding 9
    wrinkle cream 406
skin-nourishing foods, A-Z of 11–14
sleep 320–26, 337, 339, 344, 363
    disturbed 322–26, 362
    stages of 321–22
    unrefreshing 386
    see also insomnia

vitamins, B-complex (*cont.*)
299, 323, 350, 359, 377–78, 383, 384,
385, 388, 421, 423, 426
B2 (riboflavin) 341, 347
B3 (niacin) 12, 79, 80, 334, 338–39,
340, 385
B5 (pantethine, pantothenic acid) 80,
257, 277, 286, 334, 336, 342, 381
B6 77, 121, 135, 178, 220, 221, 290,
308, 327, 334, 337, 339, 350, 384,
386, 411, 421, 430, 432
B12 121, 135, 145, 146, 345, 365–66,
369, 377, 381, 400, 425
C 10, 12, 33, 38, 73, 112, 126, 127,
129–30, 143, 144, 148, 150, 151,
152, 163, 164–66, 178, 213, 216,
256, 258, 259, 276, 277–78, 287,
288, 291, 296, 297, 423, 425, 430
and Alzheimer's 317
and brain 305–6, 308, 334, 349
and cognitive function 345
and contraceptive pill 428
and drug addiction 330
for energy 361–62, 383, 384, 388
and menstrual problems 431–32
and mitochondrial organelles 359
and quercetin 340–41
seizures 351
and sex 410, 417, 420, 422, 425
D 167, 182, 218–19, 423
E 10, 11, 24, 37, 97, 131, 148, 151,
154, 158, 214, 259, 317, 336, 341,
359, 384, 400–401, 417–18, 420,
423, 425, 435, 439
K 12, 144, 150, 152, 178, 219, 220,
221, 233, 423
multivitamin supplements 268
P 223
U 13
see also folic acid
voice, deepening 248
vomiting 192, 413

wakame 71, 73
walnuts 153, 154, 219, 289, 341
warfarin 130, 131, 318, 333, 408, 435
warts, genital 431
water
drinking 363
retention 72, 111, 157
watercress 155, 223, 342
watermelons 125, 290, 342, 385
Wechsler memory scale 343
weight gain 111, 116, 140, 349, 362, 399,
403
weight loss 72, 86–91
and fertility 397
West, Zita 433
Natural Pregnancy 398

wheat 75, 80, 93, 290, 328, 386
sprouted 222
wheat bran 127
wheatgrass 70, 80, 155, 291, 298, 342
white willow 186, 375
wholegrains 99, 151, 152, 218, 221, 288,
290, 340, 382, 386, 420, 421, 423
wholewheat 125, 152
wild Chinese violet 35
wild oregano 189
wild yam 405, 406–7
Wilkie, David 217
wind 78, 79, 94
wine, red 153, 341
winter squash 223, 290
wolfberry 224
women, and autoimmune conditions
372–73
wound healing 277, 299
wrinkles 27
wrists, exercises 240–41

X-rays 291
xanthine oxidase 232
xylitol 13, 183, 197–98, 223

Yale University 196
yams *see* sweet potatoes
yarrow 83–84
yeast 96
infections 437–38
products 231, 366
yoga 29, 88, 104–8, 137–38, 168,
171–75, 177, 200, 205, 211, 224,
234–43, 260, 268, 270, 313, 352–56
anti-arthritic exercises 237–43
asanas 49–51, 105–8, 138, 172–75,
227, 230, 233–37, 300–303, 390–92,
439–42
Astanga 88, 390
mudras 173, 352–56
Sivananda 270
Vini 51–52, 270, 390
yoghurt 220, 222, 342, 424
bioactive 80
non-fat 125
yucca 186

zeaxanthin 39
Ziment, Dr Irwin 143
zinc 9, 10, 14, 31, 34, 36, 56, 80, 97,
155, 178, 204, 209, 225, 233, 289, 291,
297, 298, 299, 328, 341, 342, 373, 388,
421, 422, 423, 429
deficiency 284–85, 342, 370, 381, 387,
418, 432
and reproductive health 400, 401,
418–19, 424, 425
zizphi fructus 409, 422